Disorders of Communication:
The Science of Intervention

PROGRESS IN CLINICAL SCIENCE SERIES

Clinical Information Technology
David Rowley and Harry Purser

Progress in the Treatment of Fluency Disorders
Edited by Lena Rustin, Harry Purser and David Rowley

Counselling Individuals: The Rational Emotive Approach
Windy Dryden

Disorders of Communication: The Science of Intervention
Edited by Margaret M Leahy

Linguistics in Clinical Practice
Edited by Kim Grundy

Progress in Clinical Science Series

Disorders of Communication: The Science of Intervention

Edited by

Margaret M. Leahy
School of Clinical Speech and Language Studies
Trinity College, Dublin

Taylor & Francis
London • New York • Philadelphia

UK   Taylor & Francis Ltd, 4 John Cherry Street, London WC1N 2ET

USA   Taylor & Francis Inc., 242 Cherry Street, Philadelphia, PA 19106–1906

First published 1989

British Library Cataloguing in Publication Data available on request

ISBN: 0 85066 432 2
ISBN: 0 85066 433 0 (pbk).

Typeset in 9/13 Bembo by
The FD Group Ltd, Fleet, Hampshire
Printed in Great Britain by BPCC Wheatons Ltd, Exeter

Contents

Contributing Authors

James H. Abbs
Speech Motor Control Laboratories
University of Wisconsin
Madison
Wisconsin   USA

Betty Byers Brown
Department of Paediatrics
University of Medicine and Dentistry
New Brunswick
New Jersey   USA
(currently Hon. Research Fellow
Department of Psychology
University of Manchester   UK)

Roxanne De Paul
Speech Motor Control Laboratories
University of Wisconsin
Madison
Wisconsin   USA

Pamela M. Enderby
Speech Therapy Department
Frenchay Hospital
Bristol   UK

Jennifer Lambert
Speech Therapy Section
Leeds Polytechnic
Leeds   UK

Margaret M. Leahy
School of Clinical Speech and
Language Studies
University of Dublin
Dublin   IRELAND

Ruth Lesser
Department of Speech
University of Newcastle upon Tyne
Queen Victoria Road
Newcastle upon Tyne   UK

Jerilyn Logemann
Department of Communication
Sciences and Disorders
2299 Sheridan Road
Evanston
Illinois   USA

Niklas Miller
Speech Therapy Department
Frenchay Hospital
Bristol   UK

John Gilbert
University of British Columbia
2211 Westbrook Mall
Vancouver
British Columbia   CANADA

Irmgarde Horsley
Department of Speech
University of Newcastle upon Tyne
Queen Victoria Road
Newcastle upon Tyne   UK

Mata Jaffe
Speech Pathology and Audiology
Pinecrest Rehabilitation Hospital
Delray Beach
Florida   USA

Alan G. Kamhi
Memphis Speech and Hearing Centre
807 Jefferson Avenue
Memphis
Tennessee   USA

Jane Russell
Speech Therapy Department
The Children's Hospital
Ladywood Middleway
Birmingham   UK

Pauline Sloane
School of Clinical Speech and
Language Studies
University of Dublin
Trinity College
Dublin   IRELAND

Joseph Stemple
St Elizabeth Medical Centre
601 Edwin Moses Boulevard
Dayton
Ohio   USA

Foreword

This book is one of a series whose primary aim is to inform the professional practice of speech and language clinicians, and their colleagues in the caring professions. The starting point for this series was a systematic review of those topics in human communication which are essential to the development of effective treatment programmes and the development of effective clinicians.

Whilst we have seen considerable advances in the scientific understanding of communication disorders in recent years much that is relevant to the practising clinician is either published in specialist scientific journals or exchanged on the conference floor. Bringing this theoretical and practical material together in book form seemed the first priority for a series of this kind. *Progress in Clinical Science* therefore aims to emphasise the scientific basis of modern clinical practice.

In addition we saw a need for texts capable of addressing broader issues in clinical practice. We wanted to provide a new resource for clinicians who wished to further their own social, interpersonal and scientific skills through further study. Topics here range from discussion of specific models of clinical intervention to the skills required for the scientific evaluation of the treatment enterprise.

Research into both the process and outcome of therapy programmes has revealed that individual therapist characteristics play a crucial role in the success or failure of treatment over a wide range of treatment approaches and client groups. Every therapist needs an injection of new stimulation in order to continue the process of evolution that characterises effective clinical practice. We need to be self-critical and we need to introduce systems of peer review in order to ensure that the work we do on behalf of our clients is of the highest possible standard. This series emphasises the need for efficacy research and the responsibility each individual clinician carries for the evaluation of their own clinical skills.

We are grateful for the help and support we have received from colleagues in many professional groups during the development of *Progress in Clinical Science*. It is our hope that the books in this series will cut across traditional disciplinary boundaries. The problems of theory construction, skill acquisition and treatment evaluation are common to every caring profession. We hope that *Progress in Clinical Science* will bring a fresh incentive for interdisciplinary collaboration at every level of professional development.

Harry Purser and Dave Rowley
Series Editors

Preface

This book is designed to introduce the clinician in training to intervention in communication disorders. The contributors are highly specialised authors drawn from both sides of the Atlantic and they present a comprehensive perspective, both theoretical and practical, on contemporary issues in clinical practice.

The book is organised into three main sections. In Section I, underlying philosophies and important aspects of the basic framework of professional intervention are discussed. The classification of communication disorders, issues regarding planning services and the development of the profession are presented, and questions about our future professional roles in these areas are raised.

Sections II and III are divided between disorders occurring in childhood and those occurring in the adult. In each chapter, topics are introduced with particular reference to their definition, possible causes and essential aspects of assessment and treatment. Relevant theoretical questions are integrated into the discussion and the vital question of therapy effectiveness is considered.

While every effort has been made to keep repetition to a minimum, some repetition is inevitable in a text of this nature. This allows for individual subjects to be considered as a whole.

The subjects of audiology and communication disorders associated with hearing and auditory disorders are considered beyond the scope of this book. This in no way undermines the significance of these topics but reflects professional boundaries that exist in some countries.

Throughout the book, the person who presents with a communication disorder is referred to variously as *the patient* or *the client,* as appropriate. This is held consistent throughout individual chapters. The speech-language pathologist or therapist is also referred to as *the speech and language clinician* or *the clinician.* It is recognised that this terminology is not without disadvantages, but it remains the most appropriate in our view.

As will be obvious from the extensive bibliography presented, there is a voluminous and challenging literature on individual subject areas. Many controversial issues are introduced — indeed the title of the book may well be controversial in itself. The overall aim in addressing these topics is not so much to provide ready answers as to stimulate an awareness and understanding of the nature of the problems facing the profession. As well as this, an objective of this book in introducing the science of intervention in communication disorders is to stimulate a questioning and searching attitude in the student while providing essential data. As the Irish proverb has it — *Doras feasa fiafraigh* — *the door to knowledge is in questioning.* If this is achieved it is due in the main to the expertise of the contributors. To them and to the series editors, Harry Purser and Dave Rowley, I express my gratitude for allowing me the privilege of working with them.

Acknowledgments

Many people helped during the final preparation of this book and I wish to express my gratitude to each one, and in particular to Pat O'Connor, Noreen Coyle and Sue Lacey; to Jim Larragy for technical assistance and to Gordon O'Connor for his drawings. The series editors, Harry Purser and Dave Rowley, provided constant support and advice and eased the transition stages enormously and I am especially grateful to them.

Margaret M. Leahy, Bealtaine, 1989.
Ollscoil Atha Cliath.
Colaiste na Trinoide.

I BASIC FRAMEWORK OF INTERVENTION

1 Philosophy in Intervention

Margaret M. Leahy

It seems appropriate to open a chapter on philosophy in intervention with an extract from Plato's writings which sets the scene for the discussion that follows. In *Laws* (720), Plato introduces two distinctive approaches to the healing process thus:

> Now there's another thing you notice. A state's invalids include not only freemen but slaves too, who are almost always treated by other slaves who either rush about on flying visits or wait to be consulted in their surgeries. This kind of doctor never gives any account of the particular illness of the individual slave, or is prepared to listen to one; he simply prescribes what he thinks best in the light of experience, as if he had precise knowledge, and with the self-confidence of a dictator. Then he dashes off on his way to the next slave patient, and so takes off his master's shoulders some of the work of attending the sick. The visits of the free doctor, by contrast, are mostly concerned with treating the illnesses of free men; his method is to construct an empirical case-history by consulting the invalid and his friends; in this way he himself learns something from the sick and at the same time he gives the individual patient all the instruction he can. He gives no prescription until he has somehow gained the invalid's consent; then, coaxing him into continued cooperation, he tries to complete his restoration to health. Which of the two methods do you think makes the doctor the better healer, or a trainer more efficient? Should they use the double method to achieve a single effect, or should the method too be single — the less satisfactory approach that makes the invalid more recalcitrant?

Plato's observations relate to a period of history long past, and there is no doubt that major advances in medical knowledge and treatment have been made since then, particularly in the present century. Nevertheless, two fundamental elements of the healing process that Plato highlights remain: the nature of the relationship in intervention and the nature of the knowledge involved.

Relationship in Clinical Intervention

Speech and language clinicians belong to a large family of health care professionals whose work centres on two basic objectives: restoring to health, and the prevention of the origins, development and recurrence of disease and disorders. The professional person involved in the process is responding to a request for help to change some problem affecting the client (or patient). In some instances, for example with children, the process may be instigated by others who are aware of and anxious about an apparent problem which may not be perceived as 'a problem' by the person. Two parties become involved in a relationship — the clinician and the client — and this relationship is considered a crucial part of the process. Relationship has been considered as a fundamental pillar of therapy or the 'soul' of casework, where other procedures, e.g. diagnosis and treatment, comprise the 'body' (Biestek, 1973).

General statements may be made about these relationships that distinguish them from other relationships in the family or community. First, by its nature the clinician–client relationship is a temporary one. Second, while the emotional component often involves the expression of attitudes and feelings, it differs fundamentally from other emotional relationships. The clinician, although acting as an individual, also acts as a representative of a profession and has a responsibility to maintain professional distance. Downie and Calman (1987, p. 84) suggest that the individual health worker represents his profession in two senses. First, he is the ascriptive representative in that the profession authorises his actions, having sanctioned his training. Second, he represents the values of the profession insofar as he acts in terms of its ethics, and its ethics are all pervasive in the actions and attitudes of the individual health worker.

Professional codes

Each profession is distinguished not only by a particular body of knowledge and a particular qualification that is acknowledged as authority to practise, but also by a code of ethics which represents the values of the profession. In general, ethical codes are expressed in deontological form — statements that concern what can and cannot be allowed in professional practice. But as Matthews (1982) points out, the ethical code is more than simply a list of do's and dont's — it serves to direct the professional worker in making decisions and allows for individuals to be censured if their professional behaviour falls below that indicated by the code. An acceptance of the code is required and each clinician should be aware of the obligations imposed by the code. Ethical codes protect the clients served by the profession as the welfare of the client is given the highest priority. Aspects of the clinician–client relationship, with the concept of professional distance either stated or implied, are defined in the code of ethics. Consider, for example, the following extracts from the codes of ethics of the College of Speech Therapists and the American Speech-Language-Hearing Association:

> Customary ethical standards of behaviour must be observed towards patients. Speech therapists must not abuse the position of trust given to them by patients and those who refer patients to them. They should not enter into disruptive personal relationships with patients during any part of the period of intervention. (CST, 1988)

> Individuals shall maintain objectivity in all matters concerning the welfare of persons served professionally. (ASHA, 1979)

Professional distance

Professional distance may also be seen by the application of other codes used by professions to signify their professional image. For example, the dress code although rapidly changing — is still maintained by many professions. Consider the dress of barristers and judges in UK courts or that of academics in universities. In hospitals, the white coat or uniform underlines the difference between the patient and the professional worker and the 'twin-set and pearls' image once distinguished the speech and language clinician. A reduction in the formality of dress may mean a move towards greater equality in the relationship between the clinician and client. Similarly, the use of first names may also encourage the realisation of such equality. However, as Kahn and Earle (1982, p. 27) point out, 'formality and tradition can be a protection in some cases to the person seeking help' as 'equality is not enough in some cases as the basis of a relationship for the supply of some kinds of needs.' In many ways, inequality exemplified by professional distance ensures the maintenance of ethical principles which protects both the client and the professional worker.

Terminology

Part of the mystique of professional activities may lie in the use of a terminology considered 'foreign' to the client. Although the naming or diagnosis of a disease or disorder may serve to reduce anxiety about the problem and bring it 'under control' ('the magic of naming', Kahn and Earle, 1982), it does not necessarily provide the client with any more information or insight into their problem than they had before. This in itself may serve to strengthen the position of the clinician, particularly when answers are unknown or explanations impossible, and it may exclude a great deal of relevant data concerning a client. Further, it implies that there is a known cause or etiology and a specific course of treatment and in many instances this is not so. However, the value of diagnosis and classification systems of diseases and disorders is not to be ignored or undermined. As Byers Brown points out in Chapter 3, diagnostic groups are subject to frequent subdivision and recategorisation as new data emerge and improved services depend on a better understanding of the nature of presenting problems. How we use the data in working with clients may justifiably be questioned.

Professional distance is also reflected in the concepts of rapport and empathy, which are important basic aspects of professional relationships.

Rapport and empathy

These concepts may seem over-emphasised to the beginning clinician, with the necessity to establish rapport in initial contact with clients stated in every treatment plan. Likewise, empathy, though not always stated, is expected to be the appropriate emotional response to a client. But they should not be under-estimated or taken for granted as they represent vital though non-scientific components of clinical interaction (Downie and Calman, 1987; Siegel and Ingham, 1987).

Although rapport implies a connection made in two directions, the responsibility for establishing it falls mainly in one — the clinician's. Initially, the clients' major role in establishing rapport is largely fulfilled by their willingness to consult with the clinician; thereafter it is up to the clinician to set the scene for developing the interaction. The clinician's responsibilities include showing warmth, interest in the client as an individual person (not a 'case' or just 'a disorder'), acceptance, willingness to help and to understand and an ability to communicate with the client, providing relevant information as well as collecting it. The concept of confidentiality about information is implied, or may be stated openly to reassure the client. The clinical setting becomes one where the client feels secure, unthreatened and assured of personal attention, and thus feels able to respond to the clinician, thereby completing the establishment of rapport. Devising appropriate intervention strategies results not only from applying theoretical knowledge to the individual but also through developing an understanding of the nature of specific problems that are presenting and through empathy, by attempting to put oneself in the place of the client and see life from the client's perspective. This idea may be referred to in different ways, e.g. 'understanding an action from the inside' (Downie and Calman,

1987, p. 37), or stepping into the shoes of the client (Kelly, 1955). Murgatroyd (1985, p. 15) stresses some points on the nature of empathy:

> Empathy involves the helper being sensitive, moment to moment, to the changing experience of the particular person one is seeking to help. Empathy is particular, not general; it is about understanding and sharing, not judging and supporting. Empathy requires you to enter the world of another person 'as if' it were your own so that you can better understand what it is like to be that person in need of your help.

Despite the fact that elements of relationships are described as non-scientific, the questioning nature of philosophy invites consideration and analysis of relationship paradigms that have helped shape the health sciences. These paradigms, which reflect fundamental views about human nature, evolved from an initial concern to explain the processes that guide human behaviour to being used as a basis for intervention. There are many competing views in this area but most have features in common that allow them to be classified in relation to the following two basic paradigms.

A subject-object paradigm

The traditional view of physical sciences stresses the empirical laws of physics and chemistry and the person is regarded as complex matter-in-motion. Symptoms are linked with changes in the physiology of the body and a course of treatment can be prescribed from expert knowledge of the laws of the traditional sciences. Such knowledge, expertise and understanding belong to the expert who is the Subject (the clinician). The Object (client) is not required to have extensive knowledge about symptoms or remedies or to acquire it. In effect there is a mysticism surrounding the process of evaluating the symptoms and assigning them to a category, as well as evaluating causal factors. The active role in the process — which is also the powerful one — is taken by the Subject who has the superior knowledge and skill to effect change in the Object. The Object takes a passive role and assumes that problems will be solved by following the given instructions. Such a paradigm is the basis of a 'bio-medical' approach (Downie and Calman, 1987) and it is shared by traditional medics and to a large degree by behaviourists.

If you refer back to Plato's Slave Doctor, some elements of his procedure can be clarified using the Subject–Object paradigm. In the first instance, the mysticism surrounding the process is held by the Slave Doctor who 'never gives any account of the particular illness . . .' Secondly, he does not 'waste time' in conversation with the patient, getting to know a different account of the problem that presents, but 'dashes off on his way . . .' And he takes the powerful active role, 'as if he had precise knowledge' . . . 'with the confidence of a dictator'. His knowledge is considered enough for him to prescribe, as is the knowledge of the Subject, who regards scientific expertise as the only basis of intervention. The approach to problem-solving is linear, following the Newtonian billiard ball model in which causality is directly linked to forces that act unidirectionally. In this instance, the treatment of the person with the problem is mechanistically linked to the etiology of the problem which is considered to have a biological basis.

A facilitative paradigm

In this instance the major role of the clinician is to understand the problem and client from the client's point of view — a phenomenological or 'first person' approach. The clinician's aim in intervening with clients is to facilitate change rather than direct it. In order to effect this, the values and motivations, perceptions and experiences of the client take precedence over those of the clinician in the process. Thus the expert in the client's reality is recognised as being himself and essentially, the direction of therapy is determined not so much by the clinician but by the client. As Keeney (1983, p. 39) puts it: 'A therapist treats a client who directs the therapist how to treat him'.

Making decisions in therapy is seen as the responsibility of both the client and the clinician with the client taking a major role. But the role of the clinician is not undermined. The expertise of the clinician is of a different nature to that of the client but it is still immensely important in many ways. First, in listening to and accepting the client as a person, active in the intervention process, the clinician recognises the expertise of the client in his own reality. Then by providing information and helping to demystify aspects of the problem, the development of the knowledge of the client about aspects of the problem that may not have been considered is furthered. The clinician plays a role in helping determine avenues for change, and ultimately, assists the client make the desired change or changes.

Plato's Free doctor fits into this paradigm, in the recognition of the importance of the patient's role, and that of his friends and family, in the process. By the fact that he 'learns something from the sick and gives the individual all the instruction he can . . .' the Free Doctor builds a relationship with the patient and, recognising the individuality of his circumstances, seeks consent in directing a course of therapy. In this way both the Doctor and the Patient are active partners in the healing process and they share their expertise to achieve a common purpose. The problem-solving process is recursive, where not just force but information and relationship become important. This inevitably moves away from the concept of diagnosis or the linear causation model as the basis of intervention. In Chapter 6, Kamhi briefly discusses how different models of intervention can be applied in working with children with language disorders.

Scientific knowledge

Plato's Slave Doctor considered that prescriptions should be based on scientific knowledge that is believed to be 'precise'. This raises the second point for discussion here: the nature of our scientific knowledge. Siegel (1987) points out that there is no single approach that qualifies as science and no single definition that will be embraced by all scientists. However, some characteristics may be shared by many, if not all sciences. Downie and Calman (1987) refer to three such characteristics which are:

1 Science is concerned with a search for patterns or uniformities which explain observable phenomena.

Classification systems derive from the perception of uniformities such as the classification of diseases, their causes and treatments (see also Chapter 3). Uniformities of change or development can also be observed, providing guidelines regarding particular phenomena, e.g. child language studies provide data on stages of acquisition of phonology and syntax (cf. Bloom and Lahey, 1978; Crystal, Fletcher and Garman, 1976).

2 The tentative nature of science is demonstrated by the use of hypotheses or suppositions used as a basis for reasoning and predicting events.

On examining a problem, an explanation may be postulated that allows for aspects of the problem to be described and verified through empirical testing. As information regarding the problem (or aspects of it) changes, new hypotheses replace those originally postulated. In this way scientific knowledge changes through research and our current knowledge is 'of its nature provisional and permanently so' (Popper, in Magee, 1973, p. 26).

3 A third characteristic is the development of paradigms which, according to Kuhn (1970), are consensually agreed-upon sets of rules about the nature of the science that define it.

Different types of paradigms may be delineated within the health sciences, e.g. there are paradigms of disease and disorders on which treatment is based (cf. Downie and Calman, 1987 re breast cancer; Crystal, 1980 and Byers Brown, 1981 re models of procedure based on linguistics and medicine). All of the caring professions involve interpersonal interaction and two relationship paradigms have already been discussed above, albeit briefly.

Speech and language clinicians as scientists

The fact that speech and language clinicians have adopted models, methods and concepts from other established professions reflects historical influences that have helped shape the profession (see Chapter 5). This in itself does not diminish our standing as an autonomous science, but it may help explain some divisions within the field and some basic differences in approaches to work. There is no doubt that the clinician has acquired scientific knowledge and expertise and that it is exploited in therapy. Neither is there doubt that the research worker knows about clinical processes and procedures. The vital non-scientific aspects of clinical work such as relationships must not be undermined when considering whether the clinician is scientist. Given the need to stimulate research in therapy, there is no reason why a well-informed clinician cannot play different roles at different times and actively contribute to the body of existing knowledge about communication disorders. In effect, practising clinicians are required by the code of ethics to evaluate the effectiveness of their work and this demands that scientific principles be exploited in the clinic. Furthermore, the clinical situation can and should become the place where hypotheses are tested and new approaches to therapy developed — in Kelly's terms (1969, p. 154), '. . . the most exciting experimental situation is the therapy room, and the most exciting colleague in the research enterprise is my client.'

A Rationale for Intervention: Altruism and Individualism

As has already been mentioned, the basic objectives of health care are restorative and preventive. Essentially the process centres on the problems of others and this provides an element of altruism that is often considered a basic feature of caring professions. Because of this, the person working in the health professions is often regarded as having a sense of 'vocation' or 'higher calling' in that self-sacrifice is implied or even required. There is no doubt that demands made often involve self-sacrifice in terms of time, effort and energy. And the rewards may be very little for some — particularly if measured in terms of money. Why then enter such a profession? There are many possible answers, but a central focus is altruism, whether as a stated and direct motivating factor or as an incidental, embedded feature of the process. In this latter sense, the 'advancement of scientific knowledge' may be a primary motivating force for an individual, but furthering knowledge of a disease or disorder ultimately is for the benefit of those affected by the problem and therefore for the benefit of all. The notion of altruism as a motivating force has been discussed by many renowned philosophers and theorists over the years. Plato (Laws, 903) discusses the individual subserving the interests of the community and emphasises altruism:

> The part exists for the sake of the whole, but the whole does not exist for the sake of the part . . . you are created for the sake of the whole and not the whole for the sake of you . . .

Although Plato's ideas on altruism may seem laudable, they have been widely criticised because individualism is largely precluded. Popper (1945, in Miller, 1983) discusses Plato's suggestion that if one is not prepared to sacrifice oneself for the common good then that individual is selfish and uncaring. In contrast, Popper cites Pericles who emphasised the right of the individual to choose his way — the right to self-determination. But he insists that individualism cannot stand alone but it must be linked with altruism: 'We are taught . . . never to forget that we must protect the injured . . .' This idea is echoed by Dryden (1987, p. 8) in contrasting 'enlightened self-interest' and selfishness following Adler's idea of social interest: 'It is recognised that decisions concerning whose interest to serve at a given moment — self or others — are complex and depend on (a) the context (b) the importance of one's own goals, and (c) the likely consequence of making such decisions.'

By pursuing a career in the health care professions, an individual can satisfy both personal interests and the interests of the community. Personally meaningful goals can be pursued by developing one's knowledge, skills and expertise and one can be satisfied that the knowledge, skills and expertise that are acquired relate directly to helping others. And so the interests of the community may be served in two ways: directly through intervention and research and indirectly, by fulfilling oneself as a caring individual

Conclusion

The objective of this chapter is to introduce the beginning clinician to questions about the nature of intervention, specifically questions regarding the professional person's role and that of the client in the process, and questions on the nature of our knowledge. Answers may not always be clear but it is important for the clinician to address such issues and develop a better understanding of themselves, their motivation and value systems as professionals and the problem solving in which they engage in the service of the community.

Acknowledgments

The author wishes to thank Clothra Ni Cholmain, Jeffrey Kallen and Mia van Doerslaer for their helpful comments on earlier drafts of this chapter.

References

BLOOM, L. and LAHEY, M. (1978) *Language Development and Language Disorders.* New York: Wiley.

BIESTEK, F.P. (1973) *The Casework Relationship.* London: Unwin.

BYERS BROWN, B. (1981) *Speech Therapy: Principles and Practice.* Edinburgh: Churchill-Livingstone.

CRYSTAL, D. (1980) *Introduction to Language Pathology.* London: Edward Arnold.

CRYSTAL, D., FLETCHER, P. and GARMAN, M. (1976) *The Grammatical Analysis of Language Disability.* London: Edward Arnold.

DOWNIE, R.S. and CALMAN, K.C. (1987) *Healthy Respect: Ethics in Health Care.* London: Faber & Faber.

DRYDEN, W. (1987) *Counselling Individuals: The Rational-Emotive Approach.* London: Taylor and Francis.

KELLY, G. (1955) *The Psychology of Personal Constructs.* New York: Norton.

KELLY, G. (1969) The language of hypothesis: Man's psychological instrument. In B. Maher, (Ed.), *Clinical Psychology and Personality: The Selected Papers of George Kelly.* New York: Wiley.

KEENEY, B. (1983) *Aesthetics of Change.* New York: Guildford Press.

KAHN, J. and EARLE, E. (1982) *The Cry for Help and the Professional Response.* Oxford: Pergamon.

KUHN, T.S. (1970) *The Structure of Scientific Revolutions* (2nd edition). Chicago: University of Chicago Press.

MAGEE, B. (1973) *Popper.* London: Fontana.

MATTHEWS, J. (1982) The professions of speech-language pathology and audiology. In G.H. Sames and E.H. Wiig (Eds), *Human Communication Disorders.* Columbus Ohio: Charles E. Merrill.

MURGATROYD, S. (1985) *Counselling and Helping.* London: British Psychological Society.

POPPER, K. (1945) Individualism versus collectivism. In D. Miller (Ed.) *A Pocket Popper.* London: Fontana.

PLATO, *The Laws,* translated by T.J. Saunders (1986). Harmondsworth: Penguin.

SIEGEL, G.M. and INGHAM, R. (1987) Theory and science in communication disorders. *Journal of Speech and Hearing Disorders,* 52, 99–104.

SIEGEL, G.M. (1987) The limits of science in communication disorders. *Journal of Speech and Hearing Disorders,* 52, 306–19.

Documents used

The College of Speech Therapists (CST), London, *Code of Ethics and Professional Conduct with Ethical Guidelines for Research* (1988).

The American Speech-Language-Hearing Association (ASHA), *Code of Ethics of the American Speech-Language-Hearing Association* (1979).

2 Aspects of the Anatomy and Physiology of Speech

Margaret M. Leahy and Joseph Stemple

Introducing the anatomy and physiology of speech allows only for an overview of the complex mechanisms and functions that help distinguish mankind from the rest of the animal kingdom. The main focus is on speech but language will be briefly considered.

This chapter will consider aspects of respiration, phonation and articulation but it must begin with a basic introduction of the nervous systems, both central and peripheral, which play the major role in the regulation of speech.

The Central Nervous System (CNS)

The CNS comprises the brain and the spinal cord which are continuous with each other at the brain stem. The brain consists of a complex network of nerve cells or neurons (grey matter) which make up its surface, the cortex. Nerve fibres (white matter) lie underneath and nuclei of neurones form the basal ganglia which lie deep in the cerebral hemispheres. The spinal cord which extends from the medulla to the second lumbar vertebra is protected by the spine. It is composed of grey matter surrounded by white matter. The grey matter is divided into ventral and dorsal columns. The ventral columns contain the cell bodies of the spinal nerves (motor) while the sensory fibres which ascend to higher levels are contained in the dorsal columns. The sensory and motor fibres synapse so that each spinal nerve carries both sensory and motor fibres.

The cortex presents a pattern of convolutions which are folded areas (gyri) divided from each other by sulci or fissures. This pattern allows for the maximum amount of neurones in the smallest possible space and provides the basic geography of the cortex (Fig. 2.1).

The longitudinal fissure divides the cortex into two main hemispheres which are connected deeply by the corpus callosum. Each hemisphere has four lobes: (1)

13

the frontal lobe which is separated from (2) the parietal lobe by the Rolandic (central) fissure and from (3) the temporal lobe by the Sylvian (lateral) fissure; (4) the occipital lobe lies posterior to the parietal and temporal lobes and superior to the cerebellum. The cerebellum also consists of right and left hemispheres and its role is important in processing data from the brain and the body that enables precise coordination of muscular movement (Hardcastle 1976).

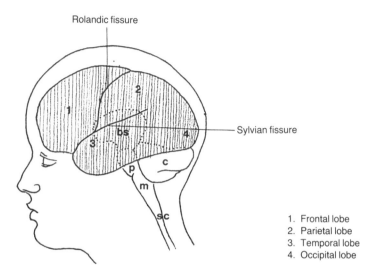

Figure 2.1: View of Cerebral Cortex in situ indicating the relative positions of Brainstem (bs), Pons (p), Medulla (m), Spinal Cord (sc) and Cerebellum (c)

Cerebral Localisation

The area of the cortex chiefly responsible for control of movement is located anterior to the Rolandic fissure. Sensory function is located posterior to this fissure. Although localisation of specific functions is a controversial issue, neurologists agree that left hemisphere dominance for the control of speech and for the control of most mental activity is the rule for the majority of individuals. The role for the right hemisphere is less certain but there is increasing evidence that it has substantial linguistic capabilities particularly in more automatic, non-propositional aspects of speech production and in aspects of comprehension (see Code, 1987).

Broca's and Wernicke's areas

In 1861, Paul Broca indicated that speech production was controlled in the third convolution of the frontal lobe of the left hemisphere. Shortly afterwards in 1874, Carl Wernicke indicated that the first convolution of the left temporal lobe was responsible for comprehension of speech. These two areas and the surrounding areas in the temporo-parietal and the posterior-inferior area of the frontal lobe have been shown subsequently to have critical importance for speech and language. In Wernicke's view of cerebral functioning, the temporal lobe receives auditory images and a memory image is deposited there. Association fibres connecting the temporal and frontal lobes are responsible for transmitting the memory image to a motor point on the occurrence of a new stimulus. A second centrifugal pathway connecting the frontal and temporal areas gives rise to movement. In normal speech the representation of movement is accompanied by innervation of the corresponding sound image which monitors the movement.

In the 1970s, this model was challenged by Jason Brown who proposed the microgenetic approach to language production in which:

1   language processing is conceived as an event which emerges over evolutionary sequential brain levels rather than across cortical areas;

2   language is processed simultaneously by complementary systems in the anterior and posterior divisions of the brain rather than by means of a rostral conveyance of nerve impulses, and

3   pathways serve to 'maintain in phase' different regions of the brain rather than to convey information (Brown and Perceman, 1987, p. 17).

The Peripheral Nervous System (PNS)

The PNS comprises the twelve cranial nerves which arise in the brain stem, the spinal nerves which are attached to the spinal cord and the autonomic nervous system which is concerned with such non-volitional activities of the body as glandular and visceral functioning.

The Cranial Nerves

The cranial nerves are named according to their primary function or in the case of the Trigeminal, because of its three main divisions. Table 2.1 provides an outline of the nerves along with their names and functions. Motor control of the speech musculature involves CN V, CN VII, CN IX, CN X and CN XII. The Auditory Nerve, CN VIII, is also of vital importance.

Table 2.1: The Cranial Nerves

CN	Name	Function/Distribution	Motor/Sensory (M/S)
I	Olfactory	smell	S
II	Optic	sight	S and M
III	Oculomotor	muscles of eye (except lat. rectus, superior oblique)	S and M S and M
IV	Trochlear	superior oblique	M
V	Trigeminal	a) face, teeth, sinuses b) muscles of mastication c) hearing (tensor tympani)	S M M
VI	Abducens	lateral rectus (eye)	S and M
VII	Facial	a) ant. two-thirds tongue and velum b) muscles of face, scalp and stepedius (hearing)	S and M M
VIII	Auditory	a) vestibular — balance; b) cochlear — hearing	S and M S and M
IX	Glossopharyngeal	post. part of tongue tonsils and pharynx	S and M
X	Vagus	heart, lungs, vocal tract, inc. laryngeal muscles lungs, bronchi, external ear	M S
XI	Spinal Accessory	upper sternocleidomastoid and trapezius muscles	M
XII	Hypoglossal	extrinsic and intrinsic tongue muscles (except palatoglossus)	M

Respiration

The process of speech depends on the breath stream. The breath is described by Borden and Harris (1980) as the 'power supply' which is converted into an acoustic signal through the movements of the larynx, and the shape of the mouth and vocal tract. Since the primary purpose of breathing is vegetative, i.e. to exchange carbon dioxide in the body for oxygen, the process has to be modified for speech production. The major changes that occur are that the inhalation phase is shortened, and the exhalation is lengthened and controlled.

 The muscles of respiration are the diaphragm, the intercostals and the costal elevators. The accessory muscles of respiration used in extreme circumstances (e.g., after running, etc.) are the muscles of the neck and shoulders. The abdominal muscles can also be considered as accessory. The diaphragm is of vital importance so it receives attention here.

The diaphragm, a large domeshaped muscle, forms the floor of the chest cavity. Its upper surface has a large tendon from which the muscle fibres radiate downwards to the ribs, sternum and vertebrae. It is attached to the sternum at the internal surface of the xiphoid process, the ribs (7–12) and the lumbar portion is formed from aponeurotic lumbo-costal arches and two crura from the lumbar vertebrae. On breathing in, the diaphragm contracts, thus enlarging the vertical dimensions of the thoracic cavity; it pulls up on the ribs and sternum as well as down on the central tendon, depressing the viscera and expanding the abdominal wall to the front and to each side. On breathing out, the diaphragm relaxes and is pushed upwards by the abdominal viscera.

The eleven pairs of external intercostal muscles running diagonally downwards between the ribs lie immediately external to the corresponding internal intercostal muscles. The costal elevators arise from the vertebrae. Their combined action is in elevating the ribs, assisting in respiration.

Reflex control of breathing is in the medulla and voluntary changes made for speech are under cortical control.

The Laryngeal Mechanism

The laryngeal mechanism consists of a complex system of cartilages, muscles and connective tissues. It is situated directly on top of the trachea which directs air to and from the lungs. Located directly above is the pharynx, the base of the tongue, the oral cavity and the nasal cavity. All of these structures form the vocal tract (Fig. 2.2).

The laryngeal framework consists of nine cartilages, three paired and three unpaired. The single cricoid cartilage is the base cartilage and it rests on the first tracheal ring which serves as the support foundation. The cricoid cartilage resembles a signet ring. Attached to its lateral sides is the thyroid cartilage which is the main body of the larynx. The thyroid cartilage, commonly known as the Adam's Apple, attaches to the cricoid at movable cricothyroid joints by two inferior arms called the inferior cornu. Two superior arms, the superior cornu, articulate with a superior supporter, the hyoid bone. The hyoid bone is the only non-articulated bone in the body as it is suspended in the neck by a series of strap muscles which are known as extrinsic laryngeal muscles.

The arytenoid cartilages are connected to the superior posterior surface of the cricoid cartilage by the cricoarytenoid joints. The arytenoids each possess a

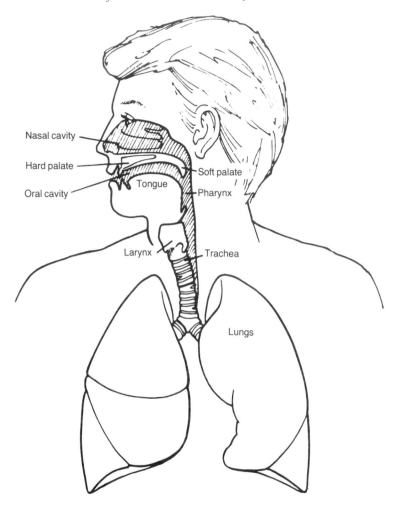

Figure 2.2: The Vocal Tract (Stemple and Holcomb, 1988, Merrill Pub. Co.)

muscular process and a vocal process and they play a very important role in the manner in which the vocal folds approximate and separate to produce voice. The muscular processes serve as the attachment points for various laryngeal muscles responsible for vocal fold movement while the vocal processes serve as the posterior attachments of the true vocal folds.

The corniculate cartilages articulate with the top of the arytenoid cartilages, forming the top of its pyramidal shape. The cuneiform cartilages are embedded in supporting laryngeal connective tissue just lateral to and above the corniculates. The leaf-shaped epiglottis cartilage attaches to the inside angle of the thyroid cartilage and is the superior most part of the larynx (Fig. 2.3).

POSTERIOR ASPECT

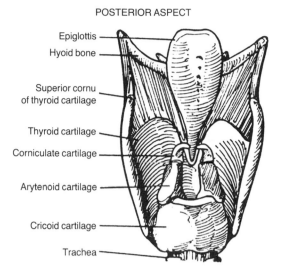

Epiglottis

Hyoid bone

Superior cornu
of thyroid cartilage

Thyroid cartilage

Corniculate cartilage

Arytenoid cartilage

Cricoid cartilage

Trachea

Figure 2.3: Laryngeal Cartilages — posterior view (Stemple and Holcomb, 1988, Merrill Pub. Co.)

The laryngeal muscles

The extrinsic muscles of the larynx (the strap muscles) comprise those that support the hyoid bone superiorly (the digastric, the stylohyoid, the mylohyoid and the geniohyoid) and inferiorly (the sternohyoid, the omohyoid) and those that support the thyroid cartilage superiorly (the thyrohyoid) and inferiorly (the sternothyroid). As well as supporting the larynx, these muscles act to raise and lower the larynx during swallowing and speech.

The functional components of the larynx are the intrinsic laryngeal muscles. Table 2.2 provides a summary of these muscles, their functions and nerve supply.

Vocal fold vibration

The most accepted theory of phonation is the Myoelastic-Aerodynamic theory (Vandenberg, 1958). This stated that following the approximation of the vocal folds, air pressure from the lungs is built up against the resistance of the adducted folds. Eventually, that pressure becomes great enough to overcome the resistance of the folds forcing them to momentarily separate, thus releasing one small puff of air. This release creates a sudden drop in air pressure directly between the vocal folds causing a suction action to begin. This suction, called the Bernoulli Effect, along

Table 2.2: The Intrinsic Laryngeal Muscles

	Attachments	Nerve Supply	Action
The True Vocal Folds: the vocalis the thyroarytenoid (+ vocal ligament)	Anteriorly: inside angle of the thyroid cartilage, close to the epiglottis Posteriorly: vocal processes of the arytenoids	recurrent laryngeal nerve	The true vocal folds are the actual vibrating bodies that produce voice
Vocal Fold Abductors: the posterior cricoarytenoids	Posterior part of cricoid cartilage and muscular processes of the arytenoid cartilages	recurrent laryngeal nerve	They cause the muscular processes of arytenoid to swivel medially which causes the vocal processes to swivel laterally thus *separating* the vocal cords
Vocal Fold Adductors: the lateral cricoarytenoids	Upper border of arch of cricoid and anterior surface of muscular process of arytenoid	recurrent laryngeal nerve	Rotation of arytenoid
the transverse arytenoids	Muscular process and lateral edge of arytenoid cartilage and lateral border of opposite arytenoid	recurrent laryngeal nerve	Slides arytenoids together
the oblique arytenoids	The summit of the arytenoid cartilage and posterior surface of muscular process of other arythenoid	recurrent laryngeal nerve	Adduction (approximation) of the vocal folds in voice production, swallowing, lifting, coughing, defecating
Vocal Fold Tensors: the cricothyroid muscles (pars rectus, pars oblique)	Antero–lateral cricoid cartilage to the inside lateral borders of the thyroid cartilage	superior laryngeal nerve	Tensening and lengthening the vocal folds (pitch changes)

with the natural static positioning of the adducted vocal folds, causes the folds to draw back together. The closer the folds draw, the greater the suction becomes, until the folds totally approximate again thus completing one vibratory cycle.

Fundamental frequency (fo)

The number of times the vocal folds complete a vibratory cycle per second is the voice fundamental frequency and is perceived by the listener as the speaker's pitch. Pitch changes within an individual are dependent on the length of the vocal folds and the amount of subglottic air pressure built up beneath the adducted folds. As the vocal folds are tensed and stretched by the actions of the cricothyroid muscles, the subglottic air pressure must be increased to counter the increased resistance of the tensed folds. Male and female voices typically vary in pitch due to mass and length of the vocal folds. Adult male vocal folds are thicker and longer than those of the adult female (15-20mm male, 9-13mm female). The average fundamental frequency for males will therefore fall within a range of 80-160 Hz while the female fundamental frequency will average 170-240 Hz.

Resonance

Before voice is perceived by others, vocal fold vibration is damped and enhanced throughout the entire vocal tract by the resonators. Appropriate coupling of the pharyngeal, oral and nasal cavities will dictate the specific characteristics of voice by determining the manner in which the fundamental and its harmonics are altered by the vocal tract. Individual resonant characteristics determine the distinctiveness of each voice.

Vocal intensity

Vocal intensity, which is perceived as loudness, is dependent on the amount of air pressure built up beneath the vocal folds and the amplitude of the vocal fold vibration. Amplitude refers to how far the vocal folds are forced open during phonation. In order to shout, it is necessary to first deeply inhale. This deep inhalation enables a greater amount of air pressure beneath the adducted folds. During the shout, the vocal folds are blown further apart than normal so that the distance the folds travel laterally is greater. This lateral excursion is the amplitude of the vibration. The resultant voice is therefore louder.

Vocal onset

The timing between the adduction of the vocal folds and the buildup of subglottic air pressure will determine the type of vocal attack or onset. This may either be breathy, hard or static. When expiration of subglottic air is begun, before the folds are fully approximated, the attack will be breathy. Adduction of the vocal folds followed by a quick, excessive buildup of subglottic air pressure will cause an explosion of sound called a hard glottal attack. A normal static attack will occur when the folds are nearly approximated just as the subglottic airflow begins.

Articulation

The structures above the larynx which are part of the vocal tract are the pharynx, the oral cavity and the nasal cavity.

The pharynx forms the posterior wall of the mouth and nose and is divided into three parts: the nasopharynx behind the nose, the oropharynx the walls of which are seen on looking into the mouth and the laryngo-pharynx which extends to the larynx. There are three pairs of constrictor muscles — the superior, middle and inferior constrictors which work together to move the bolus of food from the mouth towards the oesophagus to the stomach. In speech, the muscles of the pharynx constrict and change the resonance of the supraglottic region. The process of articulation results from changes made in the shape of the vocal tract, produced by movements of the jaw tongue lips and velum.

The oral cavity

The palate forms the roof of the mouth and is divided into a bony hard palate that extends from the upper teeth (three quarters way back) to the muscular soft palate or velum which is attached to the hard palate and to the lateral walls of the oropharynx. The soft palate presents a projection centrally which is called the uvula (Fig. 2.4). The muscles of the soft palate elevate and retract it to close the nasopharynx from the oropharynx during swallowing (preventing regurgitation upwards to the nose). These muscles are the levator palatini, the tensor palatini, the glossopalatal and the pharyngopalatal.

The tongue is a muscular body or corpus which is attached to the hyoid bone. Its anterior end, the apex lies behind the closed incisor teeth at rest. Its upper surface, the dorsum is mottled with buds.

The extrinsic muscles of the tongue are: the genioglossus, the hyoglossus and the styloglossus. These muscles, with their origins outside the tongue change its

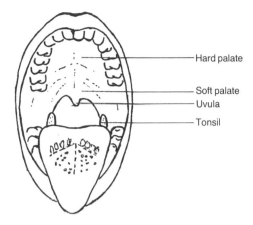

Figure 2.4: The Oral Cavity

shape and positioning. The intrinsic muscles are: the superior and inferior longitudinal muscles and the transverse and vertical muscles. The superior and inferior longitudinal muscles act to shorten the tongue and to bulge it upwards. The transverse and vertical muscles narrow and flatten the tongue.

Conclusion

This introduction represents some basic aspects of the anatomy and physiology of speech production which could only be considered as the 'tip of the iceberg' of the data available. It is important to recall that information about the processes involved in the production of speech and language is continually expanding and that much has yet to be learned about these complex processes which are delicately balanced yet highly resistant. Although many speech and language disorders do not have organic origins, many do. In both events, the clinician needs to understand as fully as possible how the balance of the functioning of the mechanism has been disturbed and what can be done to correct it.

References

BORDEN, G.J. and HARRIS, K.S. (1980) *Speech Science Primer.* Baltimore: Williams and Wilkins.
BROWN, J.W. and PERCEMAN, E. (1987) Neurological basis of language processes. In

R. Chapey (Ed.), *Language Intervention Strategies in Aphasia*. Baltimore: Williams and Wilkins.

CODE, C. (1987) *Language, Aphasia and the Right Hemisphere*. Chichester: Wiley.

HARDCASTLE, W.J. (1976) *Physiology of Speech Production*. London: Academic Press.

VANDENBERG, J. (1958) Myoelastic–aerodynamic theory of voice production. *Journal of Speech and Hearing Research*, 1, 227–44.

3   The Classification of Communication Disorders

Betty Byers Brown

The term *communication disorders* has come into use as a convenient way of referring to a number of clinical entities. It is only recently that it has become part of common professional parlance and it has yet to be adopted by the general public. It represents a field of clinical and research activity which has outgrown the concepts and classification on which it was founded. As a unitary concept, it has yet to generate a classification system which is internationally acceptable.

Prior to the emergence of the term *communication disorders,* reference was made only to its component parts: speech, hearing and language. In Britain, the adoption of the title *Disorders of Communication* for the journal to replace *Speech Pathology and Therapy* in 1966, acknowledged the need for a new vision. It was stated in the editorial that 'it has become increasingly apparent that the scope of speech therapy is wider than was initially conceived, and that we are concerned with that aspect of human behaviour which enables one individual to maintain contact with another' (Morley, 1966).

The United States, while retaining the terms speech, hearing and language in the title of its professional association and official journals, now supports the use of the term communication disorders for the discipline (Siegel and Ingham 1987). The Canadian professional association has named its new journal Human Communication, Canada but guidelines for practice are generated for Language-Speech Pathology and Audiology (Canadian Department of Health and Welfare, 1982). Clinicians in different countries practise under the titles of audiologist, speech-language pathologist or speech therapist but there is no clinical title using the term communication disorders since that would signify a field too broad to be mastered by one individual.

The expansion of the field of professional activity is shown, not only in the subdivisions of different specialties but in the incorporation of entirely new procedures. Once a skill has been mastered it may be put to other uses than the primary one. Speech pathologists who have training and experience in the control of the speech mechanism to produce articulate utterance, are now making use of their skill to attack primary, noncommunicative disabilities such as feeding and swallowing disorders.

Clinicians who have developed a special interest in the pragmatic functions of language and its basic structure are changing the media through which they work to include visual symbolic systems. This has generated the rapidly growing field of augmentative communication which is also the offshoot of a greatly expanded technology. The original classifications through which professional bodies set out to explain and clarify their procedures are no longer comprehensive enough, even though they have been subjected to continuing revision.

The Need to Classify

Clinical classification systems are built into the concept of clinical practice. If such practice is to develop in a rational and cohesive manner, a framework has to be employed which will allow conditions to be grouped together. Since new information is being gathered all the time, these diagnostic groups are subjected to frequent subdivision and recategorisation. A frequent impact of new information upon a diagnostic group is to show that it was not so homogeneous as was originally thought. If the heterogeneous elements have a sufficient amount in common with each other, they may form a subgroup. This may be seen with conditions of oral–motor impairment where the dyspraxic group has emerged with characteristics which give it an individual status within the larger group of neurologically based conditions affecting movement of the articulators (Edwards, 1984).

Examination of common characteristics within original diagnostic groups will not only lead to the creation of new groups but to the reclassification of former group members. For example, the conventional production and use of consonants and vowels was first perceived to be an articulatory process. Increased knowledge of linguistic development in children revealed that impairments may show themselves in failure to master the sound system of the language. Further examination revealed that some children who had not achieved the systematic acquisition of vowels and consonants did not have difficulty in individual sound production. The term Disorders of Articulation was therefore not appropriate for this group which was then reclassified as Linguistic/Phonological Disorders.

The lack of a suitably comprehensive conceptual framework at the time of the first taxonomies led to the *ad hoc* adoption of terms from a number of other disciplines. The basic and best developed model was the medical one, but the strong subsequent influence of the behavioural sciences was soon reflected in both categories and terms. The behavioural influence on communication disorders has not, however, led to an international classification system such as those generated by the earlier medical models. Attempts have been made to look at communication disorders as disruptions of the communication process rather than basing them upon individual pathologies of organs or systems. This has led to the creation and propagation of models which are necessarily abstract. The utility of such models in drawing together medical and behavioural components is thoroughly discussed by Crystal (1980).

The Communication Chain

Drawing upon the earlier work of Denes and Pinson (1973) who first introduced the idea of combining different properties, acoustic, biological, informational into the speech chain, Crystal uses the communication chain to cover a larger number of components. This would appear to provide a useful framework for a classification system. However, other developments within the professions concerned have redirected attention to those functional, clinical aspects which dictate the nature and extent of remedial procedures. While one aspect of professional growth is reflected in the search for a unifying theory of communication disorders, another is concerned with the clear delineation of diagnostic groups for the purpose of treatment and professional accountability. These aims are not necessarily incompatible but they may be difficult to reconcile. The more advanced the status of communication disorders as a discipline in any one country, the more its classification and terms reflect the attempt to support a conceptual framework by the use of a logically derived terminology. In countries where professional activities are intensive and wide ranging, a suitable framework for the classification of disorders and procedures is required for the following purposes:

1 Clinical Practice: to establish a code of practice
                       to determine methods of prevention, identification
                       and intervention
                       to determine treatment efficacy

2 Education: to train professional personnel
               to share information across professions
               to inform the public

3 Research: to describe subjects in research studies including
              epidemiological studies
              to provide interdisciplinary investigations

4 Remuneration: to establish scales of fees for services.

In developing their classification systems different countries make different compromises. Given the choice between major reconsiderations or rationalisations of existing states, the balance at the moment is in favour of rationalisation. To see how this has come about we must look at early ideas.

Historical bases for classification

The first classification within the field of communication disorders came with the division of speech and hearing. Professionals working with the hearing-impaired developed categories appropriate to measurement, causation and educational and medical management. The new professions, which developed for the purpose of studying and treating speech disorders, found it necessary to develop a category of basic terms which essentially operated as a classification system for the next forty years. It consisted of the following elements:

1 Voice and Resonance: abnormalities   of   phonation   and   vocal modulation
2 Articulation: abnormalities in the production or use of the sounds of speech
3 Language: abnormalities in the comprehension and/or use of verbal or written symbols
4 Fluency or Rhythm: abnormalities in the rate, timing and flow of speech.

Two principal modifiers were then introduced; the division into:

ORGANIC   FUNCTIONAL
the cause lying in   where the mechanism appears
pathology   to be capable of working normally
of organs or systems   but fails to do so

and the division by

ACQUIRED   DEVELOPMENTAL/CONGENITAL
where established function is   where the disorder is present at
lost or impaired   birth or becomes apparent
                                 during development.

The interrelation of the four basic categories and the two basic modifiers allowed for a useful and flexible form of classification with an increasing number of subclassifications and then cross classifications. At the time of this development, the professions concerned with communication disorders were dominated by the medical model of diagnosis. The categories of voice, articulation, language and fluency adopted diagnostic terms which were already in medical practice (e.g., aphonia, loss or absence of phonation; dysphasia, impairment of language resulting from cerebral damage). As a consequence, the categories have crossed into medical international classifications which exist to promote a common language among a number of diverse bodies (ICD-9, WHO 1978).

These basic categories have proved to be surprisingly robust. They were used by the Committee of Enquiry into Speech Therapy Services for England and Wales to discuss the manner in which disorders of communication were perceived and treated by the profession of speech therapy. As was stated in the committee's report (1972, p. 21), the terms Voice, Articulation, Resonance and Language are part of the basic vocabulary of speech therapists. The committee substituted the term Disorders of Rhythm for Disorders of Fluency in classifying stammering (stuttering) but the definition remained the same: 'characterized by abnormal hesitation, blocking or repetition of sounds, syllables or word'.

The same terms provide the basic categories for the classification of language-speech disorders used in the Canadian Department of Health and Welfare Guidelines (1982) where they constitute a five-fold taxonomy for the diagnosis and treatment of communication disorders. They are still used in major student texts (Shames and Wiig, 1982) and come up for discussion in most serious attempts to achieve a rationale for diagnosis and intervention (Crystal, 1980; Byers Brown, 1981). When an attempt has been made to base a classification system upon a different concept of speech and language it has proved less durable. For example, Mysak's attempt to relate speech disorders to the pathologies of different physiological systems (1976) had logic but introduced too many new terms to be acceptable to practitioners.

As a consequence of their durability and utility, there is obviously a case to be made for the retention of the basic categories of Voice, Articulation, Language and Fluency in any further revision of the subject. This has been acknowledged in the recent revision by the American Speech-Language-Hearing Association of its classification of Speech-Language Pathology and Audiology Procedures and Communication disorders (ASHA, 1986). In the first section of speech-language pathology procedures, the categories language, speech articulation, speech rate, fluency, voice and resonance are included as focal points of assessment to determine the nature of a problem. The aim of this classification was to provide a coding system to permit diverse, comprehensive analysis of professional services data. It came about in response to the perceived inadequacies in the conceptualisation of speech, language and hearing disorders and misapplication of procedures in such international systems as the International Classification of Diseases-Clinical Modification (ICD-9CM) and the Diagnostic and Statistical Manual of Mental Disorders (DSM III).

International classification systems

The International Classification of Diseases was developed as a statistical tool to enable comparison between countries at the same point in time and between countries over time. It was neither intended to be a clinical classification of medicines nor a nomenclature of diseases. This is made clear in a recent directive from the World Health Organization (WHO) concerning the tenth revision of the classification (ICD-10) which will come into effect from January 1, 1993. The outline for revision groups together disease and the factors which influence its progress. Disorders of communication have been represented in past editions under the chapter headings Mental Disorders and Diseases of the Nervous System, and scattered references may be found in other sections. While this representation is unsatisfactory to those professions which are entirely concerned with communication disorders, it is not unreasonable in regard to the first purpose of the classification and the fact that the WHO has a basic interest in conditions affecting mortality and in the spread of disease. The proposed revision (ICD-10) indicates the groups which would be involved in Speech-Language Hearing Classification. Mental Disorders; Developmental Disorders; Diseases of the Ear; Symptoms, Signs and Abnormal Clinical Laboratory Findings not classified elsewhere. Within these categories, individual components are coded in more than one way to allow for specific reference (e.g., aphasia has a number which indicates that it is associated with the nervous system and hoarseness has a number which indicates that it relates to the respiratory system).

It is inevitable in a classification of this nature that many communication disorders are going to be classified under such headings as 'Not classified elsewhere'.

Clinical modifications

The United States Health Department has published its clinical modifications to ICD-9 with the recommendation that this be used in all clinical settings. Its coding is required for reporting diagnoses and diseases to all US Public Health systems. This clinical modification does not make any real change in the status of communication disorders and many of them find their way into the category Symptoms, Signs, and Ill defined Conditions (e.g., voice disturbances and other speech disturbances). Many conditions are unsuitably classified under Mental Disorders because that appeared to be their nearest medical affiliation.

International Classification of Impairments, Disabilities and Handicaps

In 1980 the World Health Organization published the above named classification in the attempt to deal with the consequences of disease, not the disease process itself. It is directed towards those concerned with health care and welfare and offers a unifying framework within which the consequences of disease can be considered. Such a classification is obviously more relevant to professions concerned with the remediation and rehabilitation of communication disorders than is the ICD. The definitions of impairment, disability and handicap which preface each division are themselves very useful.

> Impairment: Any loss or impairment of psychological, physiological or anatomical structure or function.

The characteristics are then given. Impairments are grouped and coded under the headings Intellectual Impairments, Other Psychological Impairments, Language Impairments, Aural Impairments, Ocular, Visual, Skeletal, and Disfiguring Impairments and Generalised, Sensory and Other Impairments. Examples of communication disorders are appropriately listed under Language Impairment with its subcategory Impairments of Speech. Impairments relate to both language structure and function and include impairments of use of other language systems, facial expression and body language. Impairments of voice production and functions are listed under speech as is impairment of speech fluency.

> Disability: Any restriction or lack of ability to perform an activity in the manner or within the range considered normal for a human being.

The characteristics are described in some detail and their relationship to impairment is drawn. In the categories of disability, Communication Disabilities constitutes a full section and comprises speaking, listening, seeing and other aspects of communication. The final section gives the definition.

> Handicap: A handicap is a disadvantage for a given individual, resulting from an impairment or a disability, that limits or prevents the fulfilment of a role that is normal.

Characteristics are again listed but an important point is added under Classification:

> It is important to note that the handicap classification is neither a taxonomy of disadvantage nor a classification of individuals. Rather it is a classification of circumstances in which disabled people are likely to find themselves, circumstances that place such individuals at a disadvantage relative to their peers when viewed from the norms of society. (p.183)

While communication is not specifically listed in the categories it must be perceived to play a part in Occupation Handicap, Social Integration Handicap, and Economic Self Sufficiency Handicap.

Diagnostic and Statistical Manual of Mental Disorders (DSM III)

DSM III is the final major classification exercise which will be discussed in this chapter. In the introduction to the manual, reference is made to the growing recognition of the principles of diagnosis in both clinical practice and research — 'Clinicians and research investigators must have a common language with which to communicate about the disorders for which they have professional responsibility' (p.1). This statement certainly holds good for communication disorders where practitioners working in educational settings may have need of the findings of highly specialised investigators into acoustical and neurophysiological processes. However, DSM III cannot be expected to meet the needs of professions concerned with communication since it was created by a different professional group, the American Psychiatric Association. It does offer a model which is nearer to the needs of professionals in communication disorders than is the ICD-9 since it places emphasis upon clinical usefulness for making treatment and management decisions in varied clinical settings; reliability of diagnostic categories; acceptability to clinicians and researchers of varying theoretical orientations; and usefulness for educating health professionals.

DSM III represents the efforts of a major professional body to modify the coding and glossary of ICD-9 to render it more suitable for use in the United States. It sets out a multiaxial system within which disorders are categorised, coded and related to each other. There are descriptions of the conditions with illustrations which support the concept of a clinically based system and give comprehensive guidance as to how to use it. Its communication codes have not, however, proved acceptable to the American Speech-Language-Hearing Association (ASHA).

The Needs of Professions in Communication Disorders

As was stated earlier in this chapter, different countries make different demands upon classifications. ASHA has concentrated upon the development of a numerical coding system. Such a system would yield information on prevalence and incidence of disorders. It will also be recommended for reimbursement purposes. Third party reimbursement sources in the United States have begun to use codes (ICD-9-CM) for billing purposes and it is obviously in the interests of ASHA to effect a change in the favour of more accurate representation of communication disorders and procedures.

The coding system which is now being advocated by ASHA is the result of several years of activity by its Task Force and Executive Board. This system is being tested in several metropolitan areas and will be submitted in its final form to the health insurance industry with the recommendation that it be used in the settlement of speech, language and hearing claims. The classifications used are independent of medical systems and thus 'assure the provision of autonomous judgement by the speech-language pathologist and audiologist' (Task Force recommendation, 1986, p. 1). This demand for autonomy could only be made by an organisation as large and powerful as ASHA. Moreover, the spur given by the need to determine its own fees for service has been lacking in other countries, such as Great Britain where the majority of practitioners are employed by the National Health Service. However, all professional organisations concerned with communication disorders must endeavour to see that the conditions which they cover are accurately described and represented within the major national and international systems. The International Association of Logopedics and Phoniatrics (IALP) is therefore under pressure from individual member countries to persuade the WHO to make changes in those systems under its jurisdiction. We may expect to see increased drive within countries to make a more accurate and comprehensive classification of communication disorders in national systems and to achieve some international consensus among these. We may also expect to see glossaries of terms revised and refined in support of these systems.

Present Status

Following the overall consideration of speech therapy procedures set out in the 1972 report, the College of Speech Therapists set up a project to review terminology. The conclusion of the principal investigator (Crystal, 1982, p. 18) was that the emphasis on terminology was misplaced 'given our present primitive knowledge of clinical linguistic symptomatology'. Not everyone agreed with this conclusion but it had the effect of reminding the profession of the need to clarify procedures and to share more clinical descriptions to provide the basis for any revision of taxonomy. It had been stated earlier that there was a fair amount of consensus among speech therapists as to the conditions requiring treatment (Byers Brown, 1981). However, this did not prove that these conditions had been clearly described within an overall professional rationale.

The Canadian guidelines were developed in support of three of the needs listed earlier in this chapter: clinical practice, education and research. Outstandingly, it testified to an interest in increasing and assessing the quality of care. In the introduction three initial definitions are given (pp. 5, 6).

Language-speech pathologist: A professional engaged in the prevention, evaluation, treatment and management of language, speech and voice disorders.

Audiologist: A professional whose primary concern is

auditory function. The principal effort is directed toward the identification, assessment and (re)habilitation of those with auditory function.

Patient: The term patient has been selected to refer to the recipients of language-speech and audiological services.

The definitions put out by ASHA are somewhat different:

Speech-language pathologist: A professional person trained in the development and disorders of human communication primarily involved in the diagnosis and remediation of speech and language disorders.

Audiologist: Specialist in the measurement of hearing and in the identification, evaluation and rehabilitation of persons with communication disorders associated with hearing loss.

The person who is the recipient of these services is referred to as the Client. The Canadian mention of prevention is in tune with current thinking in Great Britain and the United States (Marge, 1984; Byers Brown, 1985) and is likely to be incorporated into future definitions of role.

Later in the introductory section the Canadian report makes the following points: 'In this document, the various disorders of human communication are described and analyzed as separate entities. However, a communication disorder is frequently bound together, not only with other disorders of communication, but also with additional handicaps which may be motorically, intellectually or emotionally based' (p. 9). They highlight the importance of a flexible classification system. Emphasis is also placed upon the practitioners' right to professional judgement (p. 14) which again militates against a rigid prescription for procedural practice.

The Essential Components of a Classification System

In any attempt to generate a new classification, professional associations concerned with communication disorders are faced with an immediate paradox. There is simultaneously a move toward professional autonomy and towards interdisciplinary co-operation. Classifications must reconcile the accurate representation of disorders and activities with their acceptability to professions outside their own. There are few definitions of the terms communication or communicative disorders, one of the most recent coming from ASHA's (1986) Glossary of terms,

> A communicative disorder is an impairment in the ability to 1) receive and/or process a symbol system; 2) represent concepts or symbol systems and/or 3) transmit and use symbol systems. The impairment is observed in disorders of hearing, language, and/or speech processes. A communicative disorder may range in severity from mild to profound. It may be developmental or acquired and individuals may demonstrate one, or any combination of the three aspects of communicative disorders. The communicative disorder may result in a primary handicapping condition or it may be secondary to other handicapping conditions.

This is not a definition which will appeal to professions other than those which ASHA represents. Even by them, it may be rejected as being too cumbersome. It is, however, extremely difficult to be both comprehensive and succinct.

The definition can be related to a simple model of communicative activity and can also be represented in chart form and extended to show how the three basic components of Communication Disorders relate to the other elements (Table 3.1).

It would be possible to extend the chart further by adding specific causal factors, e.g., encephalitis may give rise to cerebral palsy with impairment of the motor component of the nervous system. This will result in absence of restriction upon articulate speech. However, there is a limit to what can usefully be added to such representations. The next step would be toward a numerical coding scheme such as is used in ICD-10, DSM-III, and now recommended by ASHA. Numbers may be used to signify the nature of the cause and also its time of onset, e.g. before or after the development of speech.

Procedures for Investigation and Management

In some classifications of communication disorders an attempt is made to relate them to the procedures by which the disorders are determined. These procedures include:

1 Case history interview: A procedure carried out to obtain all the information relevant to the patient's condition.
2 Screening: A procedure to identify whether the person is in need of further investigation.
3 Assessment: A procedure carried out to establish the nature of a problem and the factors which are contributing to it.

Table 3.1: Communicative Disorder

Anatomical Site	Functional Site	Resulting Impairment	Category
Failure of Reception or Processing			
Outer, middle and inner ear auditory nerve	Auditory receptive mechanism	Absence, loss or restriction of auditory acuity	Hearing disorder
Inner ear, auditory nerve temporal cortex of brain and associated areas	Auditory processing mechanism	Absence, loss or restriction of selection, retention and comprehension of auditory signal	Language disorder
The eye and visual nerve	Visual receptive mechanism	Absence, loss or impairment of visual acuity	Visual disorder
Visual nerve, occiputal cortex of brain and associated areas	Visual processing mechanism	Absence, loss or restriction of selection, retention and comprehension of visual signal	Visual/language disorder
Failure of Representation			
Cerebral cortex and associated areas of brain	Central processing and generating mechanisms	Absence, loss or restriction of ability to communicate through symbols	Language disorder
Failure of Transmission and Use			
Central nervous system (motor)		Absence, loss or restriction of articulate speech	Fluency disorder
Peripheral nerves			Speech or articulation disorder
Larynx	Speech production mechanism	Absence, loss or restriction in use of voice	Voice disorder
Tongue, lips, palate		Absence, loss or restriction of ability to produce sounds of speech	Articulation disorder Resonance disorder

Screening and assessment may be directed to the basic categories of hearing, voice, articulation, language and fluency. The most comprehensive assessments may be carried out across all categories and the most selective will relate only to one category or to a specific condition within that category, e.g. the assessment of dysarthria.

The classification systems of Canada, Great Britain and the United States also include remedial and rehabilitation procedures which may be called 'intervention procedures'. These too, are related to the basic communication categories. In the ASHA system both classification and assessment procedures are listed under the headings Audiology Procedures and Speech-Language Pathology Procedures. In the Canadian Guidelines, Assessment and Treatment are given separate sections. The placing of the items and the amount of description given in their support depends upon the purpose of the classification. Where the classification makes use of numerical coding for reporting and remuneration purposes, the entries are as succinct and economical as possible since the numbers carry major information. Where the classification is used as guidelines of practice it is necessarily more explanatory.

New Categories

It is also necessary to find a place for those new procedures which have grown up around the skills of the professional and the increased scope of the subject. We may therefore find 'speech related procedures' which will include assessment of swallowing and feeding disorders. Also requiring a place are those assessments aimed at providing for the use of communication aids or augmentative communication devices.

A number of professionals now work with very young children who are at risk for communication disorders. Assessment and management are at the level of precursors rather than skills. The treatment is essentially prophylactic rather than remedial or rehabilitatory. We have yet to see clear guidelines emerging in this area though classifications of emergent language are now coming forward (Stark and Bond, 1985; Byers Brown, Bendersky and Chapman, 1986).

It will be apparent from the preceding discussion that an attempt to generate a classification of communication disorders to suit every purpose, is highly unrealistic. Different systems will be devised for different purposes. A classification which clinicians will use to help them apply or devise the most efficacious form of treatment will not be the same as that devised to assist in costing. More than one system can be used professionally so long as the aims of each are clearly understood. The overall aims of any exercise in classification will remain the same, namely to maintain order and to increase understanding.

References

BYERS BROWN, B. (1981) *Speech Therapy: Principles and Practice.* Edinburgh: Churchill Livingstone.

BYERS BROWN, B, (1985). Evidence upon which to act: the identification of communication disorders. *British Journal of Disorders of Communication*, 20, 3–18.

BYERS BROWN, B., BENDERSKY, M. and CHAPMAN, T. (1986) The early utterances of pre-terms infants. *British Journal of Disorders of Communication*, 21, 307–19.

CRYSTAL, D. (1980). *Introduction to Language Pathology.* London: Edward Arnold.

CRYSTAL, D. (1982). Terms, time and teeth. *British Journal of Disorders of Communication*, 17, 3–19.

DENES, P.B. and PINSON, E.N. (1973). *The Speech Chain: The Physics and Biology of Spoken Language.* New York: Anchor Books.

EDWARDS, M. (1984). *Disorders of Articulation.* New York; Wien: Springer-Verlag.

MARGE, M. (1984). The prevention of communication disorders. *ASHA*, 26, 29–33.

MORLEY, M. (1966). Editorial, *British Journal of Disorders of Communication*, 1, 1.

MYSAK, E.D. (1976). *Pathologies of Speech Systems.* Baltimore: Wilkins and Wilkins.

SHAMES, G.H. and WIIG, E.H. (Eds) (1982). *Human Communication Disorders.* Columbus, Ohio: Merrill.

SIEGEL, G.M. and INGHAM, R.J. (1987). Theory and science in communication disorders. *Journal of Speech and Hearing Disorders*, 52, 99–104.

STARK, R.E. and BOND, J.L. (1985). *Pre-linguistic Speech Development of Young At-risk Children.* Paper presented at the annual convention of the American Speech-Language-Hearing Association, Washington.

Reports and Manuals

American Speech-Language-Hearing Association (ASHA) (1986). *Classification of Speech-Language Pathology and Audiology Procedures and Communication Disorders.* Report of the task force on classification.

American Psychiatric Association. (1980). *Diagnostic and Statistical Manual of Mental Disorders DSM III.* Washington.

Canadian Department of Health and Welfare. Institutional and Professional Services Division. Health Services Directorate. (1982). *Guidelines for the Practice of Language-Speech Pathology and Audiology.* Ottowa, Canada.

U.S. Department of Health, Human Services, Public Health Service. Health Care Financing Administration. DHHS Publication No. (PHS) 80–1260. (1980). *International Classification of Diseases* (2nd ed., fourth revision).

World Health Organization. *International Classification of Impairments, Disabilities and Handicaps* (ICD9, 1978; ICD10, 1980). Geneva WHO.

Report of the Committee of Enquiry. Her Majesty's Stationery Office. *Speech Therapy Services* (1972). London.

4   The Epidemiology of Communication Disorders

Pamela M. Enderby

Services for the speech and language impaired in the United Kingdom, along with many other countries, is noticeably disparate. This is probably related to the fact that the service has grown on the basis of local argument and history rather than on objective studies and information. If there is to be efficient planning in the health care process it is essential to be informed with regard to the size and needs of the population to be served and the professional skills and abilities required to serve those needs. This chapter will offer one approach to calculating the number of speech and language clinicians required to provide an equitable service. The chapter reviews information regarding the size of the speech and language impaired population. Information relating to the role of the speech and language clincian with different client groups will be analysed.

It is recognised that there are weaknesses in the methodology of collating a mixture of information, some of it sound, some of it less sound, and then adding philosophy. Despite this the author feels sure that this approach is more appropriate than the traditional *ad hoc* way of deciding on service levels. Finally the figures will call into question some of our basic premises regarding the provision of service, suggesting that inability to offer an equitable service in one way should lead to consideration of different forms of provision to meet the needs of the speech and language disabled population.

Method

Speech and language disorders form a heterogenous group as they are often either secondary to a variety of underlying medical or surgical problems, or else part of a general or specific developmental disorder. There is little detailed information on the size of the speech and language impaired population and less information with regard to those with speech and language handicap. For the purposes of this paper the terms 'impairment', 'disability' and 'handicap' will not be used indiscriminately, but as defined by the World Health Organization (WHO) in 1980, thus:

> impairments are concerned with the loss of abnormalities of body structure and appearance and with organ or system function resulting from any cause; disability reflects the consequence of impairment of functional performance and activity by the individual; handicaps represent the disadvantages resulting from an impairment or disability that limits or prevents the fulfilment of normal roles in life.

A review of the literature (Enderby and Philipp, 1986) was used to assist in estimating the number of persons in the United Kingdom with speech and language disorders associated with underlying disease. In this report the main groups of medical, developmental and congenital problems are listed, and, where possible, the size of the speech and language handicapped population has been estimated from population studies and case series cited in the literature. It is recognised that the list is not exclusive. In some conditions where several studies are cited the median incidence and prevalence rate have been selected to estimate the number of speech and language disabled people.

This method of study is similar to that used in the report to the committee of enquiry into the UK speech therapy services (1972) commonly referred to as the Quirk Report. Incidence and prevalence estimates are difficult to derive for several reasons: definitions are not always uniform, available information is sparse, and information is often based on specific populations rather than community-based studies. Thus the findings must be considered as an approximation. It is expected that the figures err on the side of caution as any difficulties in interpretation have led to exclusion rather than inclusion. The study is based on the 1983 estimated mid-year population of the United Kingdom (56,377,000 persons) which was produced by the Office of Population, Census and Surveys, England and Wales (OPCS).

Clinical experience has led to an opinion, albeit subjective, of the proportions of 'severe' and 'moderate' speech handicap represented in different population groups. In this report the term 'severe' has been applied to persons who have difficulty in making themselves understood by anyone other than their immediate family. This group also includes the non-vocal. The term 'moderate' includes those persons whose speech defect is noticeable to the lay person, but who may nevertheless remain intelligible.

Information on clinical intervention has been gathered in two ways. First, from studying the text books and relevant journals with regard to current thinking about speech and language therapeutic intervention; second, an analysis of intervention by speech and language clinician within one district health authority has been conducted. The data have been collected on a time recording sheet which allows analysis not only of the clinicians' input, but also the amount of intervention each patient from each client group receives. In addition some arbitrary decisions have been made with regard to what seems 'reasonable'. The chapter will try and be clear about what is fact and what is philosophy.

Numbers of patients with speech and language handicap

The study of the literature supports a widely held view that the true incidence and prevalence of speech and language disorders is much higher than previously estimated. The data that has been gathered are deficient in many respects, but suggest a revised estimate for the size of the speech and language handicap population in the United Kingdom to be 2.3 million persons (severe communication disorders — 800,000 persons). These estimates are probably conservative as some groups of speech and language disorders have not been included. For example, there is no readily available data from which to estimate the likely number of persons with autism, mutism, psychological speech losses, familial dystonias, psychiatric speech disturbances, etc. The estimates nevertheless suggest that the speech impaired population quoted in the Quirk Report (1972) of 324,180 persons is, in 1989, an underestimate.

Time analysis: the clinicians' input

The computer-based time analysis system of speech and language clinicians showed that Senior II and Senior I Clinicians make an average of 5.3 face-to-face contacts each day. Their working day has a mean of seven hours and the length of treatment sessions is forty five minutes. Thus the contact time with patients per clinician day is 3.9 hours. Non face-to-face contact time shows a mean of 0.85 hours. This includes individual patient directed activities, such as telephone calls, liaison with associated professionals, discussions with relatives, analysing test results, writing reports etc. These clinical duties involve general patient directed activities, such as organising treatment materials, attending case conferences, teaching groups of staff, and so on. Non-clinical professional duties include collection of statistics, ordering equipment, and attending professional staff meetings, accounting for 0.70 hours. If we assume that the working year is forty-six weeks for each speech and language clinician it is easy to deduce that there is the possibility of 897 face-to-face hours per clinician if we continue to pursue this approach to intervention.

Provision of Services

Children requiring speech therapy

In the Quirk report on speech therapy (1972) the available literature concerning children with speech and language disabilities was discussed. This report cited many studies, including the pioneering work of Morley (1972), which reported that 14 per cent of young children were unintelligible to their teachers.

Taking into consideration the social class and age variations between populations that have been studied Quirk suggested that between 2 and 3 per cent of the normal school population have a specific speech defect. However, Ingram (1972) cautions readers that in the United Kingdom a number of studies of different population samples have become available, but that the criteria for defining a speech problem were remarkably crude. 'Before estimates of the prevalence of disorders of speech in childhood are accepted the criteria of what constitutes a speech defect and the methods of selection should be reviewed with care . . .' Fortunately detailed information has since become available from the National Child Development Study (Peckham 1973: Butler, Peckham and Sheridan, 1973). This study was based on a longitudinal survey of over 15,000 seven-year-old children, born in one week in 1958. A survey of these children has shown that at the age of seven years between 10 per cent and 13 per cent of the children had some degree of speech impairment. These speech impaired children were more often males and often from manual social backgrounds. Teachers reported 10.7 per cent of the children to be difficult to understand because of poor speech.

Clearly the prevalence of language delay is dependent on the definitions used and the reports vary considerably: 0.07 per cent (Ingram 1963) 5.3 per cent (Morley, 1965), 8.4 per cent (Silver, 1980). It is interesting that increasing prevalence has been shown in a chronological fashion; this may reflect the fact that recently more sensitive ways of assessing delayed or abnormal speech and language have been perfected, possibly resulting in improved detection.

The Office of Population Census and Surveys (OPCS) indicate that children aged between nought and four years old account for 6.37 per cent of the general population and children aged between five and fourteen years old account for 13.09 per cent of the population. A mid-point of the prevalence figures would suggest that there are 1,091 children per 100,000 population with specific speech and language disorders. The referral of these children to services will tend to bunch at certain ages, usually at three years and then at five years. We would therefore expect 369 referrals per annum per 100,000 population. Most children require at least two hours face-to-face contact with the speech and language clinician so that she can observe general behaviour, interaction in play and assess the communication disorder, both formally and informally. Thus, 738 hours of assessment would be required per annum to service the estimated population. The average amount of time spent with a child and family following assessment in order to explain, reassure and to plan a programme of help, is on average 1.5 hours per child.

A significant proportion of the children will not require further intervention from the clinician, thus accounting for the apparently low mean figure of 0.5 hours for reassessment. Thirty per cent of the population referred to Speech Therapy would therefore require a mean of thirty hours direct intervention, be it individually or in a group situation.

Clinicians will not be surprised that there is a broad range of treatment lengths running from two hours to over a hundred hours. For the population we are discussing this would account for 3,690 hours of intervention. Ten per cent of the children referred have profound problems requiring lengthy and regular involvement accounting for a further 3,394 hours of contact. Thus it is possible to deduce that children's services will require 8,169 hours' clinical contact which, when divided by the 897 hours available to each speech and language clinician indicates that 9.10 clinicians per 100,000 population should be available to provide an equitable service for this group.

It should be pointed out that the level of intervention proposed here is not extravagant. If one considers a child who is not speaking by the age of three, or is speaking in a way that is not intelligible to others, it would seem reasonable that he requires a two-hour assessment. In addition it would seem reasonable that his parents are given at least 1.5 hours' counselling and advice and it does not appear to be extravagant to offer the child on average thirty hours' treatment to try and remedy the problem.

Mental Handicap

Although mental retardation constitutes the largest disabled population with associated communication disorders (Ingram 1972) it is one of the most problematic to review. There is no sharp dividing line between intellectual normality and sub-normality; persons with mental handicap are not impaired equally in functions and may have concomitant specific impairments. At least 2.5 per cent of children have intellectual handicap (IQ less than seventy) and 'over half of these show a severe language deficiency or an articulation defect or both' (Rutter, Tizard and Whitmore, 1970). If we consider again the percentage of children in the population as was done in the previous section and calculate that 2.5 per cent of these will be intellectually handicapped and of these 50 per cent will have problems with communication, we arrive at a figure of 243 children up to the age of fourteen per 100,000 population who will require the speech and language clinician's consideration. The referral rates again tend to cluster at three-years-old, seven years and fourteen years, leading to an average approximation of fifty referrals per 100,000 population.

Mentally handicapped patients are notoriously difficult to assess, requiring indepth, formal and long term informal observation to establish whether communication development is out of line with mental development. Thus these fifty mentally handicapped persons will require, on average, a five-hour assessment, resulting in 250 hours of time spent on this activity. Of these half will require full intervention which, for the purposes of this paper, has been defined as one hour a day for five days a week for forty-six weeks a year.

Commitment to intervening with the mentally handicapped needs to be complete as efforts to change the behaviour of those with learning disabilities is only possible if treatment is delivered with sufficient intensity to ensure that not only the behaviour is learned, but that it is generalised and used. Thus speech and language intervention could lead to 5,750 hours of face-to-face contact with these clients. The other twenty-five patients referred will usually require reassessment, guidance, advice and support. Additionally there is a great deal of training that goes on for those who care for the mentally handicapped in order to ensure that the environment promotes communication.

This general training and advice is difficult to quantify but we have suggested that one hour twice a week for forty-six weeks appears to be a reasonable average for each of these twenty-five clients. In reality the intervention is provided in a group context with teaching programmes being conducted by speech and language clinicians for groups of caring staff and/or relatives. Thus for the purposes of this calculation and to reflect reality rather than idealism I shall allot 1,150 hours to these clients rather than the 2,300 hours which would be required for individual fact-to-face input.

Re-appraisal, participation in case conferences and emphasis on changing the general culture towards communication are difficult to divide up, and as this is not classified in this study as being 'face-to-face time' I shall omit these separate figures. Thus the speech and language clinician is directly involved for 7,150 hours. If we divide this by the 897 hours available for each clinician for face-to-face time then we can deduce that we require 7.97 whole time equivalents per 100,000 population to deliver this level of service.

This accounts for only one section of the mentally handicapped population and ignores the fact that the non face-to-face component is larger for this group than others, thus these figures are recognised to be another low estimate.

Adult services

The adult services can be divided into four main areas: stroke, the progressively ill, head injury and dysphonia (including laryngectomy).

Cerebral Vascular Disease. Some 2 persons per 1,000 population have a stroke each year (Whisnant, 1976). The survival rate is suggested to be between 63 and 77 per cent (Carter, 1964; Marquardsen, 1969). Excluding those who die, or those whose speech recovers quickly, stroke has an annual incidence of between 0.03 per cent (Bonita and Anderson 1983) and 0.02 per cent (Gresham and Phillips, 1979; Wade, Langton-Hewer, David and Enderby, 1986). Prevalence rates are cited between 0.04 per cent (Gresham and Phillips, 1979) and 0.05 per cent (Hopkins, 1975; Matsumoto, Whisnant, Kurland and Okasaki, 1978) thus we would expect 30 referrals annually with stroke-related speech and language disorders per 100,000 population. A further fifteen patients may be re-referred or referred following a second stroke or deterioration. Thus there will be forty-five patients to be assessed by this service.

Assessment of aphasia on average takes 2.5 hours requiring 112.5 hours to be spent on this activity. Many of the patients with persisting speech and language disorder will require one of three kinds of intervention:

1 *Regular therapy.* This is defined as 1.5 hours treatment (including re-assessment) per day for four days per week for six months.
2 *Guidance.* This covers the group of patients requiring support, reassurance, reassessment amounting to one hour per week for six months.
3 *Stimulation.* Some patients will require exposure to a socially stimulating environment to promote communicative effectiveness. These patients are often seen in a group situation and it would account for five hours intervention per group per week for forty-six weeks.

Stroke studies within this district over the last five years have shown that approximately 33 per cent of the forty-five patients fall into one of the treatment categories outlined above. Thus regular therapy for fifteen patients will require 2,340 hours of intervention per year. Fifteen patients will require guidance accounting for 390 hours of intervention, and the final fifteen patients who would benefit from stimulation account for 230 hours of involvement. Therefore the total face-to-face time for stroke population offering this degree of flexibility would add up to 3,072.5 hours, this divided by the 897 hours available to each clinician would suggest that 3.42 whole time equivalents are required to offer this level of service consistently for stroke patients.

Some studies have suggested that intensive intervention for some stroke dysphasic patients is efficacious (Wertz, Collins and Brookshire, 1978; Basso, Capitani and Vignolo, 1979; Vignolo, 1964). A study by Leigh-Smith, Denis, Enderby, Wade and Langton Hewer (1987) indicated that between five and fourteen patients per 100,000 per year would meet criteria suggested as being appropriate for inclusion in this form of therapy (four hours a day for five days a week for three months). If intensive therapy is to be pursued then it is suggested that a further whole time clinician is allowed even when accounting for removing that particular group from the regular therapy sessions.

Progressively Ill. Many of the progressive neurological diseases may lead to a concomitant speech and language disorder. Parkinsons Disease has an incidence rate of twenty cases per 100,000 population and a prevalence rate of 100 to 150 cases per 100,000 (Brewis, Pozkanzer and Rolland, 1966). The proportion of patients suffering from speech disorders associated with Parkinsons Disease has been reported as low as 3.8 per cent (Hoehn and Yahr, 1967) to 50 per cent in more detailed studies (Logemann, Fisher and Blonsky, 1978; Merritt, 1979). Gibberd, Oxtoby and Jewell (1985), found that 36 per cent of patients with Parkinsons Disease considered that they had no speech difficulty.

The incidence of Multiple Sclerosis in Britain has been suggested to be three per 100,000 population (Kurtzke, 1982) however the incidence rate of this disease with uncertain onset is difficult. Prevalence rate may be more accurate and is considered to be between 0.06 and 0.08 per cent within the United Kingdom. Approximately half have some degree of speech and language disorder and of these one third have great difficulty (Darley, Brown and Goodstein, 1972).

Motor Neurone Disease has an incidence of 1.6 per 100,000 population (Kurland, 1977) the prevalence rate is indicated to be six per 100,000. In 25 per cent of cases dysarthria and dysphagia are the first symptoms of motor neurone disease (Garfinkle and Kimmelman, 1982), however all patients will finally have some degree of speaking and swallowing difficulty as the disease progresses (Bobowick and Brody, 1973).

Patients with Freidrichs Ataxia, muscular dystrophy, myasthenia gravis and Huntingdons chorea may also have quite severe communication problems. The suggested incidence and prevalence rates are seen in Table 4.1.

Due to the insidious nature of many neurological diseases and the slow onset of speech problems the time of referral to speech therapy varies noticeably from district to district according to the services available and the knowledge of the consultants with regard to the role of speech and language clinicians with such disorders.

In one health district studied for this chapter sixteen patients were referred per 100,000 population per annum with speech language and swallowing problems associated with progressive neurological disease. These sixteen patients required assessment for a mean of 2.5 hours and they had an average of one hours intervention per week for six months. Six of these patients required communication aids, each of these patients required an average of fifteen hours' direct intervention time. Reassessment plays a high role in the speech clinician's intervention with the

Table 4.1: Estimates for the size of the UK speech and language handicapped populations associated with certain medical problems.* 1985 (Listed in order of decreasing prevalence of the disorder.)
Reproduced by kind permission of the *British Journal of Disorders of Communication:* 21, 151–165, 1986 (Aug.)

Disorder	Incidence of disorder per 100,000 population	Prevalence of disorder per 100,000 population	Percent with disorder causing speech or language problem	Number of speech/lang handicapped per 100,000 population	Number of severely handicapped speech/lang per 100,000 population	Number with moderate speech/lang handicap 100,000 population
Mental handicap (all ages)	NK	2,500.0	55.0	1375.0	800.0	575.0
Stammering	3495.0	1,070.0	100.0	1070.0	70.0	1000.0
Pre-school age speech & lang.**	NK	691.2	100.0	691.2	230.4	460.8
School age speech & lang.**	NK	400.0	100.0	400.0	200.0	200.0
CVA	200.0	500.0	30.0	150.0	70.0	80.0
Deafness	1.6	200.0	60.0	120.0	45.0	75.0
Cerebral Palsy***	2.0	175.0	60.0	105.0	20.0	85.0
Cleft Palate***	2.0	NK (>142.0)	40.0	57.0	19.0	38.0
Parkinson's Disease	20.0	125.0	55.0	69.0	23.0	46.0
Multiple Sclerosis	3.0	60.0	55.0	33.0	10.0	23.0
Dysphonia	28.0	28.0	100.0	28.0	10.0	18.0
Muscular Dystrophy	1.2	20.0	25.0	5.0	2.0	3.0
Motor Neurone Disease	1.6	6.0	57.5	3.5	1.2	2.3
Myasthenia Gravis	3.0	6.0	25.0	1.5	0.5	1.0
Huntington's Chorea	0.4	5.0	60.0	3.0	1.0	2.0
Laryngectomy	0.9	3.0	100.0	3.0	2.0	1.0
Friedreich's Ataxia	0.4	2.0	60.0	1.2	0.6	0.6
Head Injury	286.0	NK (800)	20.0	NK (160)	NK (60)	NK (100)

*   *Many of the figures in this table are estimated from references cited in the text. They should be used as a guide rather than a definitive statement.*

**   *The incidence and prevalence estimates are derived from the number of pre-school children per 100,000 general population.*

***   *Based on the numbers per 100,000 new born population.*

NK   *Not known.*

progressively ill in order for her to report back to the medical consultants any change in status and on which to base advice. A further 2.5 hours per patient should be set aside for this. This time is used in different ways so that there may be many short reassessments or a few longer reassessments according to the type of the disorder. Accordingly a speech clinician can account for 586 hours of face-to-face contact time resulting in a requirement of 0.65 of a whole time equivalent speech and language clinician per 100,000 population to offer this basic level of intervention.

Head Injury. It is difficult to establish the morbidity associated with head injury. The numbers of patients suffering head injury is large; in 1972 there were 142,000 admissions to hospital in England and Wales of patients suffering the effects of head injury (Field Research, DHSS 1975). Fortunately the majority of patients suffering head injury make a full recovery, but there is a small percentage who remain severely and permanently handicapped. Data from the OPCS suggest an annual incidence rate in England and Wales of 1.1 per cent for persistent dysphasia from intra cranial injury without skull fracture, and an incidence of 1.5 per cent following a fractured skull. The prevalence rate may be estimated broadly as being 160 people per 100,000 who have some degree of dysphasia as the result of head injury. Of course the prevalence rate covers a very long span of years and therefore it is difficult to speculate what a reasonable referral rate would be.

However, studies of one particular district suggest that a referral rate of twenty patients per 100,000 population is a fair expectation. All patients referred require an assessment and the mean time for assessing head injury patients has been found to be three hours. The range of speech therapy intervention available to these patients is again varied, some require little input following assessment and guidance, others require literally hundreds of hours of therapy. Again the broad range in the standard deviation of intervention time suggest that the means are not particularly useful, but it does give some impression of the services that may be needed. The mean of treatment of the head injured population is twenty three hours per case. This would lead to 460 hours to cover the referral rate per year. Thus the total care of this population would require 520 hours' face to face contact time leading to 0.57 of a whole time equivalent speech and language clinician per 100,000 population to offer this basic level of intervention.

Dysphonia (including laryngectomy). Phonatory problems may be a symptom of neurological, organic or functional disorders. Some of the neurological and organic dysphonias have been included in other sections. This section includes those dysphonias related to polyps, nodules, oedema of the vocal cords and dysphonia associated with functional disorders. Aphonia associated with laryngectomy should also be considered. A review of the literature and a study of patterns of referral are detailed by Enderby and Philipp (1986). This and other studies concludes that there is annual incidence of dysphonia of 28 per 100,000. The incidence of laryngectomy per 100,000 population is estimated to be 0.9 and the prevalence 3.0. There appear to be some regional variations with regard to these figures which are possibly associated with the time of detection and availability of radiotherapy. The amount of treatment that dysphonic patients and laryngectomy patients require is again very varied. The different approaches available, the different philosophies underlying the treatments have an effect on the intervention. For the purposes of this article we would suggest that there will be twenty eight referrals per year per 100,000 of people with dysphonia, and one referral per year per 100,000 population for laryngectomy. The speech clinician will be involved with the laryngectomy patient pre- and post-operatively and this will lead to sixty hours of intervention.

Of the dysphonic patients following a 1.5 hour assessment, ten will require limited therapy and guidance averaging two hours each, and eighteen will require ten hours of direct treatment, be this to do with counselling, relaxation or direct voice therapy. Thus dysphonic patients require 142 hours of intervention. This along with the hours required for laryngectomy requires 0.22 whole time equivalent speech and language clinician.

Care of the Elderly

Some 14 per cent of the population are over 65 years of age. Many of those requiring therapy will already have been covered in previous sections, however increasing age gives rise to a greater likelihood of acquiring speech and language disorders associated with neurological illness or disease or psychological deterioration. Study of one care of the elderly unit showed that we would expect fifty new referrals per year per 100,000 population. These required on average 2.5 hours of assessment. Twenty had specific treatment on average twice a week for three months leading to 480 hours. A further thirty required support, stimulation, guidance leading to 0.5 hours per week for a year. To offer this flexibility of service we would require 1,295 hours leading to 1.4 whole time equivalent speech and language clinicians.

Conclusion

Quirk (1972) suggested that the speech therapy service should be based on six clinicians per 100,000 population. When considering his suggestion that 324,180 persons in the United Kingdom had a speech and language handicap as compared to the present projected figures of 2.3 million it is not surprising that the profession does not feel that his indications are now valid. One way of speculating how many speech clinicians we require would be to multiply Quirk's figure of six clinicians by seven indicating the acknowledged increase in speech and language handicap in the community. Thus, one could argue for forty-two speech and language clinicians per 100,000 population; however, this figure should be questioned as the sparse information on incidence and prevalence of speech and language disorders available to the Quirk Commission was only matched by the sparse information on the role of the speech clinician. Further, we must be aware that there are many more people with speech and language impairment, disability and handicap who do not require the service of speech clinicians. Thus the analysis that has been discussed here is another way of speculating how to develop speech therapy provision. If an equitable service is to be implemented and if current methods of intervention are to be pursued then it would appear that at least 23.37 speech and language clinicians per 100,000 population is justified. Without this level of staffing, service provision is spread thinly and the allocation is not usually done on a rational basis.

Considering the needs of the population and the reality of funding difficulties it may be necessary for us to question whether there are other alternatives to solving the provision of services to the speech and language disabled. We must consider whether continuing in our present mould is justified, whether it is practical, and whether it is likely to be resourced.

We have a choice between offering the model of service presently available in an inequitable way and rationing our provision to the clients, or we change our concept of the provision dramatically, redefining the role of the speech clinician and the way that relates not only to patients and their relatives but also to other professionals.

By looking at the position now in some detail and the implications that it poses for the future we have more information to fuel discussions of the future of the profession.

References

BASSO, A., CAPITANI, E. and VIGNOLO, L. (1979) Influence of rehabilitation on language skills in aphasic patients: A controlled study. *Archives of Neurology,* 36, 190–6.

BLONSKY, E. (1975) Comparison of speech and swallowing function in patients with tremor disorders and in the normal geriatric patients. *Journal of Gerontology,* 30, 299–303.

BOBOWICK, A.R. and BRODY, J.A. (1973) Epidemiology of motor neurone disease. *New England Journal of Medicine,* 288, 2047–55.

BONITA, R. and ANDERSON, A. (1983) Speech and language disorders after stroke: An epidemiological study. *New Zealand Speech and Language Therapy Journal,* 38, 2–9.

BREWIS, M., POZKANZER, D.C. and ROLLAND, C. (1966) Neurological disease in an English city. *Acta Neurological Scandinavia Supplement,* 42, 24, 1–89.

BUTLER, N.R., PECKHAM, C. and SHERIDAN, M. (1973). Speech defects in children aged 7 years: A national study. *British Medical Journal*, 3, 253–7.

CARTER, A.B. (1964) *Cerebral Infarction*. New York: Macmillan.

DARLEY, F., BROWN, J. and GOLDSTEIN, N. (1972) Dysarthria in multiple sclerosis. *Journal of Speech and Hearing Research*, 15, 229–45.

ENDERBY, P.M., PHILIPP, R. (1986) Speech and language handicap: Towards knowing the size of the problem. *British Journal of Disorders of Communication*, 21, 151–65.

FIELD RESEARCH DIVISION OF DHSS (1975) *Epidemiology of Head Injuries in England and Wales*. London: DHSS.

GARFINKLE, T.J. and KIMMELMAN, C.P. (1982) Neurologic disorders: Amyotrophic lateral sclerosis, myasthenia gravis, multiple sclerosis, and poliomyelitis. *American Journal of Otolaryngology*, 14, 204–12.

GIBBERD, F.B., OXTOBY, M. and JEWELL P.F. (1985) The treatment of Parkinsons Disease: A consumer view. *Health Trends*, 17, 19–21.

GRESHAM, G. and PHILLIPS, T. (1979) Epidemiology profile of long term stroke disability: The Framingham study. *Archives of Physical Medicine and Rehabilitation*, 60, 487–97.

HOEHN, M.M. and YAHR, M.D. (1967) Parkinsonism: Onset, progress and mortality. *Neurology (Minneapolis)*, 17, 427–42

HOPKINS, A. (1975) The need for speech therapy for dysphasia following stroke. *Health Trends*, 7, 58–60.

INGRAM, T.T. (1963) Report of the Scottish Dysphasia Subcommittee of the Scottish Paediatric Society. (Unpublished).

INGRAM, T.T. (1972) Classification of speech and language disorders in young children. In M. Rutter and J. Martin (Eds), *The Child with Delayed Speech*. London: Spastics International Medical Publication.

KURTZKE, J.F. (1982) The current neurological burden of illness and injury in the US. *Journal of Neurology*, Nov., 1207–14.

KURLAND, L.T. (1977) Epidemiology of amyotrophic lateral sclerosis with emphasis on antecedent events from case control comparisons. In D.F. Rose (Ed.), *Motor Neurone Disease*. New York: Grune and Stratton.

LEIGH-SMITH, J.A., DENIS, R., ENDERBY, P.M., WADE, D. and LANGTON-HEWER, R. (1987) Selection of aphasic stroke patients for intensive speech therapy. *Journal of Neurology, Neurosurgery and Psychiatry*, 50, 1488–92.

LOGEMANN, J., FISHER, M. and BLONSKY, E. (1978) Frequency of cooccurrence of vocal tract dysfunction in a large sample of Parkinsons patients. *Journal of Speech and Hearing Disorders*, 43, 41–57.

MARQUARDSEN, J. (1969) The natural history of cerebrovascular disease. *Acta Neurologica Scandinavia Supplement*, 45, 90–188.

MATSUMOTO, N. WHISNANT, J., KURLAND, L. and OKASAKI, H. (1978) Natural history of stroke in Rochester Minnesota, 1955–1969. *Stroke*, 4, 20–9.

MERRITT, H. (1979) *A Textbook of Clinical Neurology* (6th ed.). Philadelphia: Lea and Febiger.

MORLEY, M.E. (1965) *The Development and Disorders of Speech in Childhood* (2nd ed.). Edinburgh: Churchill Livingstone.

MORLEY, M.E. (1972) *The Development and Disorders of Speech in Chidhood* (3rd ed.). Edinburgh: Churchill Livingstone.

OFFICE OF POPULATION CENSUSES AND SURVEYS ENGLAND AND WALES (1984) *Population Trends.* 38, 37.

PECKHAM, C.S. (1973) Speech defects in a national sample of children aged 7 years. *British Journal of Disorders of Communication,* 8, 2–8.

QUIRK, R. (1972) *Speech Therapy Services.* London: HMSO.

RUTTER, M., TIZARD, J. and WHITMORE, K. (Eds) (1970) *Education, Health and Behaviour.* London: Longmans.

SILVER, P.A. (1980) The prevalence, stability and significance of developmental language delay in pre-school children. *Developmental Medicine and Child Neurology,* 22, 768–77.

TOMSEN, I.V. (1976) Evaluation of outcome of traumatic aphasia in patients with severe verified focal lesions. *Folia Phoniatrica,* 28, 362–77.

VIGNOLO, L.A. (1964) Evolution of aphasia and language rehabilitation: A retrospective exploratory study. *Cortex,* 1, 344–67.

WADE, D.T., LANGTON-HEWER, R., DAVID, R.M. and ENDERBY, P.M. (1986) *Stroke: A Critical Approach to Diagnosis, Treatment and Management.* London: Chapman and Hall Medical.

WALTON, J. and NATRASS, F. (1954) On the classification, natural history and treatment of the myopathies. *Brain,* 77, 169.

WERTZ, R.T., COLLINS, M.J. and BROOKSHIRE, R.H. (1978) The Veterans Administration Co-operative study on aphasia: A comparison of individual and group treatment. *Journal of Speech and Hearing Research,* 21, 4, 652–67.

WHISNANT, J.P. (1976) *Ninth Pfizer Symposium: Stroke.* Edinburgh: Churchill Livingstone.

WORLD HEALTH ORGANIZATION (1980) *International Classification of Impairments, Disabilities and Handicaps.* Geneva: WHO.

5 The Profession at Work

Betty Byers Brown and John Gilbert

Professional activities in communication disorders are devoted to one main end, that of providing the best possible care for those who suffer from communication handicaps. To this end, the individual practitioner offers guidance, diagnostic assessments, remedy, support and information for the benefit of those who suffer and those who care for them. The history of professional care can be traced back to devoted and sensitive people in every country who have devised special programmes and services. Professionals who want to work with the communication handicapped child or adult have to devise some way of doing so within programmes of health care or education which will give patient/client access and continuity. They are responsible not only for finding a place for their services within these larger care systems but for helping to shape those systems. Through their skills and knowledge, the practitioners should be able to recommend and promote changes which will result in more effective treatment for more people.

Communication disorders will be more or less handicapping depending upon the importance which society attaches to a particular communication skill. Communication handicaps are therefore in a very real sense the products of the whole community not simply the person who has the disorder. Professionals must also see their role as one of helping society to understand and accept its members and to make it easier for them to contribute. As soon as the total role of the professional is perceived to include the care of the individual, the shaping of the system and the education of the community, it becomes apparent that a professional organisation is needed. This will allow individual practitioners to combine their strengths to make a more effective work force. It will also offer professional support and resource. The organisation will carry responsibility for trying to bring about increased service provision for the communication handicapped. The stronger the professional organisation, the more impact it will have upon the service provision.

It has been suggested (Byers Brown and Monkhouse, 1983) that across the globe there are three levels of professional activity with the following characteristics.

1　Countries where the profession of communication disorders has been developed and established. Here at least one professional organisation or association exists: there are structured services and a variety of work settings; there are training programmes which are recognised and supervised; there is epidemiological data available and there is a high degree of professional autonomy together with a strong sense of professional identity.

2　Countries where the profession is in the process of developing. Here a training programme is at least contemplated if not started: an estimate of need has been made; an interested person in a high place has been found; there are demands for a service coming from those in other professions who have been trained or have visited abroad and seen what a service can offer. Professional identity is only starting to be perceived and there is no professional autonomy. The lead is coming from individual professionals in speech and hearing who have been trained abroad.

3　Countries where the profession is awaiting development. Here a first start is being made to identify problems; an official or influential individual has shown interest; the state of the education is such that 'different' children can be identified.

This chapter is concerned with the first level, that of full professional development. This usually takes a long time to achieve, as may be seen by viewing the progress of three countries.

Professional Development in the United Kingdom

In the United Kingdom the major professional association concerned with communication disorders is the College of Speech Therapists. This is a more circumscribed organisation than those of the other two countries to which reference will be made. The College only admits to full membership those who are eligible to practice clinically in speech pathology and therapy. It does not embrace the practice of audiology although courses in the subject are required for all who are entering the profession of speech therapy. A number of speech therapists hold additional qualifications in audiology but this number is small.

The first movements towards a speech therapy service began in Manchester in 1906, to be shortly followed by developments in Glasgow. Children who stammered were given special help within the school system. Developments in London started in two major teaching hospitals which set up special clinics for children with speech problems. One of these became a teaching clinic for students trained at the Central School of Speech and Drama. Steady though sporadic development occurred in both schools and hospitals between the two world wars. Two professional associations were formed, one from a nucleus of remedial teachers and another with a more medical orientation. The amalgamation of these two societies was not able to take place until after the end of the second world war. The College of Speech Therapists came into being in 1947 with a clearly defined set of aims which included standardised examination procedures leading to a diploma. The Diploma of the College of Speech Therapists remained the sole means of entry into the profession for the next twenty years. Diplomates worked in the school or hospital services with a small number engaging in private practice.

The development of the speech therapy profession under the leadership of its College Council proceeded concurrently with the development of the National Health Service (NHS) which came into being in 1948. The many arrangements which were worked out to accommodate speech and language clinicians within the NHS are chronicled in the report of the Committee of Enquiry into Speech Therapy Services (1972). This committee was set up by four departments of state 'to consider the need for and the role of speech therapy in the field of education and medicine, the assessment and treatment of those specially concerned in this work and to make recommendations'. Among the most important recommendations were (1) that all future training of speech and language clinicians should be at degree level and (2) that the organisation of speech therapy services should be unified and administered under the health authorities. The committee's report was accepted and acted upon by the Government. As a direct consequence, some 90 per cent of all those who practice speech therapy are employed by the NHS. This gives the United Kingdom a unique position with regard to the management of communication disorders. All persons from infancy to old age are entitled to speech therapy if the need is demonstrated and this is provided without direct cost to the patient or his family. However, such provision is still dependent upon funding being available at the level of the health districts. In view of high demands and dwindling resources this cannot be guaranteed.

With the change to degree programmes of training, the College adopted a professional rather than a training role. It regulates professional entry through its power to recognise graduates as being qualified to practise. Courses that offer speech therapy qualifications must be recognised by the College and are subject to its requirements with regard to course content and to clinical practical training. The College has been empowered, as of 1985, to issue a certificate independent of membership to those who meet its requirements. The certificate is now required as a condition of employment in the NHS. Thus the College maintains control of the academic and clinical standards of the profession through its impact upon training and upon employment. As with all such professional bodies, the College has a code of ethics which must be supported by its members. Statutory Registration is under active consideration by the College which now has a membership of some 5,000 (as of May 1987).

Professional Development in Ireland

The situation in the Republic of Ireland is different to that in the United Kingdom and is probably best considered under the second level of professional activity described above. (It should be noted that six counties in the North of Ireland are part of the United Kingdom.) A training course was established in 1969 which The College of Speech Therapists (London) monitored; graduates were awarded the Diploma of the College of Speech Therapists. A degree programme replaced the diploma course in 1977 and the College of Speech Therapists continues to play its role in monitoring course requirements and in recognising graduates as qualified to practise. A separate autonomous body, the Irish Association of Speech Therapists, was instituted in 1971 and has a membership of 101 as of June 1987. Close links with the United Kingdom remain and Ireland is regarded as a 'region' of the College of Speech Therapists.

Although there is general acceptance of the profession within the health services in Ireland, speech therapy is still very much in its infancy there and the practice of therapy is directly affected by the major rationalisation programme for health care currently in progress.

Professional Development in Canada

In Canada, speech-language pathology and audiology is a young profession whose numbers of practitioners are few relative to the needs of the population. Although these practitioners have been trained in Canada, England, France, United States, Australia, Belgium, or elsewhere, they have responded to Canada's specifically multicultural needs. The development of university programmes in Canada has been influenced by both British and American training philosophies. The profession of speech-language pathology and audiology has been organised at the national level since 1964, although professional associations were formed in some provinces prior to this time. In 1987, the membership of the Canadian Association of Speech-Language Pathologists and Audiologists numbered close to 2,200 individuals.

The first provincial speech and hearing associations were established in the western and central provinces in the late 1950s. The eastern provinces, initially united in the 'Atlantic Provinces Speech and Hearing Association', formed independent associations in the late 1970s. In 1964, when fourteen Canadians met to found a national association, certification was considered a major necessity. Although the first bylaws were written in 1967, the CSHA was not incorporated until 1975 — approximately two decades after the formation of the first provincial speech and hearing associations. At that time, with only 283 full members and 78 student members, the national association struggled to develop its identity in the presence of the older and more established provincial associations.

Certification

In addition to the roots of the profession being firmly entrenched at the provincial level, the first seeds for professional regulation were also seen at this level. As a result, divergent requirements for practice existed from province to province although divergence between requirements for membership in provincial associations are fast decreasing. Two provinces have non-statutory registration; two provinces have statutory legislation under a licensing bill; and in at least three provinces some form of statutory regulation of the profession is actively being sought at this time (May 1987).

In 1981, a milestone in the history of the profession was reached when the then Canadian Speech and Hearing Association revised its bylaws in an attempt to bring the provinces closer together at a national level. Under its current bylaws, the governing body of the CASLPA is the National Council which comprises an Executive Committee and ten Councillors — one representative from each province. Audiologists and speech and language clinicians across Canada are represented at a national level and a forum exists where issues of national concern can be discussed and direction taken by the CSHA, or other bodies. This Committee conducted a national survey of a stratified, randomly selected sample of CSHA members. An analysis of the results indicated that 91.7 per cent of the respondents were in favour of self-regulation (i.e., certification) and its pursuit by the national association.

Given the mandate by its members to proceed with the establishment of guidelines for the certification of practitioners, in 1982 the CSHA approached the Department of National Health and Welfare for assistance to establish a Task Force on Certification. This Task Force, convened to discuss and prepare guidelines for the certification of Audiologists and Speech and Language Clinicians, first met in 1983 and dealt specifically with the issue of 'input regulation' (i.e, regulation of the 'producers' of service). The issue of 'output regulation' (i.e., regulation of the services produced) had been addressed previously in a 1982 Department of National Health and Welfare's Report entitled, 'Clinical Guidelines in Speech-Language Pathology and Audiology'.

The Task Force selectively reviewed literature in the area of professional regulation. Discussion centred around the need for regulatory intervention, types of regulation, advantages and disadvantages, and possible models. It also reviewed the *status quo* with respect to professional regulation of the profession of speech-language pathology and audiology in the ten Canadian provinces; of the profession in selected countries; and of other selected health disciplines in Canada.

Following publication of the Task Force Report, the CSHA established an *ad hoc* Committee on Certification, which developed a core-curriculum for both Audiology and Speech-Language Pathology. The implementation of Certification was then placed in the hands of a Standing Committee on Examinations, which revised the core-curriculum and renamed it Scopes of Practice in Audiology and Speech-Language Pathology and developed the first examination for Certification, given to all 1987 graduating students in April 1987. The Committee is actively working on the development of a programme for (a) continuing clinical competency and (b) monitoring of clinical practice during training.

Thus, in a relatively short period of time (thirty years) the profession has developed: (1) a sound academic base in the Universities, (2) an effective network of provincial associations, and (3) a dynamic national association. That it has been able to develop in this time frame is due largely to the strong influence of immigrant Speech and Language Pathologists and Audiologists into Canada from the United States, the United Kingdom, Europe and Australia.

Professional Development in the United States

The profession in the United States has developed more slowly than that of Canada, the timescale being similar to the United Kingdom. Its professional association, the American Speech-Language-Hearing Association numbers 52,000 (May 1987) with about 70 per cent of the members being engaged in clinical practice. The work of individual specialists in speech correction started at approximately the same time as in the United Kingdom with the Chicago public schools employing about ten speech correction teachers in 1910. Detroit, Boston, and San Francisco began to follow this example with the state of Wisconsin showing eight cities with speech correction programmes by 1916. Wisconsin was also responsible for generating the first university speech clinic providing practical training for students taking courses connected with communication skills. A Ph.D. in the field of communication disorders was awarded to Sara M. Stinchfield in 1921. The University of Wisconsin stimulated other universities in the mid-west to follow its example. As a consequence, the study of speech, hearing and other aspects of communication disorders was at degree level from inception.

In 1952, the first national professional association was formed and given the name of the American Academy of Speech Correction. Subsequent changes were made in 1927 (The American Society for the Study of Disorders of Speech); in 1934 (The American Speech Correction Association); in 1947 (American Speech and Hearing Association); and in 1978 the association assumed its present name with the useful acronym ASHA retained. ASHA's status as a nonprofit organisation allows it to engage in lobbying efforts with Congress and state legislatures to effect laws and regulations befitting professionals and those with communication disabilities. Speech–language and hearing associations exist in all of the individual states of the union. These associations are independent of ASHA although that organisation provides formal recognition for those state associations which seek it. ASHA recognition largely rests on the basis of membership requirements for individual affiliation with the state associations (i.e., the master's degree or equivalent for voting membership). ASHA's executive director, writing in 1987 (Spahr, 1987), emphasised that good working relationships between ASHA and the state associations are critical to the vitality of the profession. Spahr then specified those areas which are most critical: (1) standards for providers of speech, language and hearing services (ASHA certification, state licensure, state department of education certification); (2) programmes that provide services to the communicatively disabled such as Medicare (federal) and Medicaid (state); and (3) state-regulated health insurance.

In addition to the highly important relations with the state associations, ASHA maintains extensive liaison activity external to the profession. This, again, is characteristic of a major professional association in communication disorders. ASHA's activities are probably the most complex of any, reflecting as they must the complexities of organisational activity existing throughout the United States in the areas of health care, education and social services.

Prospective speech–language pathologists and audiologists must complete their course work and clinical practicum in an institution approved by ASHA. ASHA also awards certificates of clinical competence which allow Master's graduates who have completed a year of supervised clinical work in the field to practice independently. They must also pass the National Examination as part of the process. This qualification will not automatically allow the professional to work in every state without state licensure. Licensing procedure is now in force in about two thirds of the states, each of which have their own requirements. The US practitioner has therefore a number of expensive and demanding steps to take in order to be able to work independently in the field. However, the level of remuneration is probably higher in the United States than elsewhere which may well compensate.

ASHA operates through a large and complex committee structure overseen by its legislative council and executive board. It has the most developed system of continuing education of any of the three countries cited and publishes three academic journals in addition to a monthly publication carrying news and information.

Standards of professional entry

The entry into the profession of speech therapy in the United Kingdom is through a university or equivalent programme leading to a bachelor's degree. The majority of these are honours degrees and all have been constructed to incorporate clinical training into the degree structure. A licence to practise can thus be granted upon graduation. Masters' degree courses may be taken for academic rather than for professional purposes. In Canada and the United States, the entry into the professions at the Master's level and the undergraduate courses do not provide the substantive work in communication disorders which is necessary for professional entry.

There are few professionals holding doctoral degrees in either Canada or the United Kingdom. In the United States this degree is not only essential for teaching or research but also for directing many of the large clinical programmes. A professional doctorate is under active consideration.

The fact that the three countries share a common language means that they use many of the same teaching texts, read the same journals and draw their clinical material from the same sources of references. The professions draw knowledge from the fields of acoustics, psychology, linguistics, medicine and education in the same fashion though the emphasis differs as does the subject's place in the curriculum. Clinically, the same goals and procedures may apply but the worksites differ because of the different systems of health care and education within which they are incorporated.

Professional Paradoxes

The strength of professional associations and the high standards of entry which they require frequently places them at variance with the demands of health care administrators. In the United Kingdom, there is a constant tendency for a number of professions to be grouped together for administrative purposes with a consequent levelling down of professional status and expertise. This tendency is strongly combatted by the individual professions. In the United States, professional organisations may have to take issue with insurance companies who pay for many aspects of health care and who put prices on procedures which may be very different from those determined by the profession. Similar negotiations may have to go on with federal and state agencies. ASHA is therefore strongly motivated to getting its own cost coding system generally accepted (see Chapter 3).

One result of all this political activity is that professional associations appear to be increasingly detached from grass roots practice and from the working lives of individuals. It is noteworthy that periods of professional optimism and trust coincide with accomplishment and visible activity. This is reflected in the Canadian statement which comes from the newest of the three professional organisations. Optimism and faith in the future both characterised United Kingdom professional activities at the time of the changes stimulated by the Committee of Enquiry (generally known as the Quirk Report after the chairman). It is important that practitioners feel that they are getting something for their money. They also need to feel that their professional organisation is readily responsive to their needs. ASHA, in spite of its power, is vulnerable to criticism since its very size and scope appear to divorce it from considerations of daily practice. However, a 'them and us' attitude occurs between a population and its governing body whatever the size. Professionals have to live and work with this paradox since they have created their associations for their own protection and advancement.

Clinical Functions

Service provision in the United States and Canada is more variable than that of the United Kingdom. However, even in the last named small country there are considerable variations between England, Scotland and Wales in the way the services are administered. There is also too much difference in provision between health districts in England relating both to the wealth of the district and the amount of money it is prepared to spend. In the United States the contrast between states is greater than the contrast between districts of the United Kingdom. A similar position exists in Canada. Procedures which might be recommended in most urban situations might be impossible to fulfil in northern Canada and other remote geographical areas where facilities or consultant specialists are available only hundreds of miles away. Moreover, the differences in health care delivery systems and in education systems among the ten provinces and the subsequent differences in registration, certification and/or licensure all affect the practising professional.

Clinical activities in all developed countries involve a large number of worksites and new areas of activity are opening up all the time. Professionals work in schools and community health clinics, hospitals, special institutions, nurseries, preschool and early intervention centres, with private agencies and in group or individual private practices. Domiciliary work is also carried out. A major development is in the early care of the high risk infant and professionals work in follow-up clinics within multidisciplinary teams. The United Kingdom has an outstanding advantage in that a child may receive continuous and interrelated diagnostic and treatment services throughout infancy and his preschool and school career. As his treatment is organised within the one system, the NHS, his notes may be transferred from one unit to another according to need. This integrated approach is impossible in most other countries. Much time may therefore be lost whenever a child, or indeed an adult, moves from state to state or agency to agency.

Clinical activities may be divided into three main groups: Screening, Assessment and Intervention. These activities have been defined in Chapter 3. The professional may carry out both screening and intervention by enlisting the aid of others and training them to carry out certain specified tasks (e.g., health visitors in the United Kingdom and Public Health nurses in the United States may carry out communication screening). Intervention is always devised by the professional practitioner who is responsible but component parts may very properly be handled by those who see the patient and client at home or on a daily basis (Warner, Byers Brown and McCartney, 1984). In some states of the United States this intervention through others is not admissible and the therapist has to give 'hands on' treatment to qualify for payment. In the United Kingdom, it has always been one of the ways in which the speech therapist works. It is not a means of saving money but a method devised because it seemed useful and retained because it proved effective. However, it has been questioned by some administrators who also consider that the therapist's main role is to give 'hands on' treatment.

In addition to working independently and to supervising the work of others, the professional in communication disorders will almost certainly work at some time within an interdisciplinary team. Communication disorders arise from a combination of factors. There is only rarely one outstanding etiology which demands a single approach. Even if there is one outstanding problem the patient may still be seen within a multidisciplinary centre since his needs may vary according to the phases of his condition. Among the professionals also involved in the management of communication disorders are paediatricians, neurologists, otolaryngologists, orthodontists, plastic surgeons, audiologists, psychologists, psychiatrists, classroom teachers and learning consultants. The teams in which they work may be large or small according to situation and need. Examples of clinical teams will occur in other chapters of this volume. A rehabilitation team, for example, may consist of a specialist in physical medicine, physiotherapist, occupational therapist, speech therapist. The team of a language unit would consist of teacher, speech therapist, psychologist, with possibly the consultant services of a clinical linguist. Interdisciplinary teams may be created for diagnostic purposes. In complex and pervasive conditions, the basic diagnostic/assessment team will be augmented and may also continue to function as an advisory body. These teams have different names and terms of reference in different countries. In the United States, the Child Study Team will assess any child thought to be at risk for handicap and will advise the parent as to the child's needs. The parent must agree in writing to the programme prescribed by the team or it cannot be carried out. The parent has also the right to ask for reassessment or to challenge the programme if the child does not appear to be responding to treatment. Different kinds of accommodations will be made in other countries but they will also reflect the rights of parents to be involved in their child's treatment.

The team concept is both practical and attractive. Not only does it allow for the full exploration of the needs of each patient or client but it provides maximum support for its members. During the development of the profession in the United Kingdom and elsewhere, there was a tendency for speech therapists to be isolated from other professionals. This was particularly true for those working in the school service. One of the steps taken to remedy this position in the United Kingdom was the creation of the integrated service. Here the speech therapy manager may develop a service structure which will allow new recruits to work in close proximity to senior members. It also allows opportunity to work in both community and hospital services so that the best general clinical grounding is given. The subsequent choice of a professional speciality may develop naturally according to preference and aptitude.

In countries such as the United States, where private practice is a notable feature, there is a marked tendency for practitioners in allied disciplines to work within the same practice. Once again, this gives maximum client care and provides support and stimulation for the practitioners.

Referral patterns

The many institutions and teams within which professionals work necessitate different referral practices. At one time it was necessry for all people requiring speech and language services to be referred by a medical practitioner. This may still be required in hospital services. School boards generally function with internal referrals after consultation with appropriate administrative authorities. A patient's physician is kept informed and (when relevant) involved in the management of communication disorders. Many communication disorders are first detected by teachers in pre-school or nursery classes or within the school environment. Teachers may make referrals individually or all referrals may be made by the principal. In the United Kingdom, an open referral policy is preferred but the need for medical examination is always recognised. Thus, if a young child is referred to the speech therapy service by parents because of delayed speech, it is important to ensure that no other problems exist. As speech and hearing services have become mature and established, their dependence upon the medical profession has decreased. However, no profession wishes to develop autonomy at the cost of patient care. Medical surveillance is essential for some conditions and co-operation desirable in most. In the United States, insurance companies may require a medical referral for reimbursement purposes.

The multiracial society

The multiracial society presents peculiar professional challenges to those in communication disorders. Whereas all professionals have to be able to work with people whose first language is different from their own, communication disorders professionals have the responsibility for establishing the nature of a problem that may occur within that language. In some kinds of disorders, assessment and management may be carried out in the official language of the country even though this is not the first language of the client. In the case of language disorders, the position is much more complicated. It is necessary to probe the first language to see whether or not the problem is one of true disorder or simply a difficulty in second language learning or use. Communication function and style are also highly culturally influenced. What might appear hesitant in one culture could simply be polite behaviour in another. In countries and states where there are immigrants from many countries, it is simply not possible for professionals to encompass all these linguistic and cultural differences. However, professional organisations have to do what they can to look after their larger immigrant or minority populations by at least providing suitable assessment and teaching materials.

Clinical functions in a bilingual environment (Canada)

Canada is officially a bilingual country with English and French having equal status in law. This presents with particular problems. It has been found, after considering successful clinical programmes which offer services in both English and French, that these separate programmes are usually run concurrently within a single clinic. Francophone therapists engage in clinical activity in French and anglophone therapists function clinically in English. Complications have been found to arise when a sole charge speech-language pathologist attempts to function in a different language within the same clinical setting. Although many professionals working in the area of language evaluation have some degree of linguistic competence in another language, Canadian professionals recognise that the evaluation of a language disorder (for example, a deficiency or deviancy in the linguistic system) requires a subtle and thorough decoding of the phonemic, syntactic and semantic system of the language. Canadian audiologists and speech-language pathologists recognise that, in evaluation, linguistic sensitivity is essential to successful examination. It is recognised that such sensitivity is difficult (though not impossible) to acquire in a second language.

In evaluation, speech-language pathologists in Canada are also sensitive to the influence of interacting languages. They are aware that this is especially significant in the evaluation of a young child's developing linguistic system.

Due to the multiplicity of languages used in Canada, many English language tests of both production and comprehension have been adapted to use in other languages. Normative data have been established for some of these adapted instruments; others are still in the experimental state. It is recognised that interpretation of these non-standard tests can only be utilised as descriptive information in the evaluative process and cannot yet yield developmental scores.

Conclusion

It will be seen that for professional activities in communication disorders to develop and prosper they must be built into the institutions of the countries which they serve. Once established, they are maintained by institutional regulation and developed by individual professional initiative. The field is an expanding and vital one in which practice is available in a wide range of settings and with a great variety of populations. There are, as have been pointed out elsewhere (Byers Brown, 1981) certain tasks which all clinicians in communication disorders have to be able to carry out. These are indicated in the definitions of role already quoted in Chapter 2. The procedures covered by the whole profession include Comprehensive Assessment: the detailed analysis of speech, voice and language systems and/or oral and pharyngeal sensori-motor competencies combined with case history. Also included may be an assessment of function and adaptation with estimation of prognosis; Treatment: the application of intervention strategies that improve, alter or compensate for conditions revealed in the assessment. Counselling will start at the assessment phase and continue throughout the therapist/patient association. In some conditions, counselling may constitute the major part of the treatment. In others it may act supportively. Without the ability to enter into the feelings of those who suffer, the clinician is unlikely to be able to help them. Professions concerned with communication disorders will therefore continue to place as much emphasis upon human insights as they will upon technical proficiency.

References

BYERS BROWN, B. (1981) *Speech Therapy: Principles and Practice.* Edinburgh: Churchill Livingstone.

BYERS BROWN, B. and MONKHOUSE, K. (1983) *Careers Across Continents: Do You Want to Work Abroad?* Paper presented at the annual convention of the American Speech-Language-Hearing Association, Cincinnati.

SPAHR, F.T. (1987) ASHA and its National Office. *ASHA,* 29, 9–14.

WARNER, J.A.W., BYERS BROWN, B. and MCCARTNEY, E. (1984) *Speech Therapy: A Clinical Companion.* Manchester: Manchester University Press.

Reports

Canada

A Survey Concerning the Audiologists and Speech Pathologists. Health and Welfare Canada. Health Manpower Report No. 1/78 (October 1978).

Clinical Guidelines in Language, Speech Pathology and Audiology. Health and Welfare Canada Report of an Expert Group convened by the Health Services and Promotion Branch. Ottawa: March 1980.

Guidelines for the Practice of Language. Speech Pathology and Audiology. Health and Welfare Canada Report of an Expert Group convened by the Health Services Directorate, Health Services and Promotions Branch. Ottawa: June 1982.

Guidelines for the Certification of Audiologists and Speech. Language Pathologists in Canada. Report of a Task Force convened by the Canadian Speech and Hearing Association and Health Services Directorate, Health Services and Promotion Branch. Ottawa: February 1985.

United Kingdom

Report of the Committee of Enquiry. Her Majesty's Stationery Office. *Speech Therapy Services.* (1987), 417, 3–4.

Registration — A Discussion Paper. *Bulletin of the College of Speech Therapists* (1972), 417, 3–4.

A Review of the Work of the College of Speech Therapists. *Bulletin of the College of Speech Therapists,* (1987) 420, 5–6.

United States

American Speech-Language-Hearing Association (ASHA) (1986). *Classification of Speech-Language Pathology and Audiology Procedures and Communication Disorders.* Report of the Task Force on classification.

ASHA (1987) Reference Issue. March 27.

Addendum

Since this chapter was written, the Government of the United Kingdom has set out proposals for radical changes to the National Health Service. These would affect the work of a number of professions including speech therapy. We may therefore see changes in the way in which speech therapy services are administered. There is likely to be an increase in private practice in all aspects of treatment for communication disorders, accelerating a process already starting to gain ground.

II   COMMUNICATION DISORDERS IN CHILDHOOD

6 Language Disorders in Children

Alan G. Kamhi

Most children acquire their native language without any formal instruction. Because no formal instruction is required, it is sometimes thought that learning a first language is not very difficult. The notion that a first language is easy to learn is, of course, false. In fact, it is arguably the most complex learning task that humans accomplish during their lifetime. The complexities involved in learning language are most readily seen in children who have difficulty learning language. In the first part of the chapter, the dimensions of language and disorders are presented. Causes and correlates of language disorders are then considered. In the second part of the chapter, some general guidelines to assess and remediate child language disorders are presented.

The Nature of Language

The way in which one defines language directly influences who will be classified as language disordered. Current definitions of language are broad-based and highly integrative. An example of such a definition was endorsed by the American Speech-Language-Hearing Association several years ago (ASHA, 1983, p. 44).

> Language is a complex and dynamic system of conventional symbols that is used in various modes for thought and communication. Contemporary views of human language hold that: a) language evolves within specific historical, social, and cultural contexts; b) language, as rule governed behaviour, is described by at least five parameters — phonologic, morphologic, syntactic, semantic, and pragmatic; c) language learning and use are determined by the interaction of biological, cognitive, psycho-social, and environmental factors; and d) effective use of language for communication requires a broad undertanding of human interaction

including such associated factors as nonverbal cues, motivation, and sociocultural roles.

As reflected in the definition, it is generally agreed that there are five dimensions of language. The five aspects of language are described briefly below.

Phonology

Phonology has to do with the way the sounds of a language are organised. It includes a description of what the sounds are and their component features (i.e., phonetics) as well as the distributional rules that govern how the sounds can be used in various word positions and the sequence rules that describe which sounds may be combined. For example, the zh sound that occurs in the word 'measure' never is used to begin an English word. Distributional rules are different in different languages. In french, for example, the zh sound can occur in the word-initial position, as in 'je' and 'jour'. An example of a sequence rule would be that /ks/ in English can occur in the middle and end of words (e.g., 'boxer', 'books'), but cannot be used to begin words.

Phonologists have also devised rules to describe how sounds are produced in certain contexts. There are three general kinds of rules or processes that govern sound changes (e.g., Ingram, 1976): (1) assimilation processes in which adjacent phonemes or features become more alike (e.g., g>g/d>g); (2) substitution processes in which one segment is substituted for another (e.g., tek/kek); and (3) syllable structure processes in which the syllable structure of the word is modified in some way (e.g., nana/banana). Chapter 7 will have more to say about phonology and phonological disorders. It is important to remember, however, that phonological disorders represent a language disorder.

Semantics

Semantics is the aspect of language that governs the meaning of words and word combinations. Sometimes semantics is divided into lexical and relational semantics. Lexical semantics involves the meaning conveyed by individual words. Words have both intensional and extensional meanings. Intensional meanings refer to the defining characteristics or criterial features of a word. A dog is a dog because it has four legs, barks, and licks people's faces. The extension of a word is the set of objects, entities, or events to which a word might apply to in the world. The set of all real or imaginary dogs that fit the intensional criteria become the extension of the entity dog.

Relational semantics refers to the relationships that exist between words. For example, in the sentence 'The Panda bear is eating bamboo', the word bear not only has lexical meaning, but also is the agent engaged in the activity of eating. Bamboo is referred to as the 'patient' (Chafe, 1970) because its state is being changed by the action of the verb. Words are thus seen as expressing abstract relational meanings in addition to their lexical meanings.

Morphology

In addition to the content words that refer to objects, entities, and events, there are a group of words and inflections that convey subtle meaning and serve specific grammatical and pragmatic functions. These words have been referred to as grammatical morphemes. Grammatical morphemes modulate meaning. Consider the sentences: 'Elmore is playing tennis', 'Elmore plays tennis', 'Elmore played tennis' and 'Elmore has played tennis'. The major elements of meaning are similar in each of these sentences. What differentiates these sentences are the grammatical morphemes (inflections and auxiliary forms) that change the tense and aspect (temporal contour) of the sentences.

Syntax

Syntax refers to the rule system that governs how words are combined into larger meaningful units of phrases, clauses, and sentences. Syntactic rules specify which word combinations and orders are acceptable and which are not. In English, the sentence 'The boy hit the ball' is a well-formed grammatical sentence, whereas 'Hit the boy ball the' is not.

Pragmatics

Pragmatics concerns the use of language in context. Language does not occur in a vacuum. It is used to serve a variety of communication functions, such as declaring, greeting, requesting information, answering questions, and so forth. Communicative intentions are best achieved by being sensitive to the listener's communicative needs and nonlinguistic context. Speakers must take into account what the listener knows and does not know about a topic. Pragmatics thus encompasses rules of conversation or discourse. Speakers must learn how to initiate conversations, take turns, maintain and change topics, and provide the appropriate amount of information in a clear manner. It has become clear recently that different kinds of discourse contexts involve different sets of rules (e.g., Lund and Duchan, 1988). The most frequent kinds of discourse children encounter are conversational, classroom, narrative and event discourse.

Defining, Classifying and Diagnosing Language Disorders

How one defines language disorders depends in part on the approach one takes to classify and diagnose language disorders. There are three general approaches to the classification and diagnosis of child language disorders: (1) an etiological (medical) approach, (2) a descriptive-linguistic approach, and (3) a processing approach.

Etiological Approach

The use of etiological typologies for classification and diagnosis of children with language disorders grew out of the early work of McGinnis (1963), Morley (1957), and Myklebust (1954). Based on Myklebust (1954), the etiologic categories used included (a) deafness and hearing impairment, (b) emotional disturbance and autism, (c) mental retardation, (d) childhood aphasia and apraxia (neurologically-based disorders). Reflecting the sociopolitical climate of the early 1960s, a fifth category of cultural or social deprivation was added.

There are several advantages to an etiological approach. Bernstein (1989) points out that etiology is a convenient way to compare and distinguish among autistic, mentally retarded, and hearing impaired children. A second advantage of the etiological approach is that it offers a diagnostic label for a child to receive services in schools and clinics. Special education programmes are often tailored to the primary etiology of the child, in that many school systems have programmes for the mentally retarded, emotionally disturbed, and hearing-impaired. A third advantage suggested by Bernstein is that etiologies provide speech-language pathologists with clues about the type of remediation that might be indicated for a particular child. For example, knowing that a child is hearing-impaired will suggest aural rehabilitation procedures and perhaps the use of alternative or augmentative systems to teach language.

The advantages of the etiological approach are more than outweighed by its disadvantages. Perhaps the most serious problem is that children in each of the etiological categories are thought to have similar language abilities. A particular diagnostic label, however, provides little information about the child's language abilities. All retarded children, for example, do not have similar language abilities. Indeed, for many years, the assessment procedures used to identify the child's etiological category did not include specific information about language performance.

Another problem with the etiological approach is that it is rare to find a child who fits neatly into one diagnostic category (Bloom and Lahey, 1978). For example, many retarded children are hearing-impaired and many autistic children are retarded. A categorical label also implies that there is only one cause for the language disorder. That is, a hearing impairment is the only cause of the language disorder in hearing-impaired children or the cognitive deficit is the only cause of language problems in retarded individuals. Although a single causal factor may be primarily responsible for a language disorder, there are always several contributing factors.

A major unfortunate outcome of the etiological approach was that it served to divide treatment domains (Aram and Nation, 1982). The mentally retarded and emotionally disturbed were considered to belong to the psychologist or special educator. Hearing-impaired children either were not served or came under the province of educators of the deaf. This left aphasic and culturally deprived children to the speech-language pathologists. Although Bernstein has suggested that different etiological labels facilitated the provision of services, determining who provides the services often depends more on the etiological label than the expertise of the professional. In most instances, speech-language pathologists are the most qualified professionals to treat language disorders regardless of etiological type.

Descriptive-Linguistic Approach

The descriptive-linguistic approach involves describing children according to the language deficit they demonstrate. Although this approach purportedly emphasises description rather than classification or diagnosis, in practice the distinction between description and classification is difficult to maintain. Unlike the etiological approach, the descriptive-linguistic approach is a developmental one. Language abilities of disordered children are compared to those of normally developing children. Children's language behaviours are described either in terms of form, content, and use (e.g., Bloom and Lahey, 1978) or in terms of the five language domains (e.g., Lund and Duchan, 1988).

The use of linguistic descriptions to describe children's language disorders can be traced to the early work of Chomsky (1957, 1965). Chomsky provided child language researchers with a powerful descriptive grammar to capture children's developing proficiency with language. Speech-language pathologists were quick to apply the new developments in linguistics and psychology to the study of language disordered children. The past 20 years have seen the development of increasingly more precise procedures to describe children's language (Crystal, Fletcher and Garman, 1976; Ingram, 1981; Miller, 1981; Stickler, 1987; Lund and Duchan, 1988).

Although the descriptive-linguistic approach has clearly placed emphasis on the language behaviours of children with language disorders, the emphasis on language has tended to obscure the etiological and non-language differences among children. Adherents of this approach sometimes base language therapy solely on the nature of the linguistic handicap without considering age, cognitive, social, and environmental factors. The descriptive-linguistic approach thus often has had a behavioural look, in that only language behaviour is considered in evaluating and treating the language disorder. For example, a syntactic delay would be treated the same way in a retarded child as it would in a child with a specific language disorder.

Processing Approaches

Processing approaches provide a means to integrate the best aspects of the descriptive-linguistic approach and the etiological approach. Generally speaking, processing approaches characterise language disorders in terms of disruptions in language comprehension or formulation processes. A variety of processes have been invoked to account for language disorders, including neurologic, sensory, perceptual, linguistic, and cognitive processes.

One popular processing view is that children with language disorders suffer from an auditory processing deficit (e.g., Eisenson, 1972). Although some children with language problems might have specific auditory processing deficits, this view has more descriptive value than explanatory value. As will be seen in the next section, few researchers now believe that a singular deficit can explain a language disorder.

Recent attempts to provide processing explanations for child language disorders have been more comprehensive and integrative. Several writers (e.g., McLean and Snyder-McLean, 1978; Hubbell, 1981; Aram and Nation, 1982) have attempted to build into their models the ways in which constitutional and environmental forces interact over time to cause language disorders. Although some of these models (e.g., Aram and Nation's Child Language Processing Model) offer considerable explanatory value, the complexity of these models can make them unappealing to most clinicians.

Definition of a Language Disorder

The different approaches to the classification and diagnosis of language disorders exemplify the problems involved in defining a language disorder. Consider, for example, the relatively simple definition proposed by Leonard (1982, p. 222): 'Children have a language disorder whenever their language abilities are below those expected for their age and their level of functioning'. Leonard notes that a broad-based definition allows one to consider children with differing etiological histories as language disordered. Adherents to the etiological approach, however, would not find this definition very useful. As was noted above, the etiological approach does not rely heavily on measures of language to make diagnostic classifications. Moreover, the fact that emotionally disturbed and mentally retarded individuals are served primarily by special educators tends to minimise the emphasis that language receives in assessment and treatment. In contrast, the descriptive-linguistic approach classifies children solely on the basis of language performance. Speech and language clinicians frequently use this approach. With such an approach, mentally retarded and autistic children would be considered to have a language disorder.

Broad-based definitions of language disorders are thus the ones preferred by speech-language pathologists. A comprehensive definition of language disorders was provided by ASHA (1980, p. 317–18):

> A language disorder is the abnormal acquisition, comprehension or expression of spoken or written language. The disorder may involve all, one, or some of the phonologic, morphologic, semantic, syntactic, or pragmatic components of the linguistic system. Individuals with language disorders frequently have problems in sentence processing or in abstracting information meaningfully for storage and retrieval from short- and long-term memory.

It should be apparent that the ASHA definition combines a descriptive linguistic orientation with a processing orientation. In the next section, the types of language-disordered children are considered. As indicated earlier, it is convenient to use etiological labels to categorise children with language disorders. As these children are being discussed, it is important to remember that the language abilities of one group of children (e.g., mentally retarded) are not unique to that group.

Types of Language-Disordered Children

Children with specific language impairment

Children with specific language impairment have received considerable attention in the literature (e.g., Leonard, 1979; Johnston, 1982). Variously labelled as developmentally aphasic, dysphasic, language impaired, language disordered, or language delayed, these children acquire language more slowly and often with less success than their age peers. These children are generally defined by the presence of a language impairment in the absence of mental deficiency, sensory and physical deficits, severe emotional disturbances, environmental factors, and brain damage.

Another important characteristic of these disordered children is that they perform within normal limits on tests of nonverbal intelligence.

A few years ago, Stark and Tallal (1981) confronted the problem of translating the definition of specific language impairment into a set of measurement criteria. These criteria dealt not only with the factors that would lead to exclusion from the group, such as hearing loss and severe emotional disturbances, but also with the degree of severity of the language deficit. Stark and Tallal considered a total of 132 children that might fit the definition of language impaired. The children eventually identified as language impaired were part of a research project investigating sensory and perceptual functioning.

The first step towards selection was to have speech-language pathologists identify language-impaired children who were between 4 and 8.5 years old from their caseloads. The clinicians were asked to include only children for whom test data and clinical impressions indicated normal hearing, normal intelligence, and adequate social and emotional adjustment. Of the 132 children initially selected, 50 were excluded because their performance IQ was too low, as measured by the revised Wechsler Intelligence Scale for Children (WISC-R) (Wechsler, 1974) or the Wechsler Pre-School and Primary Scale of Intelligence (WPSSI) (Wechsler, 1963). No child whose performance IQ was less than 85 was considered to have a specific language deficit. An additional five children were eliminated because of hearing impairment (3), neurological impairment (1), and severe emotional disturbance (1).

Language abilities were tapped by a variety of tests. A receptive language age score was calculated by averaging age-related scores obtained on the Test of Auditory Comprehension of Language (Carrow, 1973), and the Token Test (De Renzi and Vignolo, 1962), and the Auditory Reception and Auditory Association Subtests of the Illinois Test of Psycholinguistic Abilities (Kirk, McCarthy and Kirk, 1968). Expressive language age was defined as the average of the age-related scores obtained from the Northwestern Syntax Screening Test, Expressive Portion (Lee, 1971), the Vocabulary Subtest of the WPPSI or WISC-R, the Grammatic Closure Subtest of the ITPA, and the Developmental Syntax Screening (DSS) procedure (Lee, 1974).

For a child to be considered language impaired, the following criteria had to be met: (1) receptive language age had to be at least six months below performance MA; (2) expressive language age had to be at least 12 months lower than performance MA; and (3) overall language age (the average of receptive and expressive language ages) had to be at least 12 months below MA as well as CA. Twenty-six of the 132 children were excluded because their receptive language ages were too high, whereas seven children were excluded because their expressive language scores were too high. An additional nine children were excluded because their scores on the Templin-Darley Test of Articulation (Templin and Darley, 1969) were more than six months below their expressive language age. Stark and Tallal reasoned that children with a phonological impairment of greater severity than their language deficit would reflect a 'mixed' disorder with a peripheral neuromuscular impairment rather than a specific language disorder of unknown etiology.

When all of the above criteria were implemented, more than two-thirds (70.5 per cent) of the children tested either (a) showed mixed disorders, such as a cognitive deficit and language delay, or (b) did not exhibit a sufficiently severe language deficit in one or more aspects of language. Importantly, the children who met the criteria were not a homogeneous group with respect to the manifestation of their language impairment. Some children showed relatively more severe deficits in expressive language than in receptive language while others showed the reverse pattern. Other children had phonological deficits in addition to a language impairment.

Stark and Tallal have clearly defined a specific subset of language disordered children. Importantly, the 93 children who did not meet their criteria of language impairment are probably no less language impaired than the 39 children who met the criteria. They just do not fall into the group of specific language impaired children. As noted earlier, the majority of excluded children (50/94) did not have performance IQs lower than 85. Most of these 50 children had performance IQ levels within the 70-84 range, that is, not low enough to be classified as retarded, but not high enough to be classified as language impaired. The children excluded because their language abilities were too high may well have had language deficits in areas not measured by the language tests. The pragmatic and discourse domain were not evaluated by Stark and Tallal's battery of tests. In addition, a severe deficit in one aspect of language, such as syntactic expression, might warrant intervention even though other areas of language are developing normally. In short, the group of children with a specific language impairment are in fact a subset of a more general group of language-impaired children whose language delay is either associated in part with other non-language deficits or not severe enough in both the receptive and expressive domains.

Mentally retarded children

The American Association on Mental Deficiency (AAMD) defines mental retardation as 'significantly subaverage general intellectual functioning existing concurrently with deficits in adaptive behaviour and manifested during the developmental period' (Grossman, 1983, p. 1). There are four categories of mental retardation based on IQ: (a) mild (52-68), (b) moderate (36-51), (c) severe (20-35), and (d) profound (below 20). Around 90 per cent of the population of retarded individuals fall into the mild range.

The degree of the language impairment in retarded individuals depends in part on the severity of the general mental deficiency. In general, the more severe the mental handicap, the more severe the language deficit. However, the relationship between language and cognition is not always perfect. Miller, Chapman and MacKenzie (1981) studied the relationship between language and cognitive abilities of 130 retarded children between the ages of seven months and seven years. The data indicated that there were individual differences among the retarded children in language performance relative to cognitive level. Approximately half of the children were functioning at or beyond the language levels expected by cognitive level. Of the remaining children, half exhibited delays in both comprehension and production and half showed delays only in productive syntax. Thus, half of the retarded children showed evidence of a specific language impairment over and above the cognitive deficit. These findings exemplify the heterogeneity of retarded children's language abilities. Recent chapters by Owens (1989) and Kamhi (1989) provide a more indepth discussion of the language and cognitive abilities of retarded individuals.

Autistic children

During the past ten years, it has become common to refer to autism as a language or communication-based disorder (e.g., Churchill, 1978). One of the major identifying characteristics of an autistic child is the failure to develop normal verbal and nonverbal communication behaviours. The other major characteristic is the difficulty autistic children exhibit in their relationships with people and objects. Interpersonal deficits are seen in their lack of eye contact, decreased physical interaction, lack of cooperative play, and so forth. Many autistic children withdraw from the approach and touch of others and often become stiff when held or cuddled (Tiegerman, 1989). Object deficits are seen in these children's limited play with toys, self-stimulatory behaviours, and nonprogressive play skills. It is also important to recognise that the majority of autistic children function within the mentally retarded range (Tiegerman, 1989).

The language behaviour of autistic children has received considerable attention during the past few years. It is common for many autistic children to go through a period of mutism sometime early in development. Many autistic children remain mute all of their lives. The indicence of mutism ranges from 28 to 61 per cent (see Tiegerman, 1989). DeMyer, Barton, DeMyer, Norton, Allen and Stelle (1973) have found that 65 per cent of the children who were mute at age 5 were still mute several years later. Eisenberg (1956) has posited that if speech has not developed by 6 years of age, there is little likelihood that it will develop at all.

The speech of autistic children who do talk is characterised by severe deficits in the pragmatic, syntactic, and semantic domains. Phonology is least impaired in these children. The speech of autistic children is also characterised by the frequent use of echolalic utterances (Prizant and Duchan, 1981). Prizant (1982) notes that 75 per cent of verbal autistic children go through a period of echolalia, and 40 per cent of the population are echolalic. Echolalia has been traditionally defined as the meaningless repetition of someone else's sentences. Prizant and Duchan, however, have found that many of the echolalic utterances of autistic children serve communicative functions and carry meaning. In many cases, these children's echoes represent their best attempts to participate in communicative exchanges.

Children with acquired aphasia

The language-disordered children discussed thus far all have language-learning problems that are noticeable at an early age. There are some children, however, who lose some aspect of their language ability due to brain damage. The most common term for this condition is 'acquired aphasia'. Several factors influence the extent of such children's language difficulties, including the severity of the head trauma, the child's age at the time of the trauma, and the child's cognitive abilities before and after the trauma.

Recent studies have found that children with acquired aphasia, like other language- disordered children, cannot be considered a homogeneous group (Miller, Campbell, Chapman, and Weismer, 1984; Cooper and Flowers, 1987). Cooper and Flowers identified fifteen brain-injured subjects between 10 and 18 years. The brain damage in these subjects occurred between 2 and 12 years of age. In general, the brain-injured subjects performed significantly more poorly on language measures than age-matched peers. They exhibited deficits in word, sentence and paragraph comprehension, confrontation naming, oral production of complex syntactic constructions and word fluency.

Learning disabled children

One of the primary characteristics of learning disabled children is a problem with oral and written language. The definition of a learning disability is similar to the definition of a specific language impairment in that both are exclusionary definitions. The definition adopted by the National Joint Committee on Learning Disabilities appears below:

> Learning disabilities is a generic term that refers to a heterogenous group
> of disorders manifested by significant difficulties in the acquisition and use
> of listening, speaking, reading, writing, reasoning, or mathematical

abilities. These disorders are intrinsic to the individual and presumed to be due to central nervous system dysfunction. Even though a learning disability may occur concomitantly with other handicapping conditions (e.g., sensory impairment, mental retardation, social and emotional disturbance) or environmental influences (e.g., cultural differences, insufficient/inappropriate instruction, psychogenic factors), it is not the direct result of those conditions or influences.

Although almost all learning disabled students have difficulty learning to read, the population of learning disabled students is clearly not a homogeneous one. One defining characteristic of learning disabled children is the extent of their oral language impairment. Studies have found that 42 to 46 per cent of children with learning disabilities have significant language deficits (Mattis, French and Rapin, 1975; Lyon and Watson, 1981). Included in this group are children who have previously been identified as having a specific language impairment. Many of the remaining 55 per cent of learning disabled children have more subtle language problems involving higher-level language forms, such as narrative and classroom discourse, figurative language, and metalinguistic judgements (Van Kleeck, 1984; Roth and Spekman, 1986).

It is important to recognise that language disorders do not go away as children get older. Instead, the manifestation of the language disorder changes with age. During the early preschool years, children have difficulty learning basic syntactic-semantic constructions and conversational rules. Early language-learning problems inevitably result in later academic difficulties (Aram, Ekelman and Nation, 1984). As indicated above, there is considerable evidence now that children without previous histories of language impairment exhibit deficits in later emerging language functions. The term 'language learning disabled' has been used (Wallach and Butler, 1984) to describe the sizeable population of learning disabled children with language learning problems.

Causative Factors

Hubbell (1981, p. 105) begins his chapter on causation in child language disorders as follows:

> If something goes wrong, it's natural to ask why. If the car won't start, you start looking for causes. Out of gas? Battery dead? If a child develops red blotches and a high fever, the physician likewise looks for causes. Similarly, if a child demonstrates impairments in the use of language, we wonder why.

Hubbell goes on to note that the search for causal factors in child language disorders has been frustratingly difficult. A primary reason for this difficulty is that many individuals have assumed that one causal factor could explain the language disorder. Causation, however, is a complex process. This complexity is best seen by contrasting three different views of the process of causation: (1) a linear cause-and-effect model, (2) an interactional model, and (3) the transactional model. These models are discussed briefly below. For a more detailed discussion, see Hubbell, (1981) or Sameroff, (1975).

Linear cause-and-effect model

In this model, often referred to as the medical model, there is a direct one-to-one relationship between cause and effect. The physician, for example, diagnoses the cause of a disease by considering its symptoms or effects. The logic of this model is that for each effect there is a cause and for each cause there is a resulting effect. The term 'linear' refers to the direct connection between cause and effect. There are two contrasting applications of the linear cause-and-effect model, one that emphasises the child's constitution and the other that emphasises the child's environment. The term 'constitution' refers to the child's neurophysical makeup and genetic endowment. As Hubbell (p. 111) notes, both views of the linear cause-and-effect model have a severe shortcoming. A language disorder does not depend solely on constitutional factors or solely on environmental factors. Both constitutional and environmental factors influence language development and thus contribute to language disorders.

Interactional model

The interactional model acknowledges that a child's development results from the interaction between constitutional and environmental factors. The example Hubbell gives (p. 111) is of a child who is born premature and then does not receive adequate medical care. Such a child is at a higher risk than one who suffers from only one of these conditions. The interactional view, however, is still an oversimplification of the process of causation. For one, it assumes that constitution and environment do not change over time. Second, it assumes that constitution and environmental factors do not influence one another. The transactional model addresses both of these concerns.

Transactional model

Unlike the previous two models, the transactional model includes change over time and acknowledges the reciprocal influences of constitutional and environmental factors (Sameroff, 1975; Hubbell, 1981). Consider, for example, two children born with Down's syndrome to two different families. Assume that the intelligence level and other constitutional factors are similar in the two children. In one family, there are two older normal siblings. The family is resentful that they now have a mentally retarded child. They specifically resent the stigma of having such a child and the trouble he will cause them throughout his development. By age five this child is not only mentally retarded, but also has significant behaviour problems. His language abilities are also about one year below his mental age.

In contrast, the family of the other Down's syndrome child have no other children. Although they are very disappointed that their child was born with Down's syndrome, they try to provide the best possible learning environment for their child. By age five their child is being mainstreamed in a normal kindergarten class. His social behaviours and language abilities are at or above his cognitive level.

This example points out the difficulty in identifying etiology and causal factors. Neither environmental nor constitutional factors alone can explain the present behaviour of the two 5-year-old Down's syndrome children. In a recent article (Kamhi, 1984), I suggested that clinicians need to generate clinical hypotheses about the different levels of cause-effect relationships that underlie a child's language disorder. To facilitate clinical hypotheses, I suggested that it is important to distinguish between symptoms that reflect the underlying or primary deficit and symptoms that reflect secondary deficits. Secondary deficits are caused by an individual's reaction to and/or compensation for the primary deficit. Pragmatic deficits, for example, are often secondary to syntactic-semantic problems (e.g., Snyder, 1984).

Although the question of causation in child language disorders is complex, it is important to recognise some of the causal factors of language disorders that have been proposed in the literature. These factors include (a) perceptual deficits (b) cognitive deficits, (c) social-interactive deficits, and (d) neurological deficits. Researchers (e.g., Tallal and Piercy, 1978; Kamhi, 1981; Johnston, 1982; Leonard, 1982; Snyder, 1984) have been especially interested in the cause of language disorders in children with specific language impairment. Recall that in these children, henceforth referred to as 'language impaired', the language deficit occurs in the absence of sensory, intellectual, emotional, or neurological deficits. Deficits in perceptual and selected cognitive abilities have received the majority of attention by researchers.

Perceptual deficits

Tallal and Piercy (1978) have looked extensively at language-impaired (LI) children's perceptual processing abilities. From a series of studies, they found that LI children had difficulty processing rapidly changing acoustic information. More specifically, LI children had difficulty responding to stimuli that incorporated brief acoustic cues (e.g., /ba/ and /da/) that were followed in rapid succession by other acoustic cues (Tallal and Stark, 1981). For example, in one of the tasks children were asked to judge which sound came first /ba/ or /da/. The stimuli were presented with varying intervals between the presentation of the first and second sound. Language-impaired children needed significantly more time to achieve 75 per cent success rates on this task.

Several questions have been raised about the causal role of low-level perceptual deficits. One problem is that difficulty processing speech sounds should have an adverse impact on phonological development. However, there are many children with language impairments who do not have associated phonological impairments. Leonard (1982), for example, notes that some of the children who perform poorly on these tasks have little difficulty using /b/ and /d/ appropriately in their speech. In contrast, some of the speech sounds with which they do have difficulty, such as /s/, are not sounds that involve rapid acoustic changes. One possible explanation for the perceptual deficits in LI children is that these deficits are the result of the language impairments rather than the cause of it.

A recent study by Bernstein and Stark (1985) also calls into question the role that perceptual factors play in the developmental language impairment. In this study, Bernstein and Stark readministered speech perception tests to a group of LI children four years after these tests revealed a significant difference in performance compared to matched controls. The children at Time 2 were between 8 and 11 years old. The older LI children performed at the same level as matched controls. In other words, these children no longer had difficulty processing rapidly changing acoustic information. Importantly, all of the LI children were still language impaired at the time of the follow-up testing. Although it is not possible to rule out completely a causal influence of perceptual deficits in young LI children's language problems, it is clear that perceptual problems do not appear to be a major causal factor in older children's language problems.

Specific cognitive deficits

It seems paradoxical that cognitive abilities have been implicated as a causal factor for a specific language impairment because LI children perform within normal limits on tests of nonverbal intelligence. However, there are many cognitive abilities not tapped by nonverbal intelligence tests. For the past 15 years or so, researchers (e.g., Kamhi, 1981; Johnston and Weismer, 1983; Kamhi, Catts, Koenig and Lewis, 1984; Savich, 1984; Roth and Clark, 1987) have attempted to find cognitive deficits that might explain the developmental language impairment. Much of this research was initially spurred by Morehead and Ingram's (1976) suggestion that LI children might suffer from a general representational deficit that affects performance on both linguistic as well as nonlinguistic tasks.

The theoretical justification for this claim emanated from the Piagetian view on the relationship between language and cognitive development. According to Piaget, language emerges as part of a more general symbolic function — a function defined as the ability to represent symbolically an external event or object in its absence. This view of language suggests that development in other symbolic behaviours, such as mental imagery, deferred imitation and symbolic play, should parallel developments in language. Children who demonstrate language disorders thus should exhibit deficits on tasks that tap nonlinguistic symbolic abilities.

The relationships between language and cognitive development has been partially supported by the research. LI children have been found to perform more poorly than MA-matched normal peers on measures of symbolic play (Terrell, Schwartz and Prelock, 1984; Roth and Clark, 1987) and anticipatory imagery (Kamhi, 1981; Johnston and Weismer, 1983; Savich, 1984). However, the LI children tend not to perform as poorly as language-age matched peers on these measures. For example, a 5-year-old LI child might perform worse than a 5-year-old normal child matched for MA, but better than a 3-year-old child matched for a language level. Thus, the deficit in nonlinguistic symbolic abilities is not as severe as the linguistic deficit, and a general representational deficit cannot account for the severity of the language impairment.

Another cognitive ability that has received some attention in the literature involves hypothesis-testing. In a recent series of studies (Kamhi *et al.,* 1984: Kamhi, Nelson, Lee and Gholson, 1985; Nelson, Kamhi and Apel, 1987), my colleagues and I have examined the ability of LI children to generate hypotheses to solve discrimination learning problems. The results of these studies indicated that LI children performed at age level when the encoding (i.e., perceptual, attentional and representational) and storage demands of the problems were minimal (e.g., Kamhi *et al.,* 1984). They performed more poorly than normal controls, however, when the encoding and storage demands were high (Nelson *et al.,* 1987).

The research clearly shows that LI children have cognitive strengths and weaknesses. Importantly, the cognitive weaknesses in these children are not limited to processing verbal information. LI children also have difficulty processing nonverbal information as well. Snyder (1984) has attempted to explain LI children's cognitive strengths and weaknesses using a multiple resource model. The basic claim is that LI children will perform better on tasks that allow them to martial multiple resources. The more a task relies on a single deficient resource, such as symbolic representation, the poorer the performance of the LI children. Multiple resource models that acknowledge parallel rather than serial processing of information hold promise for explaining the language and cognitive deficit in LI children.

Assessment Considerations

Much has been written about the assessment of children's language skills (e.g., Hubbell, 1981; Miller, 1981; James, 1989; Lund and Duchan, 1988). There is general agreement that the purposes of assessment are to (1) identify children with language disorders, (2) design appropriate language intervention programmes, and (3) monitor changes that result from intervention (James, 1985). There is some disagreement, however, concerning the distinction between the assessment and diagnostic process.

Some theorists, such as Nation and Aram (1977), view assessment procedures as a part of the diagnostic process. The end products of the diagnostic process are clinical hypotheses about pertinent causal factors and recommendations for services based on these hypotheses. Other theorists place little emphasis on diagnosis in their assessment procedures (e.g., Naremore, 1980; James, 1989). Lund and Duchan take a middle ground by including a question about causal factors as one of the five questions that should be answered in assessment. The five questions are:

1 Does the child have a language problem?
2 What is causing the problem?
3 What are the areas of deficit?
4 What are the regularities in the child's language performance?
5 What is recommended for the child?

As James (1989, p. 157) accurately states: '. . . the task of assessing children's language would be relatively simple if language were easily quantified like height or weight.' Language, however, is a multidimensional, complex, and dynamic entity involving many interrelated processes and abilities. Although it is possible to group children according to their overall pattern of language performance, to a certain extent every child presents a unique pattern of language abilities. One of the major challenges in assessment is thus to describe the unique pattern of language behaviours that each language-disordered child presents.

In the sections to follow, two basic assessment questions are addressed: what to assess and how to assess it? It is important to keep in mind while reading these sections that no assessment test or procedure is a substitute for an informed speech-language pathologist. As Siegel and Broen (1976, p. 75) have stated: '. . . The most useful and dependable *language assessment device* is an informed clinician who feels compelled to keep up with developments in psycholinguistics, speech pathology, and related fields, and who is not slavishly attached to a particular model of language or of assessment.'

The assessment of a child with a presumed language disorder includes more than just an evaluation of language and communication abilities. Because language is dependent on cognitive, social and physiological factors, these areas need to be assessed as well. Indeed, it is best to think of assessment of the whole child rather than assessment of specific language skills. Each of these areas is considered in more detail below.

Cognitive abilities

Cognitive development can be viewed from several perspectives, including a Piagetian perspective, an information processing perspective, and a psychometric perspective. These perspectives provide different models for the assessment of cognitive abilities. The Piagetian perspective focuses attention on the sensorimotor precursors and correlates to language, such as object knowledge, means–ends behaviour, imitation, and symbolic play (see Miller, Chapman, Branston and Reichle, 1980; Lund and Duchan, 1983). It is relatively common in the assessment of young children to include assessment of these early developing cognitive abilities. The Piagetian perspective, however, provides little guidelines for the assessment of cognitive abilities in children much beyond the sensorimotor period.

The information processing perspective considers attentional, memory, and metacognitive processes. The assessment of auditory perceptual processes is consistent with an information processing perspective. The ITPA (Kirk *et al.,* 1968) with its emphasis on discrete auditory and visual processes reflects such a perspective.

Recently, there has been considerable interest in the kinds of problem-solving strategies children use to solve cognitive tasks. Assessment of problem-solving strategies often involves determining how impulsive-reflective a child is in solving problems. The Matching Familiar Figures Test (Kagan, 1966) was designed to evaluate what has been referred to as 'cognitive style' in the literature. Another important aspect of problem-solving behaviour is children's ability to monitor and evaluate the effectiveness of their problem-solving strategies. The recent interest in children's metalinguistic abilities grew out of a more general concern with children's metacognitive abilities. Metalinguistic abilities involve reflecting on language performance, such as the ability to make judgements about grammatical accuracy. The assessment of metalinguistic competence has become an important part of the language assessment process (see Van Kleeck, 1984).

The psychometric perspective is the one associated with intelligence testing. Intelligence tests, such as the Stanford-Binet and the WISC, measure verbal as well as nonverbal abilities. Because intelligence tests directly assess language abilities, the relationship between language and the psychometric construct IQ is confounded. This is why LI children are defined by their performance on nonverbal intelligence tests. Commonly used nonverbal intelligence tests include the Leiter International Performance Scales (Arthur, 1952), The Columbia Mental Maturity Scale (Burgemeister, Blum and Lorge, 1972), and the Test of Nonverbal Intelligence (Brown, Sherbenou and Johnsen, 1982).

Social abilities

The social bases of language have been well documented in the literature (e.g., Bates, 1979; Bruner, 1975, 1977; Sachs, 1985). These investigators have proposed that language develops from the early social interactions between infants and their parents. Early social behaviours include eye contact, mutual gazing, smiling, imitative routines, ritualised games (e.g., peek-a-boo), and sharing. Early social behaviours represent some of the early communicative behaviours that infants demonstrate. Others include crying, laughter, pointing, and reaching.

Although considerable research has focused on the social bases of early language development, social factors are an important aspect of language development throughout development. The social aspects of language include not only interpersonal relationships but also motivational, attitudinal and emotional factors. Assessing these aspects of behaviours through observation and interview techniques is an important component of evaluating overall communicative competence.

Physiological factors

Physiological factors present a broad category of behaviours that include sensory, physical, neurological and genetic contributions to development. Speech-language pathologists are most comfortable evaluating hearing sensitivity and the structural integrity of the oral mechanism. Information about a child's medical and developmental history is usually obtained by interviewing the parent or from medical records and other referral sources.

Language abilities

The actual assessment of language abilities is, of course, the major part of the assessment process. Children's knowledge of language is reflected in their ability to comprehend and produce language. In order to understand and express language, children must have knowledge of the linguistic rules in the five language domains: phonology, syntax, morphology, semantics, and pragmatics. An important consideration in assessing language knowledge is familiarity with the course of language development in normal children. The specific aspects of language that get assessed will necessarily change as children get older. For example, there is no need to evaluate early communicative behaviours in a 5-year-old child. Similarly, the language forms and structures produced by a 10-year-old are not the same as those produced by a 5-year-old.

Procedures for obtaining information about a child's language behaviours are generally divided into two categories: standardised and nonstandardised. Standardised tests of language provide a specific set of stimuli to elicit behaviour from the child and specific standards to interpret the elicited behaviours (Hubbell, 1981; James, 1989). Most standardised tests are norm-referenced, meaning that a particular child's performance can be compared to a normative sample. Standardised tests are most useful in identifying children that might be eligible for speech-language services. They provide a widely accepted means for certifying that a child meets specific eligibility criteria. In contrast, standardised tests are least useful in providing the detailed information necessary for developing an intervention plan (Hubbell, 1981). Another shortcoming of standardised tests is that they do not assess all aspects of language. Pragmatic aspects of language are not easily adapted to a standardised test format.

James (1989, pp. 176–7) has compiled a list of selected standardised tests used to assess language. The table includes information about the abilities and components assessed, the age ranges specified, and the type of score derived. Some of the tests included in the list are the Preschool Language Scale (Zimmerman, Steiner and Evatt-Pond, 1979), the Test of Language Development-Primary (Newcomer and Hammill, 1982), the Peabody Picture Vocabulary Test-Revised (Dunn and Dunn, 1981), and Developmental Sentence Analysis (Lee, 1974).

Nonstandardised procedures are sometimes referred to as informal or unstructured as opposed to formal or structured tests (e.g., Hubbell, 1981). Such procedures, however, are quite formal and can be highly structured. James (p. 179) notes that nonstandardised procedures are different from standardised procedures in that they do not have a standard set of stimuli or instructions that must be followed, nor do they have well-established norms for interpretation. One of the major advantages of such procedures is that they are flexible and can be adapted to the specific child being evaluated.

Nonstandardised procedures include collecting and analysing spontaneous language samples, eliciting production of particular language structures, and the use of specific probes to evaluate comprehension of selected language forms. The best way to evaluate children's language production is to obtain a sample of their language and to analyse it. In recent years, a number of analytic procedures have been described in the literature (e.g., Crystal, Fletcher and Garman, 1976; Miller, 1981; Stickler, 1987; Lund and Duchan, 1988). I find Lund and Duchan's approach to assessment the most appealing because they offer the most comprehensive and up-to-date procedures to evaluate discourse abilities. Beginning clinicians, however, might prefer Miller or Stickler, both of whom provide straightforward guidelines for assessment as well as normative guidelines.

Computer programs have also been developed to perform linguistic analyses. Among the more widely used programs are SALT (Miller and Chapman, 1983), Lingquest 1 (Mordecai, Palin and Palmer, 1982), and Computerized Profiling (Long, 1986). Clinicians must be familiar with the language structures they wish to analyse before using computerised language sampling procedures. It is also important to remember that computers do not interpret data. Clinicians interpret data.

Theoretical Basis of Intervention

It should be apparent by now that designing and implementing an intervention program for a language-disordered child is no easy task. As with language assessment, the best language intervention is provided by an informed clinician who feels compelled to keep up with developments in psycholinguistics, speech pathology, and related fields, and who is not slavishly attached to a particular model of language or of intervention.

Language disorders are associated with a variety of causal factors, involve different aspects of language, and vary in their severity. Faced with such variety, clinicians need to have some basic organisational framework to aid in identifying intervention goals and procedures. At the core of this framework is a theory about what language is, how it is learned, and how it can be taught.

In recent years, there has been much written about the theoretical bases of therapy (e.g., Craig, 1984; Johnston, 1983; McLean, 1989). Johnston and McLean take issue with clinicians who say things like, 'I want something practical — not a lot of theory.' What these clinicians fail to recognise is that all therapy is theoretically based. Some clinicians, however, do not acknowledge the theoretical bases of their therapy. Providing treatment without knowledge of the theoretical bases that underlie it is akin to being a technician who fixes things without understanding how they work.

Acknowledging the theoretical bases of one's language intervention does not mean there is necessarily one proven theory of language and learning. It is not uncommon for clinicians to feel overwhelmed by the technical writing and the complexity of theoretical models. Although having some working knowledge of theoretical models is important, it is more important for clinicians to be able to express and defend the theoretical models that motivate their assessment and intervention programs. For many clinicians this might mean working backwards, that is, determining what their theory of language and learning is based on how they assess and remediate language disorders. A clinician, for example, whose assessment procedures focus solely on language behaviours has a different theory of language than the clinician whose assessment procedures include the evaluation of cognitive, social, and physiological behaviours. In the same vein, the clinician who uses non-directive, client-oriented therapy procedures (see Fey, 1986) might have a different theory of learning than the clinician who uses clinician-oriented approaches.

One's theories about language and learning often lead to a set of principles that guide the intervention process. Theories and principles directly influence the actual therapy program. Johnston (1985, p. 132) has written that language intervention is best understood as a set of principles that apply for all language-disordered children rather than as a set of lesson plans or program descriptions. In her article (p. 132) she provides ten principles of language intervention:

1   Teach language that expresses the child's available meanings
2   Teach language that accomplishes the child's desired purposes
3   Teach language that the child can interpret given his current knowledge about the language and the world
4   Teach language recognizing the child's preferred strategies
5   Teach language while seeming to pursue some other goal
6   Teach language by providing concentrated, salient examples of a single pattern
7   Teach language in context which clarify meaning
8   Teach language in natural as well as contrived transactions
9   Teach language while communicating real messages
10 Teach language in the child's world.

Perhaps the underlying principle of language intervention is that it is a problem solving process, both for the child learning language and for the clinician who must determine how best to teach language. As Hubbell (1981, p. 197) has written: 'The use of language involves active problem solving. Children have to decide what the utterances they hear mean; in addition, they have to decide what to say themselves, and how to say it.' Language intervention also is a problem solving task. The clinician has to identify language learning problems, determine the factors that are contributing to these problems, and design an intervention program to treat these problems.

The actual therapy treatment programme has three general components: content, context, and procedures (e.g., McLean, 1985). Content refers to the goals of the therapy. Context refers to the setting, participants, and materials of therapy. Procedures are the actual ways or activities used to teach language. These components of therapy are described in more detail below.

Content

Deciding what it is we want children to be able to do is the question that underlies decisions about language goals (Rees, 1983). Rees adds that oftentimes clinical goals are determined by the availability, attractiveness, or popularity of published tests and materials. For example, for many years it was common to administer the ITPA, teach the skills tapped by the various ITPA subtests, and readminister the test. Although many children presumably became more adept at solving auditory and visual discrimination tasks, there was often not a corresponding improvement in communication skills.

It has also been common practice for clinicians to target certain language forms because use of these forms is easily measured by pre- and post-test instruments. A good example of this practice involves the teaching of auxiliary forms, such as auxiliary *is* in present progressive sentences (e.g., 'He is running'.) Language-impaired children have been shown to have considerable difficulty acquiring auxiliary forms (e.g., Johnston and Schery, 1976; Johnston and Kamhi, 1984). Although these forms add little or no meaning to a sentence (compare 'John is running' with 'John running') and have little communicative value, clinicians spend inordinate amounts of time teaching children to use these forms.

The determination of appropriate language goals is the final step of the assessment process. An important criterion in judging the appropriateness of a goal is the extent to which the attainment of the goal will enhance communicative effectiveness. For young language-disordered children, increasing the frequency with which a child initiates topics or teaching a child how to request clarification clearly enhances communicative effectiveness. In contrast, teaching a young child to use auxiliary forms or to say 'caught' instead of 'catched' has little communicative value and would not be an appropriate language goal if the child has more basic communicative deficits. Teaching auxiliary forms or past tense markers is more likely to be an appropriate language goal for an older language-disordered child (e.g., past 5 years of age) who lacks some of the grammatical niceties of language.

As reflected in Johnston's first three principles, language goals should be determined by the child's available meanings, desired purposes, and conceptual level. In general, therapy with young children should focus on increasing the range of meanings and functions expressed, whereas therapy with older children should place more attention on the well-formedness of the structures used to express various meanings and functions and the ability to use these structures in different discourse contexts.

Context

The physical setting of therapy is probably the most frequent aspect of context discussed in the literature (cf. Bernstein and Tiegerman, 1989). The influence of physical setting on language therapy, however, seems to be vastly overrated. The principles of language intervention, selection of therapy goals, and procedures should not vary according to the setting in which therapy takes place. In other words, language therapy in the schools should not be very different than language therapy in a hospital or clinic. Settings do, however, differ in terms of the clients they attract, administrative factors, co-workers, and the extent to which a particular therapy aproach is endorsed. Note that the last factor can vary within similar setting types (i.e., clinics) as well as between settings.

To underscore these points about therapy settings, students might find it worthwhile to read Nelson's (1989) chapter on language intervention in school settings. Some parts of the chapter address issues that are relevant only to school settings, such as the development of Individual Educational Plans (IEP's) and interactions with classroom teachers. Other parts of the chapter, however, present more general principles of therapy (e.g., integration of content, form and use, individualisation, and involvement of others) that are not specific to school settings.

Another aspect of context is the social context or the participants in the therapy settings. Clinician-child dyads and group therapy with one clinician and several children are the most typical interactive contexts. With infants and very young children, parents are sometimes part of the therapy context. The social context has an obvious impact on the therapy process. For example, the child receives more focused and relevant input in individual therapy than in group therapy. In group situations, attentional skills receive considerable emphasis.

The importance of materials is often overlooked in discussions about therapy context. The materials used in therapy constrain what children will talk about and how they will talk about it (Miller, 1981). Using picture books, for example, will encourage the use of descriptive phrases linked by and (e.g., There's a fire engine, and here's a fireman, and this is a policeman.). Games tend to elicit phrases such as, 'It's my/your turn' or a narrow set of questions (Miller, 1981). Activities that involve physical manipulation, such as puzzles, drawing, often stifle talking because children become too involved performing the physical activity.

Another concern about materials is that clinicians sometimes begin believing that it is the materials that are doing the teaching rather than the clinician. One way to dispel this belief is to conduct therapy without the usual set of materials. An exercise such as this provides some indication of one's reliance on therapy materials rather than knowledge of language and the therapy process.

Procedures

I find it useful to think about the actual teaching of speech-language forms in terms of a three-part sequence: (a) the clinician provides a model of communicative behaviour, (b) the child responds in some way to the model, and (c) the clinician provides some kind of feedback to the child about the response. Each of these parts of therapy is discussed below in some detail.

Although there are many different approaches to therapy, ranging from clinician-oriented approaches to child-oriented approaches (see Fey, 1986), and different terminology used to describe the therapy process, the language models children are exposed to during therapy determine what they will learn. In most cases these models are verbal, although nonverbal communicative behaviours (e.g., gestures) and alternative communication system (e.g., sign language) can also serve as language input. Models can vary in terms of their content and structure as well as in the frequency with which they are produced. The specific language objective determines the structure and content of the language models. The frequency with which a model is produced can be viewed as a continuum that ranges from highly repetitive and systematic modelling of a particular structure (i.e., focused stimulation) at one end to low levels of repetition and unsystematic modelling of structures (general stimulation) at the other end.

Focused stimulation is often used to teach progressive forms. The clinician might have a series of ten picture cards depicting actions that can be described by the same phrase structure rule (NP + Aux + V + ing). The actual models might include sentences such as 'He is running,' 'He is jumping,' and 'He is swimming'. With general stimulation there is no focus to the language input. Particular language structures are not repeated in any consistent manner. Instead, clinicians attempt to model language forms approximately one level above the child's current level of language functioning. Models at the same level or below the child's current level will not teach the child anything, whereas models more than one level above the child's current level will be too difficult to learn (Kuhn, 1972). For example, if a child is currently producing mostly two-word utterances, the clinician should model three-constituent utterances that expand the child's two word utterances (e.g., child says 'Mommy sock' and clinician responds 'Yes, Mommy has a sock').

The child's response to the clinician's model can also be viewed on a continuum. In this case the continuum ranges from an elicited exact repetition of the model to no response. Operant approaches often require exact imitations of the models (e.g., Gray and Ryan, 1973; Stremel and Waryas, 1974). An approach to therapy that has come to be called 'modelling' initially requires no response from the child (Leonard, 1975). The child is asked to listen to ten language models before he is given the opportunity to respond. It is important to note that it is the response required from the child that differentiates the operant and modelling approaches rather than the language models provided.

In certain forms of play therapy no response is ever required from the child. The clinician makes no attempt to elicit repetitions of language models. Instead, the clinician might follow the child's lead and comment on what the child is playing with or talking about. Alternatively, the clinician might engage in parallel play and comment on her own activities (see Fey, 1986). The theoretical rationale for this kind of therapy approach is that language is a mental activity that involves rule induction and other reasoning processes. Learning language is thus not necessrily facilitated by repeating language models. The child must induce a language rule from these models and this rule induction is more likely to occur 'off-line' when the child has time to think about language rather than 'on-line' when the child is actually repeating language forms. Connell (1987), however, recently reported that an imitative approach was more effective than a modelling approach in teaching a group of language-impaired children an invented morphological rule. One possible explanation for this finding was that the imitative approach helped to focus attention on the language models to be learned.

In general, the younger the child, the less stringent the response demands should be. Infants and very young children are often not very responsive to highly directive clinician-oriented approaches that require elicited imitative responses. As children get older and their comprehension and metalinguistic competence increase, they can be more easily directed to produce specific responses.

The final component of therapy sequence is the clinician's response to the child's response. There are two kinds of feedback clinicians can provide to children: evaluative feedback and communicative feedback. Evaluative feedback is when the clinician offers an appraisal of the appropriateness or accuracy of the child's response. Comments that reflect evaluative feedback include, 'Good,' 'Good talking/words', 'I like the way you said that', 'No, that wasn't so good'. Clinicians are more likely to give positive evaluative feedback than negative evaluative feedback. For evaluative feedback to be meaningful, however, positive evaluations should follow only appropriate child responses. There are a variety of ways to handle inappropriate responses, including direct negative evaluations (e.g., 'That was not too good', 'You missed that one'); corrective feedback (e.g., 'You said "catched" instead of "caught"'), and neutral feedback (e.g., 'Let's try that one again later').

Importantly, it is not necessary nor desirable for clinicians to evaluate the appropriateness of every response or utterance a child makes. Responding to children's utterances in communicative rather than evaluative ways also provides feedback to the child. For example, a child might say, 'Hey, there's a spider on the floor' to which the clinician responds 'Yeah, it's a really big one. Do you like spiders?' Not only is communicative feedback more in line with the kinds of discourse children will encounter outside the therapy context, but expansions and recasts have been shown to facilitate language learning in normal children (Nelson, 1987).

Therapy approaches differ in the extent to which they advocate evaluative and communicative feedback. Operant approaches are usually associated with well-defined schedules for providing evaluative feedback. In contrast, client-oriented therapy approaches, such as play therapy, tend to place more emphasis on communicative feedback.

I think it is important to mention why I have avoided using the term 'reinforcement' in this section on feedback. It is, of course, common practice for clinicians to talk about reinforcement schedules and the different types of reinforcements used. There are two basic reasons why I think the term 'reinforcement' should be expunged from one's clinical vocabulary. First, the term is associated with a behaviorist theory of language learning that holds that reinforcement plays a major role in language learning. This theory has been shown to have little merit (e.g., Chomsky, 1965). Indeed, even Skinner who proposed the theory no longer believes it can explain language acquisition. Use of the term reinforcement thus creates a theoretical mismatch between one's theory of language and therapy procedures (see Craig, 1983). The second problem is that reinforcement plays three roles in therapy not just one. The child might be reinforced to pay attention to language models, to sustain attention throughout the therapy session, and to provide evaluative feedback about the appropriateness of a response. The term reinforcement thus not only evokes outdated and incorrect theoretical notions of language learning, but is also ambiguous.

Effectiveness of Therapy

One way to approach questions about therapy effectiveness is through clinical studies in which a specific therapy approach (e.g., modelling vs. imitation) is evaluated in terms of its effectiveness on one or more clients (e.g., Connell, 1986; Courtright, 1976). Clinical research, however, generally has not examined the effectiveness of a broader treatment regimen. As Schery and Lipsey (1983) point out, a complete treatment regimen consists of many specific therapy treatments and, therefore, its overall effects are probably somewhat different from the effects of any one therapy technique. In a review of clinical treatment studies, Leonard (1981) found that researchers rarely addressed questions about the generality or duration of treatment effects and the range of clients for which a specific approach was appropriate.

Another approach to the question of therapy effectiveness is to consider general programme evaluation, the basic function of which is to provide information for decision making at local, state and federal levels. To do this, Schery and Lipsey (1983) suggest that programme information is needed in four areas: 1. accountability; 2. programme premises; 3. management and administration and 4. planning. Accountability is usually interpreted as having readily accessible complete records of clients served, along with a justifiable rationale to document need for service. Other accountability issues involve demonstrating that a particular programme serves a need and should continue to be funded. Programme premises include basic assumptions that govern the provision of service, e.g., the assumption that speech-language clinicians with graduate degrees can deliver services more effectively and efficiently than individuals without professional training. As Schery and Lipsey point out, assumptions such as these help determine the programme model under which school and clinic operate.

Management and administration refers to the process rather than the outcome of providing services. The process component of programme evaluation involves keeping track of key operations and activities that constitute the programme (Schery and Lipsey, 1983, p. 263). A comprehensive programme evaluation would include questions about access, equity and efficiency (Schery and Lipsey, 1983, p. 264). Programme planning involves foreseeing trends and needs so that the programme can adapt to the changes that might occur in the future.

The last approach to therapy effectiveness that will be considered is reflected in a recent article by Siegel (1987) on the limits of science. Siegel argues that the most important question to ask about therapy is not whether it works, but rather whether it makes sense. Siegel begins with the assumption that it does work. There is no experiment that would convince him otherwise because the definitive treatment experiment cannot be done, there being too many uncontrollable variables relating to the client, clinician setting, therapy method, measures used and so forth. Efficacy studies, therefore, are not needed to demonstrate that therapy works, although they might help influence programme funding decisions. The accountability issue is different and relates to funding decisions and programme evaluation. It is not appropriate to conclude that because a particular programme is not accountable, therapy is ineffective. As Siegel (p. 310) states, 'It seems incontrovertible that all human behaviour is potentially malleable, and that none of us, client or therapist, is working to the absolute limits of his or her ability'. In other words there is no doubt that speech-language clinicians are capable of changing a client's communicative behaviour. Moreover, it is difficult to imagine a speech-language clinician who would knowingly use a therapy procedure that was ineffective in modifying communitive performance.

In light of these points, clinicians should begin with the assumption that therapy works. Good record-keeping will allow the clinician to address outcome and accountability questions about specific programme effectiveness. The more interesting research questions, however, are those that address the process of therapy and behaviour change. Clinicians who seek answers to these questions will develop a better understanding of the behavioural processes in therapy and, in turn, be better able to develop therapy plans that are tailored to individual client needs.

Conclusion

I began this chapter by noting that learning a first language is the most complex learning task humans accomplish during their lifetime. These complexities are best seen in children who have difficulty learning language. What this means is that there are no easy answers to the questions most frequently raised about these children, namely: What is a language disorder? What causes it? How are language abilities assessed? How are language abilities taught? In this chapter, I have provided answers to each of these questions. Some of my answers might be more satisfactory to you than others. I am least satisfied with my answer to the question about causal factors. Perhaps you would have liked more information about the interpersonal aspects of therapy, augmentative communication, teaching adolescents, or a better description of language analysis procedures. The information provided in this chapter, however, was meant to whet the appetite, not satiate it. Indeed the complexity of language learning and language disorders ensures that even the most voracious appetite will never be satisfied.

References

ARAM, D. and NATION, J. (1982) *Child Language Disorders.* St. Louis, MO: Mosby.

ARAM, D., EKELMAN, B. and NATION, J. (1984) Preschoolers with Language disorders: 10 years later. *Journal of Speech and Hearing Research,* 27, 232–44.

ARTHUR, G. (1952) *The Arthur Adaptation of the Leiter International Performance Scale.* Washington, DC: Psychological Service Center Press.

ASHA COMMITTEE ON LANGUAGE, SPEECH AND HEARING SERVICES IN THE SCHOOLS. (April 1980) Definitions for communicative disorders and differences, *ASHA,* 22, 317–18.

ASHA COMMITTEE ON LANGUAGE (June, 1983) Definition of Language, *ASHA,* 25, 44.

BATES, E. (1979) *The Emergence of Symbols.* New York: Academic Press.

BERNSTEIN, D. (1989) The Nature of Language and its Disorders. In L. Bernstein and E. Tiegerman (Eds), *Language and Communication Disorders in Children* (2nd ed.). Columbus, OH: Merrill.

BERNSTEIN, D. and TIEGERMAN, E. (1989) (Eds) *Language and Communication Disorders in Children* (2nd ed.). Columbus OH: Merrill.

BERNSTEIN, L. and STARK, R. (1985) Speech perception development in language-impaired children: A 4-year follow-up study. *Journal of Speech and Hearing Disorders,* 50, 21–31.

BLOOM, L. and LAHEY, M. (1978) *Language Development and Language Disorders.* New York: John Wiley and Sons.

BROWN, L., SHERBENOU, R. and JOHNSEN, S. (1982) *Test of Nonverbal Intelligence.* Austin, TX: Pro-Ed.

BRUNER, J. (1975) The ontogenesis of speech acts. *Journal of Child Language,* 2, 1–19.

BRUNER, J. (1977) Early social interaction and language acquisition. In R. Schaffer (Ed.) *Studies in Mother-Infant Interaction.* New York: Academic Press.

BURGEMEISTER, B., BLUM, L. and LORGE, I. (1972) *Columbia Mental Maturity Scale* (3rd ed.). New York: Harcourt Brace Jovanovich.

CARROW, E. (1973) *Test for Auditory Comprehension of Language* (5th ed.). Boston: Teaching Resources Corp.

CHAFE, W. (1970) *Meaning and Structure of Language.* Chicago: University of Chicago Press.

CHOMSKY, N. (1957) *Syntactic Structures.* The Hague: Mouton.

CHOMSKY, N. (1965) *Aspects of the Theory of Syntax.* Cambridge, MA: MIT Press.

CHURCHILL, D. (1978) *Language of Autistic Children.* New York: Wiley.

CONNELL, P. (1987) An effect of modeling and imitation teaching procedures on children with and without specific language impairment. *Journal of Speech and Hearing Research,* 30, 105–14.

COOPER, J. and FLOWERS, C. (1987) Children with a history of acquired aphasia: Residual language and academic impairments. *Journal of Speech and Hearing Disorders,* 52, 251–63.

COURTRIGHT, J.A. and COURTRIGHT, I.C. (1976) Imitative modeling as a theoretical base for instructing language-disordered children. *Journal of Speech and Hearing Research,* 19, 655–63.

CRAIG, H. (1984) Applications of pragmatic language models for intervention. In T. Gallagher and C. Prutting (Eds), *Pragmatic Assessment and Intervention Issues.* San Diego: College Hill.

CRYSTAL, D., FLETCHER, P. and GARMAN, M. (1976) *The Grammatical Analysis of Language Disability: A Procedure for Assessment and Remediation.* London: Edward Arnold.

DEMYER, M., BARTON, S., DEMYER, E., NORTON, J., ALLEN, J. and STELLE, R. (1973) Prognosis in autism: A follow-up study. *Journal of Autism and Childhood Schizophrenia,* 3, 199–216.

DERENZIE, E. and VIGNOLO, L. (1962) The token test: A sensitive test to detect receptive disturbances in aphasics. *Brain,* 85, 665–78.

DUNN, L. and DUNN, L. (1981) *Peabody Picture Vocabulary Test — Revised.* Circle Pines, MN: American Guidance Service.

EISENBERG, L. (1956) The autistic child in adolescence. *American Journal of Psychiatry,* 112, 607–12.

EISENSON, J. (1972) *Aphasia in Children.* New York: Harper and Row.

FEY, M. (1986) *Language Intervention with Children*. San Diego: College Hill.

GROSSMAN, H. (1983) *Classification in Mental Retardation*. Washington, DC: American Association on Mental Deficiency.

GRAY, B. and RYAN, B. (1973) *A Language Program for the Nonlanguage Child*. Champaign, IL: Research Press.

HUBBELL, R. (1981) *Children's Language Disorders: An Integrated Approach*. Englewood Cliffs, NJ: Prentice Hall.

INGRAM, D. (1976) *Phonological Disability in Children*. New York: Elsevier North-Holland.

INGRAM, D. (1981) *Procedures for the Phonological Analysis of Children's Language*. Baltimore, MD: University Park Press.

JAMES, S. (1989) Assessing children with language disorders. In D. Bernstein and E. Tiegerman (Eds), *Language and Communication Disorders in Children* (2nd ed.). Columbus, OH: Merrill.

JOHNSTON, J. (1982) The language disordered child. In N. Lass, J. Northern, D. Yoder, and L. McReynolds (Eds), *Speech, Language and Hearing*. Philadelphia: W.B. Saunders Co.

JOHNSTON, J. (1983) What is language intervention? The role of theory. In J. Miller, D. Yoder, and R. Schieflebusch (Eds), *Contemporary Issues in Language Intervention*. ASHA Reports 12, Rockville, MD: ASHA.

JOHNSTON, J. (1985) Fit, focus and functionality: An essay on early language intervention. *Child Language Teaching and Therapy*, 1, 1125–35.

JOHNSTON, J. and KAMHI, A. (1984) The same can be less: Syntactic and semantic aspects of the utterances of language-impaired children. *Merrill-Palmer Quarterly*, 30, 65–85.

JOHNSTON, J. and SCHERY, T. (1976) The use of grammatical morphemes by children with communication disorders. In D. Morehead and A. Morehead (Eds) *Normal and Deficient Child Language*. Baltimore: University Park Press.

JOHNSTON, J. and WEISMER, S. (1983) Mental rotation abilities in language-disordered children. *Journal of Speech and Hearing Research*, 26, 397–404.

KAGAN, J. (1966) Reflection-impulsivity: The generality and dynamics of conceptual tempo. *Journal of Abnormal Psychology*, 71, 17–24.

KAMHI, A. (1981) Nonlinguistic and conceptual abilities of language impaired and normally developing children. *Journal of Speech and Hearing Research*, 24, 435–45.

KAMHI, A. (1984) Problem solving in child language disorders: The clinician as clinical scientist. *Language, Speech, and Hearing Services in Schools*, 15, 226–34.

KAMHI, A. (1989) Language and cognition in the mentally handicapped: Last rites for the difference-delay controversy. In M. Beveridge, G. Conti-Ramsden, and I. Leudar (Eds), *Language and Communication in the Mentally Handicapped*. London: Croom Helm.

KAMHI, A., CATTS, H., KOENIG, L. and LEWIS, B. (1984) Hypothesis testing and nonlinguistic symbolic abilities in language impaired children. *Journal of Speech and Hearing Disorders*, 49, 169–77.

KAMHI, A., NELSON, L., LEE, R. and GHOLSON, B. (1985) The ability of language-disordered children to use and modify hypotheses in discrimination learning. *Applied Psycholinguistics*, 6, 435–52.

KIRK, S., McCARTHY, J. and KIRK, W. (1968) *The Illinois Test of Psycholinguistic Abilities*. Champaign, IL: University of Illinois Press.

KUHN, D. (1972) Mechanisms of change in the development of cognitive structures. *Child Development,* 43, 833–44.

LEE, L. (1971) *Northwestern Syntax Screening Test.* Evanston, IL: Northwestern University Press.

LEE, L. (1974) *Developmental Sentence Analysis.* Evanston, IL: Northwestern University Press.

LEONARD, L. (1975) Modeling as a clinical procedure in language training. *Language, Speech, and Hearing Services in Schools,* 6, 72–85.

LEONARD, L. (1979) Language impairments in children. *Merrill-Palmer Quarterly,* 25, 205–32.

LEONARD, L. (1981) Facilitating linguistic skills in children with specific language impairment. *Applied Psycholinguistics,* 2, 89–119.

LEONARD, L. (1982) Early language development and language disorders. In G. Shames and E. Wiig (Eds), *Human Communication Disorders: An Introduction.* Columbus, OH: Merrill.

LONG, S. (1986) *Computerized Profiling.* Arcata, CA: Steve Long.

LUND, N. and DUCHAN, J. (1983) *Assessing Children's Language in Naturalistic Contexts.* Englewood Cliffs, NJ: Prentice-Hall.

LUND, N. and DUCHAN, J. (1988) *Assessing Children's Language in Naturalistic Contexts* (2nd ed.). Englewood Cliffs, NJ: Prentice-Hall.

LYON, G. and WATSON, B. (1981) Empirically derived subgroups of learning disabled readers: Diagnostic characteristics. *Journal of Learning Disabilities,* 14, 256–61.

MATTIS, S., FRENCH, J. and RAPIN, I. (1975) Dyslexia in children and young adults: Three independent neuropsychological syndromes. *Developmental Medicine and Child Neurology,* 17, 1150–63.

MCGINNIS, M. (1963) *Aphasic Children: Identification and Education by the Association Method.* Washington, DC: Alexander Graham Bell Association for the Deaf.

MCLEAN, J. (1989) A language-communication intervention model. In D. Bernstein and E. Tiegerman (Eds), *Language and Communication Disorders in Children* (2nd ed.). Columbus, OH: Merrill.

MCLEAN, J. and SYNDER-MCLEAN, L. (1978) *A Transactional Approach to Early Language Training.* Columbus. OH: Merrill.

MILLER, J. (1981) *Assessing Language Production in Children.* Baltimore: University Park Press.

MILLER, J., CAMPBELL, T., CHAPMAN, R. and WEISMER, S. (1984) Language behavior in acquired childhood aphasia. In A. Holland (Ed.), *Language Disorders in Children.* San Diego: College-Hill.

MILLER, J. and CHAPMAN, R. (1983) *SALT: Systematic Analysis of Language Transcripts.* Madison, WI: Language Analysis Laboratory, Waisman Center, University of Wisconsin.

MILLER, J., CHAPMAN, R., BRANSTON, M. and REICHLE, J. (1980). Language comprehension in sensorimotor stages V and VI. *Journal of Speech and Hearing Research,* 23, 284–311.

MILLER, J., CHAPMAN, R. and MACKENZIE, H. (1981) Individual differences in the language acquisition of mentally retarded children. Proceedings from the Second Wisconsin Symposium on Research in Child Language Disorders. University of Wisconsin.

MORDECAI, D., PALIN, M. and PALMER, C. (1982) *Lingquest 1: Language Sample*

Analysis. Columbus, OH: Merrill.

MOREHEAD, D. and INGRAM, D. (1976) The development of base syntax in normal and linguistically deviant children. In D. Morehead and A. Morehead (Eds), *Normal and Deficient Child Language.* Baltimore: University Park Press.

MORLEY, M. (1957) *The Development and Disorders of Speech in Childhood.* Edinburgh: Churchill Livingston.

MYKLEBUST, H. (1954) *Auditory Disorders in Children: A Manual for Differential Diagnosis.* New York: Grune and Stratton.

NATION, J. and ARAM, D. (1977) *Diagnosis of Speech and Language Disorders.* St. Louis: Mosby.

NAREMORE, R. (1980) Language disorders in children. In T. Hixon, L. Shriberg, and J. Saxman (Eds), *Introduction to Communication Disorders.* Englewood Cliffs, NJ: Prentice-Hall.

NELSON, L., KAMHI, A. and APEL, K. (1987) Cognitive strengths and weaknesses in language-impaired children: One more look. *Journal of Speech and Hearing Disorders,* 52, 36–43.

NELSON, N. (1989) Language intervention in school settings. In D. Bernstein and E., Tiegerman (Eds), *Language and Communication Disorders in Children* (2nd ed.). Columbus, OH: Merrill.

NELSON, K. (1987) Some observations from the perspective of the rare event cognitive comparison theory of language acquisition. In K. Nelson and A. Van Kleeck (Eds), *Children's Language,* Volume 6. Hillsdale, NJ: Erlbaum.

NEWCOMER, P. and HAMMIL, L.D. (1982) *The Test of Language Development-Primary.* Austin, TX: Pro-Ed.

OWENS, R. (1989) Mental retardation: Difference or delay. In D. Bernstein and E. Tiegerman (Eds), *Language and Communication Disorders in Children* (2nd ed.). Columbus, OH: Merrill.

PRIZANT, B. (1982) Speech-language pathologists and autistic children: What is our role? Part I. *AHSA,* 24, 463–8.

PRIZANT, B. and DUCHAN, J. (1981) The functions of immediate echolalia in autistic children. *Journal of Speech and Hearing Disorders,* 46, 241–9.

REES, N. (1983) Language intervention with children, In J. Miller, D. Yoder and R. Schiefelbusch (Eds), *Contemporary Issues in Language Intervention.* ASHA Reports, 12. Rockville, MD: ASHA.

ROTH, F. and CLARK, D. (1987) Symbolic play and social participation abilities of language-impaired and normally developing children. *Journal of Speech and Hearing Disorders,* 52, 17–29.

ROTH, F. and SPEKMAN, N. (1986) Narrative discourse: Spontaneously generated stories of learning-disabled and normally achieving students. *Journal of Speech and Hearing Disorders,* 51, 8–23.

SACHS, J. (1985) Prelinguistic development. In J. Berko-Gleason (Ed.), *The Development of Language.* Columbus, OH: Merrill.

SAMEROFF, A. (1975) Early influences on development: Fact or fancy? *Merrill-Palmer Quarterly,* 21, 267–94.

SAVICH, P. (1984) Anticipatory imagery ability in normal and language-disabled children. *Journal of Speech and Hearing Research,* 27, 294–502.

SCHERY, T. and LIPSEY, M. (1983) Program evaluation for speech and hearing services, in J. Miller *et al.* (Eds), *Contemporary Issues in Language Intervention.*

ASHA Reports, 12. Rockville, MD: ASHA.

SIEGEL, G. and BROEN, P. (1976) Language assessment. In L. Lloyd (Ed.), *Communication, Assessment and Intervention Strategies*. Baltimore: University Park Press.

SIEGEL, G. (1987) The limits of science in communication disorders. *Journal of Speech and Hearing Disorders*, 52, 306–13.

SNYDER, L. (1984) Communicative competence in children with delayed language development. In R. Schiefelbusch and J. Picker (Eds), *The Acquisition of Communicative Competence*. Baltimore: University Park Press.

STARK, R. and TALLAL, P. (1981) Selection of children with specific language deficits. *Journal of Speech and Hearing Disorders*, 46, 114–23.

STICKLER, K. (1987) *Guide to Analysis of Language Transcripts*. Eau Clair, WI: Thinking Publications.

STREMEL, K. and WARYAS, C. (1974) A behavioral-psycholinguistic approach to language training. In L. McReynolds (Ed.) *Developing Systematic Procedures for Training Children's Language*. ASHA Monographs, No. 18. Rockville, MD: ASHA.

TALLAL, P. and PIERCY, M. (1978) Defects of auditory perception in children with developmental aphasia. In M. Wyke (Ed.) *Developmental Dysphasia*. New York: Academic Press.

TALLAL, P. and STARK, R. (1981) A re-examination of some non-verbal perceptual abilities of language impaired and normal children as a function of age and sensory modality. *Journal of Speech and Hearing Research*, 24, 351–7.

TEMPLIN, M. and DARLEY, F. (1969) *The Templin-Darley test of Articulation*. Iowa City, IA: Bureau of Educational Research and Service.

TERRELL, B., SCHWARTZ, R. and PRELOCK, P. (1984) Symbolic play in normal and language-impaired children. *Journal of Speech and Hearing Research*, 27, 424–30.

TIEGERMAN, E. (1989) Autism. In D. Bernstein and E. Tiegerman (Eds) *Language and Communication Disorders in Children* (2nd ed.). Columbus, OH: Merrill.

VAN KLEECK, A. (1984) Assessment and intervention: Does 'meta' matter? In G. Wallach and K. Butler (Eds), *Language Learning Disabilities in School-Age Children*. Baltimore: Williams and Wilkins.

WALLACH, G. and BUTLER, J. (1984) *Language Learning Disabilities in School-Age Children*. Baltimore: Williams and Wilkins.

WECHSLER, D. (1963) *Wechsler Preschool and Primary Scale of Intelligence*. New York: The Psychological Corp.

WECHSLER, D. (1974) *Wechsler Intelligence Scale for Children — Revised*. New York: The Psychological Corp.

ZIMMERMAN, I., STEINER, V. and EVATT-POND, R. (1979) *Preschool Language Scale*. Columbus, OH: Merrill.

7 Childhood Phonological Disorders

Jennifer Lambert

In the past twenty years there have been significant developments in the description and the explanation of phonological disorders in childhood. As Kamhi points out in Chapter 6, phonology is integral to language and phonological disorders represent a language disorder. Grunwell (1988) describes a phonological disorder as 'an abnormal, or inadequate or disorganised system of patterns evidenced by deviations in the spoken language', and advances the hypothesis that the dysfunction is 'at the phonological level of cortical representation and organisation of the language system'. When the speech and language clinician sees a child referred with speech that is not readily intelligible, the major objective is to describe and analyse the child's speech patterns, and to formulate an appropriate management programme. This involves making distinctions between the possible reasons for the lack of intelligibility which in turn guide the choice of management techniques employed.

Phonological Disorders

Discussion between speech and language clinicians as to how they *manage* childhood phonological disorders is likely to lead to a heated debate. In the past twenty years there have been considerable developments in the description and more recently in the explanation of such disorders although the implications of such developments have not always been adopted by practitioners.

The application of linguistic theory to the study of language development and childhood pronunciation has enabled detailed analysis of speech behaviour. What has emerged from such analysis is an understanding of predictable patterns of development and the rule-governed nature of child speech, as well as recognition of the occurrence of individual differences for example in the order of acquisition of phonemes. Knowledge of these patterns helps us to make distinctions between

103

those children whose speech is childlike and normally immature and those whose speech patterns show differing types of atypical development.

When children are acquiring spoken language there are two major components involved. First, they have to achieve mastery of the motor abilities necessary to produce a range of speech sounds, and second they have to learn the organisational patterns in which those sounds are used in their particular language. So it is not only important to be able to articulate /t/ and /s/, but to understand that in English these sounds are used contrastively. They also need to understand the possible sequences of sounds which are acceptable in the language and also what constraints are placed on the position of sounds and the effect of the phonetic context on their production. The study of child phonology considers both of these components. A child whose pronunciation development is delayed may have problems with either the articulatory or the phonological component or both.

The process by which such acquisition occurs has been the subject of much interest for linguists, psychologists and speech pathologists. The roles of perception and production constraints, the relationship between adult and child speech, and the relationship between phonology, other levels of language development and cognitive abilities are three issues which have been central in the attempts to develop a model of phonological development. Early structuralist models accounted for some of the general patterns which occur and assumed a relatively passive role on the part of the child focusing on linguistic universals (Jakobson, 1968).

Natural phonology (Stampe, 1969, 1979) established the concept of phonological processes defined by Stampe as mental operations which adapt phonological intentions to phonological capacities. The effect of a process is to allow for a simplification in pronunciation for example producing stops instead of fricatives. As fricatives begin to be incorporated into the system, the child is seen as 'suppressing' the stopping process. Whilst the deterministic nature of these so called operations is questioned the descriptive and possibly explanatory value of natural processes is eminently applicable to analysis and remediation of phonological disorders.

Most recent cognitive theories stress a much more active role on the part of the child, recognising the ability to form and test hypotheses about the phonological system. This view highlights the differences amongst individuals and the creativity of the language process. Cognitive phonology may well be able to offer explanations for the process of the phonological acquisition (see for example Leonard (1985), Yeni-Komshian, Kavanagh and Ferguson (1980), Macken and Ferguson (1983), Schwartz (1984), Stoel-Gammon and Dunn (1985), and Fletcher and Garman (1986) for reviews and developments in language acquisition theory).

The differing theoretical approaches have emphasised different basic units in the acquisition process. These in turn have influenced clinical concepts and the development of clinical procedures. Contrastive analysis of phonemes, distinctive features and processes are the three which are consistently used in current procedures.

Until the 1960s it was usual in clinical practice to refer to disorders of speech sound production as articulation disorders. A further distinction was made between those speech disorders of organic causation and those of unknown aetiology (functional). Disorders which are primarily articulatory usually result from structural or neurological deficit and manifest their linguistic effect at a phonetic level that is in the child's ability to produce sounds accurately or consistently (see Chapters 8 and 11). There is currently debate on the need to make a further distinction in the category of phonetic disorder between phonetic and articulatory disorders (Hewlett, 1985), thus making a clearer distinction between a phonetic programming disorder such as apraxia of speech and a motor disorder (phonetic realisation disorder) such as dysarthria.

The term 'functional' was applied to those disorders of speech sound production where no identifiable cause could be discerned. The term 'functional' is no longer in general use and the terms phonological delay and disorder have replaced it, being more useful as descriptions of the problem, though it must be noted that these terms are not in themselves explanatory and need to be accompanied by appropriate pathological information.

Linguistically, such disorders manifest their main effect at a phonological level where the child has problems in developing the sound system and structure of the language. Children with phonological delay do not normally have problems with the articulation of sounds though there is a range in the levels of difficulty experienced. At a phonological level the child's unintelligible speech may be characterised by a reduced range of sounds within the language and also by the range of processes which are used to describe the differences between child and adult speech. Such processes may have an effect on both the sound system and the structure (Ingram, 1976; Leonard, 1985; Grunwell, 1988). Table 7.1 summarises the processes observed in normal development and employed in Phonological Assessment of Child Speech (PACS — Grunwell, 1985).

Table 7.1: Phonological Processes (after Grunwell, 1985)

Structural Simplifications	Systemic Simplifications
Weak syllable deletion:	Fronting: /k/--[t]
Final consonant deletion: cat[ka]	Stopping: /s/--[t]
Vocalisation: /-1/--[u]	Gliding: /r/--[w]
Reduplication: bottle [bobo]	Context-sensitive
Consonant Harmony:dog [gog]	Voicing:party [badi]
Cluster Reduction:/sp/--[p]	Glottal replacement:
/bl/--[b]	Glottal Insertion

Children with disordered phonological development may present with a set of persisting processes which are similar to those observed in normal development. Other patterns may present:

Chronological mismatch
Unusual/idiosyncratic processes
Variable use of processes
Systematic sound preferences   (Grunwell, 1985)

The therapist then is faced with the prospect of distinguishing between normally developing but immature speech, delayed phonological development, atypical phonological development and articulatory incompetence. In addition to those children whose primary problem is at a phonetic or phonological level, there are many conditions (e.g., mental retardation, hearing impairment) where phonological problems occur, but are not the primary presenting problem. A further problem exists in that phonetic and phonological level difficulties can co-exist, again exemplified in the case of hearing impairment and also in structural disorders such as cleft palate.

The principles and techniques described in this chapter are applicable to phonological development across this wide range of disorders, but are essentially directed at the management of phonological disorder as the primary problem.

Causative Factors

The distinction between articulatory (phonetic) and phonological disorders has been referred to above and the observation made that often there is no clear indication of the aetiology of a phonological disorder. There is some indication from the difference in response to treatment that a number of factors may be involved. Research into the nature of phonological development has contributed much in the way of suggesting what some of the variables may be (Fee and Ingram, 1982; Compton, 1976; Menyuk, Menn and Silber, 1986).

A number of aetiologies have been considered. These have considered breakdown at different points in the processing of speech and predominantly from two perspectives; linguistic and motor-acoustic. A failure to perceive and discriminate speech sounds accurately was thought to be of primary importance in some research (Beresford and Grady, 1968; and see Rees, 1973 for a summary of earlier work in this area). This has now been developed as part of a more general cognitive/linguistic view of the disorders — a lack of knowledge about the sound system and/or structure; such a failure might have perceptual or productive effects. The other major variable which has received focus is the child's articulatory skill —

a failure in the ability to produce speech sounds accurately postulated as causative. There is some evidence that some children who have no readily discernible organic damage may show a degree of ariculatory incompetence (Hewlett, 1987). For some children a combination of factors may be in operation. Traditional approaches of therapy tend to make use of the perceptual and motor components, though neither fully explains the level of breakdown.

More recently, attention has been drawn to metalinguistic ability (Howell and Dean, 1985). This is the ability to analyse and talk about language. This facility develops alongside other aspects of language acquisition and is apparently less well developed in children with language impairment. Training in this cognitive awareness can help the child develop repair strategies — the ability to self-correct.

The relationship between phonetic, phonological levels and other levels of language ability cannot be ignored. Phonological disorders and syntactic disorders co-exist for many children and this may extend into later problems in reading development (Vellutino, 1979; Klein, 1985). A speech and language clinician can make use of phonological output assessment and training to help both children and adults with reading difficulties (Stackhouse, 1985; Coltheart, 1987).

Assessment Considerations

'An accurate assessment and characterisation of the speech sound problem is the first and perhaps most essential component in the clinical treatment of children with speech disorders' (Elbert and Gierut, 1986). The clinician's concern is to produce an analysis which can be used as a basis for remediation. What is required is a detailed knowledge of normal spoken language development with reference to a number of perspectives including linguistic, pathological and psychological. In addition a detailed description of the phonetic and phonological capabilities exemplified in the person's speech is required. In time it will become more possible to compare this capability with those of other people with disabilities. At the present time there are few published accounts of such differences.

Goals of analysis

The analysis at a phonological level forms part of an overall assessment of language behaviour. The emphasis on which is the appropriate linguistic level for management will depend on the pattern presenting. If a child of four years is producing single words only, the focus of concern is unlikely to be at the phonological level. However, if a 4-year-old is producing a wide range of sentence structures, but is generally unintelligible then phonology probably will be the focus.

The assessment components which need to be considered in any evaluation of phonological development will include auditory behaviour, cognitive abilities, the phonological analysis, neuromotor skills. The role of assessment is fundamental to the clinician's ability to make treatment decisions (see Ingram, 1982 for summary of issues; also Stoel-Gammon and Dunn, 1985; and Grunwell, 1983). It is worth distinguishing at this point between investigative and rehabilitative therapy. It is quite reasonable to undertake some therapeutic intervention during the assessment process which is primarily concerned with probing the child's abilities and will help in the overall evaluation.

Assessment of disordered phonology: content

In order to gain a representative sample of system, structure and processes it is necessary to have a relatively large corpus of items. Ideally, 200-250 provides a useful corpus size (Grunwell, 1985). Realisticallly it may be appropriate to collect a shorter sample, say 75-100 utterances and then check the development and its variability. It should then be possible to carry out further assessment on a more focused sample.

Different methods are used in available procedures to collect this data sample. Many tests and assessments have traditionally elicited naming responses to picture stimuli: e.g., Edinburgh Articulation Test (Anthony, Bogle, Ingram and McIsaac, 1971); Sheffield Articulation test and Fisher-Logemann (Fisher and Logemann, 1971). There are advantages to this sampling, in that the therapist knows what the target item is and that it can be carried out fairly rapidly. The disadvantage of such a method is that the context effects cannot be measured and patterns that are representative for a child may not occur.

Some assessment procedures make use of both elicited single word and continuous speech samples: e.g., Newcastle speech assessment (Beresford, 1981), Goldman-Fristoe (Goldman and Fristoe, 1972) and PACS (Grunwell, 1985), which may have specific modes of elicitation. Procedures such as these provide the most comprehensive corpus for analysis. The effects of phonetic context can be taken into account as can suprasegmental features such as stress. The relationship between segmental and suprasegmental behaviour is an area of developing research and may in the future provide a better understanding of segmental errors.

When the child has particularly unintelligible speech then delayed imitation procedures may be useful for eliciting data: e.g., Phonological Process Analysis (Weiner, 1984). Recording the sample at the time of data collection is important as well as a gloss of the utterances.

Transcription

Most clinicians use a broad phonemic transcription and for many children with delayed phonology this may be adequate. However, in many cases it is necessary to use a narrow transcription in order to adequately describe the phonetic variability. Such a transcription would require the use of diacritics and PRDS (Phonetic Representation of Disordered Speech) symbols. This is particularly the case for children when articulatory or programming disorders are suspected.

Organisation of sequence of analysis

Several frameworks have been postulated. These have been developed from different theoretical standpoints and may consider units of different size. Distinctive feature analysis and generative phonology theories have been applied to phonological analysis with differing degrees of success (Compton and Hutton, 1978; McReynolds and Huston, 1971; McReynolds and Engmann 1975). The current trend is to apply natural phonology and its development to the analysis (see Grunwell, 1988 for a review of some current procedures). The traditional framework of analysing speech sound errors in terms of substitutions, omissions and distortions has been replaced in current education programmes with a two part analysis.

The first part consists of consideration of the range of phones produced and their distribution in terms of place in syllable structure and the constraints which affect the sequence of phones. In some frameworks this approach is referred to as an independent analysis (i.e., analysis as a self-contained system without reference to the adult target). A similar form of analysis is included in PACS and the Newcastle speech assessment. The second approach is referred to as a relational or contrastive analysis in which the child's pronunciation is compared with the adult model in terms of phonological processes, and ability to signal contrasts in meaning usually by some form of 'model and replica' table or distributional chart and additionally in the case of PACS by a developmental profile. The terms static and dynamic have been applied to these two approaches, implying a phonemic as opposed to a process view. Analysis of clusters and syllable and word structures (phonotactic possibilities) is also included in the Newcastle assessment and PACS. The therapist may therefore make a choice in the procedure by which the data is handled, although the explanatory power of individual procedures varies. What is important is that phonological principles are applied as these offer considerable benefit in describing the speech sound distribution and contrastive patterns.

All of the assessments referred to so far make use of perceptual observation by the therapist and this will continue to be the prime clinical mode of assessment. The use of non-linguistic, acoustic and physiological measurements (e.g., measurement of Voice Onset Time and the use of Visispeech to construct a prosody profile) have primarily had research applications, but their clinical use will probably increase with increased availability of equipment (Edwards, 1983).

An examination of the oro-facial complex should accompany the phonological analysis including the child's ability to imitate speech sounds. Canning and Rose (1974), and Kent, Kent and Rosenbek (1987) provide baseline measurements on speed of movement. This is usually extended to a level of stimulability testing (i.e., the ability to produce sounds after appropriate cueing including articulatory instruction). The results of this testing can be used as treatment indicators (see Fleming, 1971 on guidelines relating to phonetic contexts for remediation and Leonard, Devescovi and Oscella, 1987 for a recent clinical paper). Other aspects of skilled behaviour relating to segmental features such as recognition of sounds, rhyming ability and segmentation may well be investigated and developed as part of the assessment and therapy processes.

Reference has already been made to the need to assess other levels of language and at this point it is valuable to consider the effect of the clinician-child interaction on the data collected. This means considering the relationship of the clinician's or parent's input — noting modelled utterances for instance and the effect of requests for clarification. This could well have implications for the way in which treatment is planned. Parents may make little use of choice strategies for example tending to rely heavily on repetition of the correct word.

The processes above are predominantly concerned with segmental features. As yet little is available in the way of assessing suprasegmental features, but information on the normal development of these features is expanding (see Schwartz in Costello, 1984 for a review). The Prosody Profile (PROP — Crystal, 1982), is one formal procedure available for considering the main prosodic patterns in clinical data.

Most assessment procedures are almost exclusively concerned with the consonantal system. It is common to find that patterns of vowel use are usually normal even for children who have severe problems with consonants. For children who are hearing impaired this is often not the case and the Royal National Institute for the Deaf assessment allows for analysis of the vowel system (Fisher, King, Parker and Wright, 1983). Reynolds (1986) in a survey of children with phonological disorders has found a number of frequently occurring processes in the vowel usage. These are: lowering, particularly affecting mid-vowels, diphthong reduction and fronting, affecting low back vowels most commonly.

Full assessment of the type described not only provides information on the level of phonetic and phonological development it may indicate the need for referral to other agencies (e.g., to the Ear Nose and Throat consultant) as well as providing the analysis from which treatment decisions can be derived. It also enables systematic measurement of progress as re-assessment will show what changes in the phonological system and structure have occurred over a period of time. This re-assessment contributes to the measurement of effectiveness. Research currently being undertaken in Edinburgh is considering the nature of this evaluation following therapy.

Evaluation

When the analysis and the other assessments have been completed, then an evaluation of the child's linguistic status can be made. This is going to consider the implications for management based on the findings. If intelligibility is seriously impaired the reasons should emerge from the analysis — there may be too few phones or the available phones may be used inadequately. Are the available contrasts used in all relevant positions of structure — is the phonetic potential exploited? For example a voicing contrast may exist, but it is not used in all places of articulation. What effect does the phonetic context have on utterance variability? Is the system and structure static? Variability in producing particular items or overlapping of phonemes may indicate that development is in progress. It has already been indicated that one of the functions of phonological analysis is to distinguish different types of disorder. The distinction between phonetic and phonological disorders is one such outcome and further distinctions can be made within the phonological group of disorders. Grunwell (1988), for instance, identifies a general clsssification of developmental disorders:

> delayed development: persisting normal processes
> uneven development: chronological mismatch — where some normal processes persist
> variable use of processes: where variability between processes from two or more stages of development occurs
> deviant development: idiosyncratic processes — systematic sound preference
> variability between normal and unusual or idiosyncratic processes from similar developmental stages occurs.

There may well be further distinctions within these groups which have clinical significance and certainly two children whose disorders are classified with the same overall label, but present with very different patterns of development. Stoel-Gammon and Dunn (1985) present the analysis of two such children. For example, final consonant deletion as a persisting process has been described as being related to a particular type of development and may sometimes be associated with hearing impairment. Children who show continued use of assimilatory processes may be particularly resistant to therapy. As more clinical data is evaluated and follow-up studies through therapy provided then such differences may be better understood.

A broad-based evaluation considering the audiological, motoric, linguistic, cognitive and psychosocial factors is constructed which then provides the basis for the individual treatment plan.

The relationship between the levels of breakdown will be summarised in the evaluation (e.g., whether there are discrepancies between the grammatical and phonological output levels). Effects of factors such as hearing status, neuromotor skills, social, cognitive and emotional maturity and other case-history information will be balanced in terms of their contribution to the problem wherever possible. Directions for the rehabilitative therapy can then be defined.

Mainstream Treatment Strategies

Principles

Therapy for phonological disorders is guided by a number of general principles and needs to take into account all the factors which may have contributed to the disorder as exemplified in the evaluation. In clinical practice it is not always possible to make clear cut distinctions between disorders and aspects of several skills and behaviours may require developing (see Stackhouse, 1984).

Therapy needs to be individualised; there is evidence perhaps more so in phonology than at other linguistic levels of idiosyncratic development (Ingram, 1976; Crystal, 1982). Early lexical development has an important influence for instance on the developing phonology.

Detailed knowledge of normal phonological acquisition is vital to the process of accurately evaluating the data (Crystal, 1987; Menyuk *et al.*, 1986). Knowledge relating to development of the sound system and structure and phonological processes will be incorporated in the treatment plan.

The constructivist theories of language development stress that the child is an active participant in the language learning process and that language emerges in contexts where there is communicative significance. This has a number of implications for the principled management of disorders. First, it is apparent that a familiar context is more likely to generate an atmosphere conducive to communication. This context is very unlikely to be a community health clinic and home-based and school-based therapy are being encouraged wherever possible. This may have further implications about who is involved in the management process.

A second impetus to strengthen the involvement of speech and language clinicians in the education process has come from the demand for support for children with language impairments in main-stream schools which has increased greatly in Britain since the implementation of the 1981 Education Act.

A further demand for increasing involvement of clinicians and linguists in the education process in the United Kingdom comes from the widening awareness of the need to develop language in the curriculum. This is highlighted in the recommendations of the Kingman report which specify the need for all school teachers to undertake a language course and to have a knowledge of the linguistic model provided in the report (Kingman, 1988). In-service education of a collaborative nature between clinicians and teacher has been developing and will need to increase if the recommendations are to be met.

Factors in speaker–listener interactions which are already firmly incorporated into speech and language therapy at other linguistic levels such as requests for clarification and expressed misunderstandings have great potential in phonology work in the development of monitoring skills. Judging the accuracy of responses is part and parcel of the child's learning to make changes. Deliberately creating situations for helping misarticulations (e.g., 'did you say cat, tat or sat') has been shown to produce more phonetic change in responses than offering a straight forced alternative (cat/tat) (Weiner and Ostrowski, 1979).

Another aspect of considering requests for clarification is in relation to parents' interactions with phonologically disordered children. There is evidence from a number of sources that parents' input to children with language impairment is significantly different at this level because the lack of intelligibility interferes with communication and parents tend to direct their clarification to particular words. Clinician/child interactions may be used to model different 'strengths' of clarification request (see Table 7.2 and McTear 1985).

Table 7.2: Hierarchical Categories of Clarification Requests

Clarification Request Categories	
Non-specific request for repetition	Weakest
Specific request for repetition	
Specific request for specification	
Potential request for elaboration	
Specific request for confirmation	
You mean + specific request for confirmation	Strongest

Another general principle concerns giving credence to different learning styles. Some children may appreciate and learn from explanations of principle, others may learn from examples and practice. Cognitive ability and age are two factors which affect learning style. Theoretically we want to move in the direction of therapy which teaches strategies enabling a child to extract rules and processes rather than just giving lots of examples of rules to practice (i.e., being knowledge based rather than practice based); though the skill elements must not be ignored.

Therapy is therefore seen as conceptual as the units on which treatment are focused are abstract — contrasting features or processes. The principles outlined above seek to guide towards a way of developing, reorganising and restructuring of knowledge of the phonological system. Phonological remediation should therefore proceed on the basis of the principles described. It is based on the systematic nature of phonology and in the procedures adopted we need to help the child to realise the underlying organisation of sound segments in the language — their contrastive use and the permissible structural possibilities.

This approach represents a major shift in emphasis from the traditional techniques adopted for 'articulation' disorders in the period before the 1970s. Therapy then concentrated its efforts on the articulatory aspects, that is on motor practice (e.g., phonetic placement techniques and systematic babble practice). The predominant technique involved the use of drills where the child practised certain target sounds, at first in isolation, then in babble syllables, followed by word and phrase practice (Van Riper and Irwin, 1958).

In the late 1960s following the development of language acquisition theories, phonological concepts began to be introduced in speech pathology literature and into the education of speech and language clinicians in the United Kingdom. (Grady, 1966; Beresford and Grady, 1968). This led to the introduction of these concepts into treatment programmes. Initially a strong dichotomy between phonetic and phonological disorders was stressed. A failure in perceptual development was seen as a specific causal factor and this was sometimes accorded the status of a specific disability rather than being envisaged as part of an overall cognitive/linguistic learning difficulty. Discrimination training based on minimal pair lexical items was very thoroughly practised with little attention initially paid to articulatory skills. The underlying assumption was that an awareness of the articulatory feature contrasts would enable the child to use such contrasts without necessarily having to be drilled in their production. Other aspects of learning were introduced; using the written system alongside the auditory and also training in recognition and segmentation skills in terms of word construction for example. Many children with delayed phonological development respond very well to this type of management, for others it was apparent that phonetic techniques needed to be incorporated into the procedures. Unfortunately very few published accounts of such treatment programmes have been available. More recently some aspects of such programmes have been described (Blache, 1982; Weiner, 1981; Neville, 1984; Jarvis, 1988).

Whilst perceptual training of minimal pairs and distinctive features was most prevalent in the 1970s and still attracts interest there has been a developing trend towards a phonological process approach. The descriptive value of processes is now widely used to select goals for treatment. The procedures involve selecting which process is to be eliminated and the prioritisation of the order of the processes which are targetted. The actual procedures may be similar to those used in the feature approach, for example eliminating the stopping process might well involve minimally paired lexical items with /t/ and /s/ being contrasted as would targeting the stop/ fricative sound class distinction. More attention is paid to the overall communicative context in the choice of treatment goals and usually more than one sound would be used to illustrate the process concerned. Stoel-Gammon and Dunn (*op cit.*) summarise the factors influencing choice of process as follows:

1   Those that contribute greatly to poor intelligibility,
2   establish sounds in a variety of sound classes and word structures,
3   are eliminated early in the course of normal acquisition,
4   typically persist in children with disordered phonology, and
5   occur more than 40 per cent of the time in the child's speech.

The underlying knowledge reorganisation is covertly recognised in aspects of such programmes, but has become much more obviously developed in the work of those seeking a metalinguistic approach (Howell and Dean, 1986). The emphasis in this approach is to give opportunities to reflect on knowledge of (a) the language and (b) individual functioning. The person is encouraged to think about characteristics of sounds which increase their underlying knowledge for example back as opposed to front, long as opposed to short. As the contrastive process starts at the non-speech sound level this 'language of language' work lends itself well to being undertaken in nursery or primary teaching contexts just as children are introduced to the language of maths.

The second phase of therapy consists of making use of this heightened awareness to make repair strategies. A number of procedures may be useful to therapists in developing these skills.

Procedures involved include listening tasks — sorting and categorising of sounds, discriminating between same/different minimal pairs, discriminating syllable final positions, and listening for shared sounds in paired words. Wherever possible these tasks should be linked to explicit teaching of alphabet knowledge. A strong relationship exists between the ability to read and spell and sound categorisation knowledge. It is useful to develop syllable and phoneme segmentation skills. The aim is to achieve recognition of phonemes within syllables and words and to show knowledge of position within the segment. The child may be asked to pick out a stimulus sound within a list of utterances and then asked whether the target sound comes at the beginning or end (Lambert, 1981). As in other levels of language development where the onus is put on the child for active involvement so in phonology training the use of role reversal is to be encouraged.

The use of homonyms has received much attention. This involves taking words which have the same realisation by the child (e.g., bow and boat), both being produced as [bo]. Tasks can be devised involving both perception and production elements. If the child is asked to produce both words together, e.g., looking at pictures, then the intention is to force a recognition that some difference needs to be made to avoid listener confusion. A word completion task can be used with older children — which sound/letter do we need to make |bo| say boat/bone etc?

Another area which can be targeted for development is that of rhyming skill. This is often deficient in both children and adults with phonological and reading difficulties (Stackhouse, 1985; Howell and Dean, 1986). Again paired words may be used but with younger children more general development work can be undertaken. There are many underpinning language tasks which should be encouraged in a pre-school or nursery environment. Work with words and non-words has been used more with adults than with children, but it may be applicable when considering structural possibilities for example.

Other strategies have been developed such as Hodson and Paden's (1983) auditory bombardment techniques where two minutes of auditory stimulation with words containing the target sound are provided at the beginning and end of each session. They also promote the idea of cycles of training where particular targets are targeted for approximately 60 minutes each during the first cycle (probably lasting twelve weeks) and then may be re-presented in different ways in ensuing cycles (Hodson and Paden, 1983).

The emphasis in these procedures outlined is very much on *facilitating emergence of speech patterns* and not on perfecting production of individual phonemes or words. The current state of the art is that in all procedures the aim will be to develop knowledge so that the phonology can be restructured by understanding the change which needs to be made in order to signal differences in meaning.

References

ANTHONY, A., BOGLE, D., INGRAM, T.T.S. and MCISAAC, M.W. (1971) *Edinburgh Articulation Test.* Edinburgh: Edinburgh University Press.

BERESFORD, R. and GRADY, P. (1968) Some aspects of assessment. *British Journal of Disorders of Communication,* 3; 1; 28–36.

BERESFORD, R. (1981) *The Newcastle Speech Assessment.* Newcastle: The University of Newcastle upon Tyne.

BLACHE, S.E. (1982) Minimal Word Pairs and Distinctive Feature Training. In M. Crary (Ed.), *Phonological Intervention, Concepts and Procedures.* San Diego: College-Hill Press.

CANNING, B.A. and ROSE, M.F. (1974) Clinical measurements of the speed of tongue and lip movement in British children with normal speech. *British Journal of Disorders of Communication,* 9, 45–50.

COLTHEART, M. (1987) The Cognitive Neuropsychology of Language In: M. Coltheart, R. Job and G. Sartori (Eds), *The Cognitive Neuropsychology of Language.* London: Lawrence Erlbaum.

COMPTON, A.J. (1976) Generative studies of children's phonological disorders: Clinical ramifications. In D.M. Morehead and A.E. Morehead (Eds), *Normal and Deficient Child Language*. Baltimore: University Park Press.

COMPTON, A.J. and HUTTON, J.S. (1978) *Compton-Hutton Phonological Assessment*. San Francisco: Carousel House.

COSTELLO, J. (Ed.) (1984) *Speech Disorders in Children*. Windsor: NFER-Nelson.

CRYSTAL, D. (1982) *Profiling Linguistic Disability*. London: Arnold.

CRYSTAL, D. (1987) *Clinical Linguistics*. London: Arnold.

EDWARDS, M. (1983) *Disorders of Articulation*. London: Springer-Verlag.

ELBERT, M. and GIERUT, J. (1986) *Handbook of Clinical Phonology*. London: Taylor and Francis.

FEE, J. and INGRAM, D. (1982) Reduplication as a strategy of phonological development, *Journal of Child Language*, 9, 41–54.

FISHER, H.B. and LOGEMANN, J.A. (1971) *The Fisher-Logemann Test of Articulation Competence*. Boston: Houghton Mifflin.

FISHER, J., KING, A., PARKER, A. and WRIGHT, R. (1983) The assessment of speech production and speech perception as a basis for therapy. In I. Hockberg, H. Levitt, and M.J. Osberger, *Speech of the Hearing Impaired*. Proceedings of the 1979 CUNY Conference on Speech of the Hearing Impaired, University Park Press, Baltimore.

FLEMING, K.J. (1971) Guidelines for choosing appropriate phonetic contexts for speech sound recognition and production practice. *Journal of Speech and Hearing Disorders*. 36, 356–67.

FLETCHER, P. and GARMAN, M. (Eds) (1986) *Language Acquisition* (2nd edition). Cambridge: Cambridge University Press.

GOLDMAN, R. and FRISTOE, M. (1972) *Goldman Fristoe Test of Articulation*. Minn AGSS Inc.

GRADY, P.A.E. (1966) Towards a new concept of dyslalia. In S. Mason (Ed.), *Signs, Signals and Symbols*. London: Methuen.

GRUNWELL, P. (1983) *Phonological Therapy: Premises, Principles and Procedures*. Proceedings XIX IALP Congress, Edinburgh.

GRUNWELL, P. (1985) *Phonological Assessment of Child Speech (PACS)*. Windsor: NFER-Nelson.

GRUNWELL, P. (1987) *Evaluation and Explanation of Developmental Phonological Disorders*. Paper presented at First International Symposium on Specific Speech and Language Disorders in Children, Reading, England.

GRUNWELL, P. (1988) *Clinical Phonology*. 2nd edition, London: Croom Helm.

HARRIS, J. and COTTAM, P. (1985) Phonetic features and phonological features in speech assessment. *British Journal of Disorders of Communication*, 20, 61–74.

HEWLETT, N. (1985) Phonological versus phonetic disorders: Some suggested modifications to the current use of the distinction. *British Journal of Disorders of Communication*, 20, 155–164.

HEWLETT, N. (1987) *Beyond Phonetics*. Paper presented in Leeds.

HODSON, B.W. and PADEN, E.P. (1983) *Targetting Intelligible Speech*. San Diego: College Hill Press.

HOWELL, J. and DEAN, E. (1986) Phonological disorders revisited. *Bulletin of the College of Speech Therapists*, 377, 11–3.

INGRAM, D. (1976) *Phonological Disability in Children*. London: Edward Arnold.

INGRAM, D. (1982) The assessment of phonological disorders in children: the state of the art. In M. Crary (Ed.), *Phonological Intervention, Concepts and Procedures*. San Diego, CA: College Hill Press.

INGRAM, D. (1986) Explanation and phonological remediation. *Child Language Teaching and Therapy*, 2, 1–16.

JAKOBSON, R. (1968) *Child Language, Aphasia and Phonological Universals*, trans. Keiler. The Hague: Mouton.

JARVIS, J. (1988) Helping the development of consonant contrasts: A case study. *Child Language Teaching and Therapy*, 4,. 46–56.

KENT, R.D., KENT, J.F. and ROSENBEK, J.C. (1987) Maximum performance tests of speech production. *Journal of Speech and Hearing Disorders*, 52, 367–87.

KINGMAN, J. (1988) *Report of the Committee of Inquiry into the Teaching of English Language*. HMSO, London.

KLEIN, H. (1985) The assessment of some persisting language difficulties in the learning disabled. In M.J. Snowling (Ed.) *Children's Written Language Difficulties*. Windsor: NFER-Nelson.

LAMBERT, J.S. (1981) *Differential Diagnosis*. In Proceedings of the seminar on language disability, University of Dublin, Ireland.

LEONARD, L.D. (1985) Unusual and subtle phonological behaviour in the speech of phonologically disordered children. *Journal of Speech Hearing Disorders*, 50, 4–13.

LEONARD, L.B., DEVESCOVI, A. and OSSELLA, T. (1987) Context-sensitive phonological patterns in children with poor intelligibility. *Child Language Teaching and Therapy*, 3, 125–32.

LOCKE, J.L. (1983) Clinical Phonology: The explanation and treatment of speech sound disorders. *Journal of Speech and Hearing Disorders*, 48, 339–441.

MACKEN, M.A. and FERGUSON, C.A. (1983) Cognitive aspects of phonological development: Model, evidence and issues In K.E. Nelson (Ed.), *Children's Language, vol 4*. Hillsdale: Erlbaum.

McREYNOLDS, L.V. and ENGMANN, D. (1975) *Distinctive Feature Analysis of Misarticulations*. Baltimore: University Park Press.

McREYNOLDS, L.V. and HUSTON, K. (1971) A distinctive feature analysis of children's misarticulations. *Journal of Speech and Hearing Disorders*, 36, 155–66.

McTEAR, M. (1985) *Children's Conversation*, Oxford: Blackwell.

MENYUK, P., MENN, L. and SILBER, R. (1986) Early strategies for the perception and production of words and sounds. In P. Fletcher and M. Garman (Eds), *Language Acquisition* (2nd edition). Cambridge: Cambridge University Press.

NEVILLE, A. (1984) Phonological therapy — from ear to mouth. *Bulletin of the College of Speech Therapists*, 390, 10–1.

REES, N. (1973) Auditory processing factors: The view from Procrustes bed. *Journal of Speech and Hearing Disorders*, 38 (3) 304–15.

REYNOLDS, J. (1986) *Phonological Disorders — Bringing the Vowels In*. Paper presented at the BAAL Seminar, Leicester, England.

SCHWARTZ, R.G. (1984) The Phonologic system: normal acquisition. In J. Costello (Ed.) *Speech Disorders in Children*. Windsor: NFER-Nelson.

STACKHOUSE, J. (1984) Phonological therapy: A case and some thoughts. *Bulletin of the College of Speech Therapists*, 381, 10–1.

STACKHOUSE, J. (1985) Segmentation, speech and spelling difficulties. In M.J. Snowling (Ed.), *Children's Written Language Difficulties*. Windsor: NFER-Nelson.

STAMPE, D. (1969) The acquisition of phonetic representation. Paper from the Fifth Regional Meeting, Chicago Linguistic Society.

STAMPE, D. (1979) *A Dissertation on Natural Phonology.* New York: Garland.

STOEL-GAMMON, C. and DUNN, C. (1985) *Normal and Disordered Phonology in Children,* Baltimore: University Park Press.

VAN KLEECK, A. (1984) Metalinguistic skills: cutting across spoken and written language and problem solving abilities. In G.P. Wallach and K.G. Butler (Eds), *Language Learning Disabilities in School Age Children.* Baltimore: Williams and Wilkins.

VAN RIPER, C. and IRWIN, J. (1958) *Voice and Articulation.* Englewood Cliffs, NJ: Prentice-Hall.

VELLUTINO, F.R. (1979) *Dyslexia: Theory and Research.* Cambridge, MA: MIT Press.

WEINER, F. (1981) Treatment of phonological disability using the method of minimal contrasts: two case studies. *Journal of Speech and Hearing Disorders,* 46, 97–103.

WEINER, F. (1984) A phonologic approach to assessment and treatment. In J. Costello (Ed.), *Speech Disorders in Children.* Windsor: NFER-Nelson.

WEINER, F. and OSTROWSKI, A. (1979) Effects of listener uncertainty on articulatory inconsistency. *Journal of Speech and Hearing Disorders,* 44, 487–503.

YENI-KOMSHIAN, G.H., KAVANAGH, J.F. and FERGUSON, C.A. (Eds) (1980) *Child Phonology, Vol 1 Production.* London: Academic Press.

8   Childhood Articulatory Disorders of Neurogenic Origin

Mata Jaffe

This chapter introduces speech disorders in childhood which result from neurologic damage. These neurogenic articulatory disorders, or neuropathologies, are the motor speech disorders of apraxia of speech (or verbal apraxia) and dysarthria, sometimes termed 'the dysarthrias' to signify a group of speech disorders rather than a single disorder.

Developmental Apraxia of Speech

There are approximately twenty terms for apraxia of speech. In children, developmental apraxia of speech (DAS) and developmental verbal dyspraxia (DVD) are used most often, although some clinicians use 'dyspraxia' when referring to a less severe form of apraxia. Apraxia is derived from the Greek, meaning 'lack of action'. Developmental apraxia of speech is defined as an articulation or phonological disorder characterised by impaired capacity to programme, or motor plan, the positions, combinations and sequences of volitional speech production. Crary (1984) adds that it is a disorder of spatial/temporal properties of speech articulation. Aram and Nation (1982) find that it is as much language based as articulatory based, and some clinicians feel that it is always accompanied by a language disorder.

While apraxia of speech is an accepted neuropathology of communication in the adult population, a current controversy surrounds DAS. Guyette and Diedrich (1981) surveyed over 100 publications on adult and childhood apraxia, and concluded that there was no evidence supporting the existence of DAS. They cited contradictory findings about characteristics of the disorder, lack of empirical evidence for reported speech and non-speech symptoms, a circularity of subject selection (i.e., selection of subjects based on behavioural characteristics that the study itself was designed to discover) and an absence of treatment studies to demonstrate specific effective treatment strategies. Deputy (1984) also outlined problems in the DAS literature: similarity of results of studies on both developmentally apraxic and phonologically disordered children known as 'syllable reducers'; inconsistency among experts regarding the defining characteristics of the disorder; research problems of subject selection, description and criteria regarding severity, concomitant problems, etc. and a problem with the scientific process itself.

Causative Factors

Brain damage is the accepted cause of verbal apraxia in adults, and the classification of DAS as a neurogenic disorder presumes brain damage. There is debate regarding cerebral dysfunction as a cause of DAS, although some researchers and clinicians make neurologic 'soft' signs (associated CNS dysfunction) a criterion for a DAS diagnosis. Guyette and Diedrich (1981) concluded that neurologic 'soft' signs to demonstrate reliability of paediatric examinations and EEG findings is poor, and that the validity of brain damage is suspect. They further argued that not all children diagnosed as DAS show neurologic 'soft' signs and that some children who have 'soft' signs are not diagnosed as DAS, precluding the presence of the signs as a distinguishing characteristic. Thus, the literature is confusing and inconclusive regarding neurologic correlates and causative factors for DAS.

Assessment Considerations

Assessing DAS is also complicated by confusion about its distinguishing characteristics. DAS is defined by a variable listing of symptoms, which are not exclusive to DAS and not one of which must be present. The disorder may coexist with a language disorder, as apraxia of speech often coexists with aphasia in adults, or may be the phonological component of an expressive language disorder. Aram and Nation (1982) view the breakdown in programming as underlying both speech and language. Ekelman and Aram (1983) demonstrated syntactic deficits in apraxic children, and Crary (1984) suggested that the child's syntactic deficits are due largely to limitations imposed by the phonological system.

In a young child, or child whose speech is significantly compromised, assessment may attempt to differentiate between a primary developmental language disorder and DAS. Some essentially non-verbal children with DAS have been diagnosed incorrectly as emotionally disturbed, so severely disrupted are their communicative interactions. In older children and in children with more intelligible speech, the distinction typically is made between a functional articulation disorder and DAS. Dysarthria and DAS may coexist, and a motor programming problem may be found in children with an anatomical problem such as cleft palate.

The clinical entity of DAS originated with Morley, Court, Miller and Garside (1955) who differentiated the syndrome by lack of intelligibility, slow response to therapy, awkward and misdirected articulatory movements, and frequent familial history of speech and language delay or disorder.

Jaffe (1986) cited thirty-three reported characteristics of DAS from twenty references within categories of developmental history and family history, non-speech and speech findings, language and prognosis. Ten characteristics listed by Aram and Nation (1982) are: difficulty in selection and sequence of phonological and articulatory movements; differences between voluntary and involuntary use of speech articulators; normal language comprehension but language formulation disorders in lexicon and syntax (i.e., significant gap between receptive and expressive language); occasional disorders in reading, spelling and writing; slow improvement with traditional articulation therapy; neurologic signs of fine and gross motor incoordination, and non-focal neurologic findings; often the presence of oral non-verbal apraxia; mixed hand laterality; predominance of males in the population; and family history of speech and language problems. Rosenbek and Wertz (1972) listed sixteen speech and language characteristics of DAS, with these additional symptoms: highly inconsistent errors; prosodic disturbances; groping trial and error speech behaviours; increasing errors with lengthier words and complexity of sound articulation; vowel as well as consonant errors; and frequent metathetic (sound reversal) errors. Other characteristics are delayed and deviant speech development, poor imitative skills, slow rate and incorrectly sequenced diadochokinesis, omission errors in all positions of words, voiced versus voiceless sound confusions, and poor oral stereognosis. As babies, there is often a history of feeding difficulties (and a later aversion to chewing), minimal and noninformative sound play, and late development of continence and motor skills. Clinicians often use the above characteristics to diagnose DAS, and sometimes make the diagnosis when no other label seems to explain the child's speech behaviour.

In recommending a diagnostic battery to assess DAS, Haynes (1985) listed the following areas: language ability; articulation, with comparison and analysis of simple and complex isolated phonemes, multi-syllabic words, and connected speech samples; oral diadochokinesis; isolated and sequenced volitional oral movements; and oral awareness and orosensory perception. A published screening tool is the Screening Test for Developmental Apraxia of Speech (Blakeley, 1980). Subtests include expressive language discrepancy, vowels and diphthongs, oral-motor movement, verbal sequencing, articulation, motorically complex words, transpositions (sound reversals) and prosody. Guyette and Diedrich (1983) pointed out several problems with the test construction, administration, scoring, standardi-sation, and validity. They also concluded that a test to diagnose DAS was premature and unjustified because of disagreement on the disorder's symptomatology.

An unpublished diagnostic evaluation of speech motor production and planning in children is Assessing Speech Motor Behaviour (Logue, 1976). The first section differentiates non-volitional from volitional oral movements. The second focuses on dominance and laterality. Section three screens the cranial nerves with speech and non-speech procedures, including diadochokinetic testing for cranial nerves V and VII. Tasks are designed for obtaining a child's cooperation through the use of meaningful material. For example, the child is directed to call to a stuffed animal: 'kitty, kitty, kitty'. The fourth section assesses competitive articulatory posturing and speech motor integration. For example, one task assesses the child's ability to talk with his teeth closed and another assesses the ability to make a postural set for a front to back articulatory sequence and vice versa. The last section uses words and phrases to detect retrial and groping errors.

The more recent phonological process analysis tests and approach may prove more useful than traditional articulation tests for assessing the speech characteristics of children suspected of DAS, especially children with poor intelligibility. However, a process analysis probably will not provide a differential diagnosis, as at least one study (Parsons, 1984) suggests that apraxic children are similar to other phonologically impaired populations.

At the close of this section, the reader should see the importance of assessing all aspects of a child's communication, not only motor speech programming and phonologic system. The clinician should obtain a detailed family history and history of the child's birth, developmental and cognitive development, language development, psychosocial functioning, and education. It is probably not useful to focus on one or two clinical speech symptoms, such as groping or prosodic disturbances. According to current thinking, it is better to consider that DAS is either imbedded in a many faceted expressive communication disorder or may be its most prominent feature in some cases. Thus, the child's receptive and expressive language system, especially length of utterance and syntactic and morphologic development, are assessed with appropriate test protocols and on-going informal observations.

Theoretical Bases of Intervention

Because of the confusion and controversy that surrounds DAS, a discussion of theoretical bases for intervention is limited to one point and implication. This author concludes that DAS rarely, if ever, exists as a single entity. While developmentally apraxic children present with a severe disorder of phonological development, DAS should probably be viewed as an asynergic disorder of communication, as suggested by Crary and Towne (1984). It is highly unlikely that any aspect or level of speech and language performance can function without some detriment to other aspects or levels, especially in the developing child. While the treatment section primarily presents ways to improve the child's motor speech programming, all parameters of the child's communication deficit must be addressed in therapy.

Mainstream Treatment Practices

Many clinicians base their diagnosis of DAS on the lengthy and arduous course of treatment as well as on speech characteristics described earlier. Therapy approaches are varied, and probably every conceivable treatment approach has been tried. As with all therapy, the age of the child, severity level, concomitant problems, and family involvement are considered. A programme for young and severely involved children emphasises language, attending, gross and fine motor imitation, and establishing voluntary control of any involuntary sounds (e.g., animal sounds, inflectional patterns, communicative utterances like 'uh oh'). The clinician encourages all expressive means, including prosody and gestures. Simple manual sign language can provide the child with a way of communicating, and the use of signs invariably decreases as verbal expression grows. The clinician may associate a favourite activity such as finger painting with 'babbling' to build and reinforce connected and sequenced vocal expression. As early as possible the clinician establishes a core vocabulary of useful words.

Some clinicians apply the Association Method (McGinnis, 1963), which begins with a phonetic or elemental approach, emphasising a precise articulatory position for each sound. There is a systematic sensory-motor association of the articulatory and sound position with the appropriate letter symbol of cursive script. A moto-kinesthetic approach is often used to teach sound placement. When determining a sequence to teach phonemes to the child, many clinicians present maximal contrast phonemes such as a bilabial stop followed by a continuant phoneme. Most clinicians express the importance of intensive and systematic drill. Some emphasise movement sequences and syllable shapes rather than sounds in isolation, and facilitate responses with systematic use of rhythm, intonation, stress and motor movements. When the clinician confronts the apraxic child's characteristic blending and sequencing problems, Chappell (1973) suggests a backward chaining procedure so that the child always emits the new phoneme first. For example, for the child who reverts to /fi/ when final /t/ is added to form the word 'feet' the clinician establishes /t/, then /it/, and finally adds /f/.

Yoss and Darley (1974) summarised these suggestions from public school clinicians: mirror work and imitation of tongue and lip movements; imitation of sustained vowels; imitation of visible consonants, then paired into CV or VC combinations; emphasis on visual or visual plus auditory input; imitation of CVC shapes, use of rhyming words combined with body movement to accent stress patterns; carrier phrases to help sequence words, and stress and intonation patterns to help the child maintain integrity of the syllables; teach self-monitoring, which may require the child to slow his rate of speech; and observe the child's behaviour for clues of effective treatment.

Total Communication

Total Communication (TC), which combines speech with all modes of communication but particularly manual communication, is considered by some (Rosenbek, Hansen, Baughman and Lemme, 1974; Jaffe, 1986) as one of the best approaches to treat moderately to severely apraxic children. In the early stages of therapy, manual communication may be the child's primary communication system: later, manual signs and alphabet augment his speech. To be most effective, a TC programme should emphasise meaning, spontaneous communication, and consequences of communicative acts and not imitation, repetition and drill. Unfortunately, verbally apraxic children often show some degree of limb apraxia, and may encounter difficulty executing sign language and finger spelling.

Jaffe (1986) discussed use of the American Manual Alphabet to establish a meaningful visuomotor and kinesthetic movement pattern to cue production of targeted phonemes and to facilitate blending and sequencing of phonemes. In a more detailed description of such a visual phoneme technique using the manual alphabet, Shelton and Garves (1985) felt that it produced earlier acquisition of a target phoneme in a pre-school apraxic child than did a more traditional auditory/visual approach.

Melodic Intonation Therapy

Another approach is Melodic Intonation Therapy (MIT), which focuses on formulation of speech through intoned sequences. MIT may be effective with apraxic children because the emphasis on movement may improve phonemic and linguistic sequencing through intersystemic organisation; prosodic alterations may improve speech production; and the reduced rate of presentation and the child's utterances may help him to plan, place and sequence the articulators and to include sounds and syllables. A commercial programme (Smith and Engel, 1984) has been developed for apraxic children and adults (language age five to fifteen) using MIT on audio cassettes. The child listens to the tape, intones the stimulus sentence of three to ten syllables, and taps along to the rhythm of the sentence. Next, the child speaks with the tape and taps along and then gradually fades the tapping. This programme also attempts to improve production of stop consonants.

Monitoring articulatory postures

Monitoring Articulatory Postures (MAP, Logue, 1978) is a speech motor training programme based on the assumption that the apraxic child needs to develop a reliable command over oral motor movements before concentrating on sound production. The programme consists of three phases. The goal of Phase I is for the child to establish, associate and maintain vowel and consonant postures. In Phase II, the clinician first presents a visual model only, but gradually fades the emphasis on the visual model and introduces the auditory model. Logue believes that considerable anticipatory and reprogramming capability is an important pre-requisite for articulate speech, and that Phase III is the programme's most critical phase. Here the child is required to assume the anticipatory posture of a vowel, consonant or word, but produce a competing vowel, consonant or word instead.

Rosenthal, Williams and Ingham (1978) conducted an experimental therapy programme with four apraxic children to establish correct articulation during slowed oral reading, gradually increase reading rates to a normal level, and then transfer this skill to monologue speech under different treatment conditions. Three of the procedure variables appeared to be effective for all four subjects: control of rate, instruction in phoneme production and highlighting of the phonemes in error.

Touch-cues

Bashir, Grahamjones and Bostwick (1984) described a 'touch-cue method' to teach speech sound sequencing, moving systematically through stages of learning consonant and vowel combinations. It is not an initial speech sound treatment approach, nor one meant to replace early language therapy. 'Touch-cues' are tactile indicators for consonants, placed on the lower face and neck. They have been developed for /b/, /d/, /g/, /ʃ/, /f/, /n/, /l/, (the recommended sequence to teach the phonemes). For example, for /b/, the index finger is placed on the lower lip; for /d/ the index finger is on the upper lip; for /n/ the index finger is on the side of the nose. The clinician or child may apply the cues.

In the early phases of therapy the touch-cues are presented simultaneously with auditory and visual cues. An additional cue for voicing may be added by placing one finger on the larynx and the other in the consonant position. The clinician can develop additional, but consistent cues for other phonemes. The programme consists of three stages, but within the same session a child may be producing complex sequences of one sound, which are higher steps and stages, while a new sound is introduced in stage I. In stage I, the goals are for the child to develop awareness of what is to be learned, to learn the topographical cues, and to produce a series of nonsense syllables. Using /b/ as an example, the first four steps in stage I are: (1) voluntary production of the phoneme in response to visual, auditory and touch-cues; (2) voluntary production of /b/ with touch-cue only; (3), /b∧b∧/ or /b∧b∧b∧/ in imitation of auditory and tactile cue; (4) /b∧b∧b∧b∧b∧/ in response to touch-cue alone.

Through steps and stages, the clinician conducts drills that incorporate previously learned sequential movements into monosyllabic CVC words and polysyllabic words, maintaining correct sequences.

PROMPT System

A similar approach to guide a child towards correct target positions and appropriate transitions is the PROMPT system (prompts for restructuring oral muscular phonetic targets, Chumpelik, 1984). This sytem uses a different PROMPT for each English phoneme. The cues are given externally to structures associated with voicing, nasality, and jaw opening. The timing of each PROMPT imposed by the clinician on the child is crucial to the system, and is especially important when moving from one sound to another.

Effectiveness of Therapy

'It all depends on the kid'. This comment accounts for such variables as the child's age, severity of the problem, and concomitant problems of developmental, emotional, sensory, motor, and sensory-integrative disabilities. Prognosis is related to these variables, as well as the intensity and quality of therapy and the family involvement. While it should be obvious that not one therapy approach can be effective for all DAS children, research regarding the effectiveness of therapy is needed.

For young, essentially non-verbal apraxic children, we have found that effective management begins with arranging a special pre-school setting for the child, family training and counselling, linking the family with a parent group or other strong support group, and arranging help for the child's other problems, such as a behaviour management programme and an occupational therapy programme. Speech-language therapy emphasises communicative interactions, elaboration of the child's existing gesture system and vocal inflection patterns, and establishment of a systematic augmentative communication system, such as manual sign language, to reduce immediate frustration of his inability to communicate.

As treatment progresses, the clinician helps the child firmly establish and integrate voluntary control over speech production through strong association of the auditory, visual and kinesthetic representation of sounds and sound patterns with whatever external cues benefit the child. One child's motor programming skills may improve by slowed auditory input and reduced rate of speech production, another by association of sound patterns with graphemes, another with prosody and movement patterns (e.g., MIT, or modification thereof), and yet another with minimal pairs contrast drills.

Our most successful therapy was with Danny, a child of above average intelligence whose speech repertoire at age 3.3 consisted of two vowel approximations. A TC Programme was initiated in a special education setting, with increasing emphasis on language development, verbal communication, phonemic placement with strong visual association cues, and reading. When Danny entered regular kindergarten at 5.2 years, his remaining speech errors were w/r, f/θ and transpositions (e.g., ephelant/elephant, whiksers/whiskers).

We have seen a variety of treatment outcomes. Some children, like Danny, acquire normal speech. Others remain severely impaired. Probably the majority continue in speech therapy throughout their school years, and even beyond, making slow gains in motor programming skills, but never attaining truly normal speech. Probably every clinician has a few children on her case load who do not respond well to traditional articulation therapy. The above suggestions and references may help these children who have difficulty associating and maintaining speech sound production combinations and sequences. While not addressed yet in the literature, some features from phonological process treatment approaches may be applied successfully with apraxic children.

Dysarthria

Dysarthria is a term used for a collection of motor speech disorders resulting from damage to the peripheral or central nervous system. While the label derives from the Greek meaning 'faulty articulation', more than articulation is affected. Respiration (breathing for speech), phonation (producing sound in the larynx), resonance (amplifying sound by modification of the size, shape and number of resonating cavities) and/or prosody (varying stress, intonation and rhythm), as well as chewing and swallowing, often are disrupted. Dysarthria is a problem of impaired muscular control, resulting in abnormal speed, range of movement, muscle tone, and coordination for speech movements. The dysarthric child usually imitates consistently within his neuromuscular limits.

Causative Factors

In contrast to DAS, brain damage unquestionably causes dysarthria in children.

Injuries to a child's CNS causing dysarthria are termed cerebral palsy (CP), a group of neurologic disorders whose etiology is damage to the motor control centres, which occurs prior to development of basic muscular system coordination. There is a high incidence (about 70–75 per cent) of dysarthria in the cerebral palsy population.

Cerebral palsy has been classified according to the presumed cause and time of cerebral insult, i.e., pre-natal hereditary and congenital, perinatal (obstetrical) and postnatal-early infancy, and a combination of factors. It is generally agreed that perinatal factors are most responsible for CP. The most common cause of CP is anoxia, or lack of oxygen in the blood supply to the brain. Hereditary causes are rare, and may be familial or progressive. More common congenital causes are those acquired in utero, which interfere with fetal and/or maternal circulation and respiration during the latter part of pregnancy and the delivery period. A common cause of foetal anoxia before onset of active labour is poor maternal blood supply. This may be caused by infections (e.g., rubella), anaemia, haemorrhage, disturbances to the placenta, toxins and drugs, and decreased foetal circulation from a twisted or kinked umbilical cord. When the birth process begins, birth complications (e.g., frank breech presentation, prolonged or precipitate labour, prematurity), inter-cranial pressure from respiratory distress, mechanical obstruction and trauma, may cause brain damage. The most common causes of anoxia during the neonatal and infancy periods are respiratory and circulatory problems, although cerebral trauma, infections, metabolic and toxic agents are often responsible.

Assessment Considerations

Assessing the speech production of school age and verbal dysarthric children does not present major difficulty, as clinicians can use standard articulation tests and assessment guidelines developed for adult dysarthric speakers. The presence of concomitant problems, such as intellectual impairment, behavioural and emotional disturbances, convulsive disorders, hearing, visual and perceptual disorders, language disorders and learning disabilities are important considerations during speech assessment and treatment of CP children of any age. These associated disorders result from brain damage imposed upon an immature nervous system.

Since the importance and efficacy of early identification and intervention with neurologically impaired children and their families is an accepted 'fact', clinicians assess younger and often more severely involved children than ever before. With these 'pre-speech' children, we assess overall postural tone and movement, head and trunk control, responses to sensory stimulation, responses to specific treatment techniques, and the interplay between mother and child. Clinicians assess the young child's feeding patterns, respiratory phonatory patterns and early sound play movements, the sensorimotor development of which presumably provides the foundation for the more complex act of speech.

At the initial evaluation of a baby or young child, the clinician's manner of asking questions, and sensitivity and respect for the child and for the mother's observations will establish the future relationship with that family. The mother and clinician should work together in the assessment, problem solving, and therapeutic management of the child.

The reader may find many descriptions of speech, pre-speech and feeding assessments and treatment of young children with sensorimotor impairment (Mueller, 1972; Schmidt, 1976; Davis, 1978; Gallender, 1979; Mysak, 1980; Campbell, 1982; Morris, 1982; Morris and Klein, 1987). Particularly useful is the Pre-Speech Assessment Scale (PSAS) (Morris, 1982), which measures pre-speech behaviours from birth through the two year developmental level. It is an excellent resource about normal and abnormal deviations of the precursors of speech. The PSAS provides a way of simultaneously observing and scoring behaviours within the normal developmental ranges of one to twenty-four months on an equal interval scale, and pathological or abnormal behaviours on an ordinal scale.

The PSAS assessment categories are: feeding behaviour, sucking, swallowing, biting and chewing, respiration-phonation, and sound-play. The PSAS assesses these feeding behaviours: length of time to eat a meal, amount and types of food eaten, and feeding position. Excessive feeding time, inadequate food intake, the need to thicken liquids, or abnormal body tone and movement, create stress between the child and feeder. The PSAS assesses the child's initiation, rhythm and separation of movements while sucking liquids from the straw, breast, cup and sucking pureed foods from a spoon. It evaluates control of drooling and primarily the oral stage of swallowing various consistencies of food and liquid.

The respiratory-phonatory system can be considered a single integrated system to produce a sound source for speech. The PSAS examines initiation, duration, loudness, pitch and intonation patterns, and voice quality during non-speech phonation (e.g., crying, squealing, laughing) and early speech phonation. Commonly present are rapid breathing rate, shallow inspiration, uncontrolled exhalation, antagonistic diaphragmatic and abdominal movements, involuntary movements of the respiratory musculature, difficulty initiating phonation, poor vocal control and quality, incoordination of respiration with phonation, and inability to generate intra-oral air pressure. Respiratory-phonatory control may break down when more demand is put on the system because of complexity of articulation and linguistic or communicative intent.

Movement patterns

Both gross motor and pre-speech behaviours of the neurologically impaired child can be divided into abnormal movement patterns, primitive movement patterns and higher developmental movement patterns. Abnormal or pathological movement patterns are due to CNS damage and are never seen in the normally developing infant. They are usually associated with abnormal posture tone and/or abnormal movement patterns in the affected parts of the body. Muscle tone may be hypertonic or hypotonic or may fluctuate with attempted movement. The abnormal movement patterns are generally stereotyped and consistent, interfering with the development of pre-speech and speech movements. Some of the abnormal and compensatory oral movements one may observe are: tongue thrust (an abnormally forceful protrusion of the tongue from the mouth), tongue retraction (a strong pulling back of the tongue to the pharyngeal space), jaw thrust (an abnormally forceful and tense downward extension of the mandible), lip retraction (drawing back of the lips so that they form a tight line over the mouth), lip pursing (a tight purse-string movement of the lips), and tonic bite reflect (an abnormally strong jaw closure when the teeth or gums are stimulated).

Primitive movement patterns occur usually during the first six months of infant development. Normally they diminish gradually and are replaced by more advanced movement patterns. Primitive movement patterns may be retained in the neurologically impaired or retarded child, interfering with the development of speech production. Some examples are: suckling (the early infantile method of sucking which involves extension-retraction of the tongue, up and down jaw excursions and loose approximation of the lips), sucking (characterised by negative pressure in the oral cavity, rhythmic up and down jaw movements, tongue tip elevation, firm approximation of the lips and minimal jaw excursions), rooting reaction (head turning in response to tactile stimulation applied to the lips or area around the mouth), and phasic bite reflex (a rhythmical bite and release pattern, seen as a series of small jaw openings and closing when the teeth or gums are stimulated).

Higher developmental movement patterns may fall anywhere on the continuum of normal development between six and twenty-four months. They are further refined in the first two or three years of life and then become refined for intelligible speech production. These movement patterns may include: munching (the earliest form of chewing which involves a flattening and spreading of the tongue combined with up and down jaw movement), chewing (characterised by spreading and rolling movements of the tongue propelling food between the teeth, tongue lateralisation and rotary jaw movements), tongue lateralisation (movement of the tongue to the sides of the mouth to propel food between the teeth for chewing), rotary jaw movements (involving the smooth interaction and integration of vertical, lateral, diagonal and eventually circular movements of the jaw used in chewing), and a controlled, sustained bite (an easy, gradual closure of the teeth on the food with an easy release of the food for chewing). The neurologically impaired child may acquire some of these higher developmental movement patterns but still be delayed compared to his chronological age.

Prior to the evaluation, the clinician usually sends the family a questionnaire concerned with feeding and sound-play behaviour. The PSAS lists questions and behaviours that the examiner should ask and observe during the evaluation. After the evaluation, which typically requires two or more sessions, the examiner transfers the recorded scores to a graph showing abnormal behaviours on one side and those in the normal developmental range on the other side. The clinician can compare the child's levels and problems within each area, compare the developmental abilities across categories, note progress or lack of progress from one evaluation to the next, and assign or revise treatment goals and priorities.

Augmentative communication systems

Most severely dysarthric children will not develop speech that meets all their communicative needs, and will require multiple communication systems. Assessment regarding augmentative communication systems begins early and is on-going. There is a large body of literature addressing evaluation, selection and use of non-speech communication systems, including communication boards, manual signing systems, and electronic communication aids (Silverman, 1980; Musselwhite and St. Louis, 1982; Capozzi and Mineo, 1986; Blackstone, 1987; Fishman, 1987).

Electronic communication systems now offer exciting options to the non-speaking or marginally speaking individual. Many different service delivery models (e.g., the itinerant specialty team and the specialty clinic model) have developed for assessing and matching people with augmentative communication systems. A multi-disciplinary team evaluates the child, matching his physical, cognitive, language and educational skills with an aid which will promote the highest possible level of personal achievement.

Theoretical Bases of Intervention

To determine the bases of intervention for dysarthria, we shall review the definition of this neurogenic speech disorder. It is characterised by impaired neuromuscular control, resulting in abnormal speed, tone, and coordination for speech movements. Aspects of respiration, phonation, resonance, articulation, prosody and eating may be affected. In children, the damage is to an immature brain. Typically this damage is present at birth and associated with cerebral palsy. The above suggest the following conclusions with regard to intervention:

1 No child with CP is like another, and therapy must be individualised and based on careful assessment and the child's responses to treatment

2 Early identification and intervention are vitally important

3 Usually there are concomitant problems which must be understood and addressed in intervention

4 Early involvement of the family is necessary to help the parents understand their child, his difficulties and the things he might be able to do if helped in the right way at any stage of his treatment and development

5 The child has a multiplicity of needs, requiring the combined efforts of many specialists, usually best accomplished in a team approach so that each member works toward the same goals rather than conflicting goals

6 Even with team support, the clinician must be knowledgeable in speech and language development, non-speech communication systems, anatomy and physiology, physical and occupational therapy, psychology, child development, education, and to some degree even computer science, engineering and design

7 Brain damage to the motor system requires physical handling to facilitate more normal movement patterns

8 The clinician must discover underlying causes for why a child cannot do something and treat the cause (e.g., the child might have difficulty producing bilabial phonemes for various reasons, such as hyper- or hypotonicity, hypersensitivity to environmental stimulation causing jaw thrusting, total extensor movement patterns, and poor head control and trunk instability preventing a stable basis for mandibular control).

Mainstream Treatment Practices

Transdisciplinary and interdisciplinary concepts of service delivery, emphasis on parent training, and strengthening the role of family members as the primary programmers for the child are all compatible with early identification and intervention. In the transdisciplinary approach, developed for early intervention by United Cerebral Palsy, each team member assumes an interchangeable role in the child's management, and is a single facilitator responsible for helping the child and parent in all activities. The transdisciplinary approach is difficult to achieve in clinical practice, and even more difficult on a training level because of the specialised and usually separated disciplines of physical, occupational, and speech-language therapy in most colleges and universities. In an interdisciplinary approach, a number of therapists and specialists, with their areas of expertise but working together as a team, interact with the child and family.

Neuro-Developmental Treatment

The Neuro-Developmental Treatment (NDT) approach (Bobath and Bobath, 1972) advocates early intervention and involvement of family members as active participants in the treatment programme. Parents must understand the goals and the steps in the programme and why they are being introduced, and learn the specific procedures. The clinician must understand the family situation and routine, and the difficulty the parents and child may have in modifying their ways of interacting, handling, feeding, etc. NDT has gained international acceptance as an effective means of treating young children with CP and has influenced the field of speech pathology more than the other major systems of physical therapy. Speech-language clinicians may acquire NDT training in eight-week basic courses, pre-speech and feeding courses, baby courses, and refresher courses. The NDT approach advocates physically handling the child to normalise muscle tone and facilitate more normal movement responses in automatic movements, handling through specific key points of control to influence movement throughout the body, and facilitating the normal movement responses, including more coordinated eating, breathing and vocalising. Therapy is incorporated into the family's daily routine and includes ordinary materials at home.

Table 8.1 shows examples of NDT based therapeutic guidelines for feeding and oral motor treatment, particularly during the first three years of the child's life. The reader is reminded that treatment is a dynamic and individualised process which does not rely on specific techniques.

Neurospeech Therapy

Neurospeech Therapy (Mysak, 1980) is another approach for treating dysarthric CP children based on an analysis of the child's motor behaviour, positioning the child to normalise tone for more normal respiration, phonation and articulation, and applying an appropriate stimulus, then initiating and guiding the expected response. To improve the child's articulation, the clinician facilitates each speech pattern with the fingers, passively moving the mandible, spreading the cheeks, shaping the lips, etc. For example, for /f/ the clinician lifts the child's upper lip with one hand, exposes the teeth, raises the lower lip against the upper incisors and requests the child to blow through the teeth. The clinician simultaneously produces the appropriate syllables. When the child can reproduce articulatory patterns, he is asked or helped to combine patterns, e.g., bilabial and labiodental patterns, then complete the series of combinations of increasing length when possible. Over-articulation, slow speech rate, and techniques to enhance sensory feedback, help improve intelligibility.

Table 8.1: Feeding and Oral Motor Treatment

Goal	Possible Intervention
1. Normal oral tactile sensitivity	1. Gradually introduce oral stimulation
2. Help the child maintain good closure around the nipple while sucking a bottle	2. Maintain hip and head flexion to break up extensor patterns that contribute to abnormal tongue thrust and jaw thrust
3. Improve spoon feeding	3. Use jaw and lip control, pressure of spoon on tongue to encourage lip closure and to inhibit bite reflex and tongue thrust
4. Facilitate chewing of solid food	4. Work first on semi-lumpy foods, provide external jaw control to help a child with poor or unstable jaw control, place strips of dried food, rare cooked meat, or bites of crisp food on the biting surfaces
5. Teach cup drinking	5. By positioning, jaw control, and by first introducing thickened liquids
6. Teach straw drinking and improve lip control and strength	6. A similar procedure to cup drinking, but only after cup drinking has been perfected
7. Facilitate normal respiration	7. By positioning, movement and pressure
8. Encourage phonation and speech	8. By inhibition of abnormal tone and with moto-kinesthetic techniques
9. Normalise responses to touch, taste, textures	9. Carefully introduce touch-pressure stimulation that is just slightly overstimulating to the child, and by balancing intensity of the stimuli and by handling, prevent any abnormal response

Augmentative Communication Systems

With the more involved child, introduction of communication systems to augment speech should begin early and be concurrent with vocal and oral motor treatment. The clinician should help the parents identify and enhance the child's non-verbal communicative interactions and strategies. At meal time, the feeder focuses not just on therapeutic handling and feeding, but on social interactions with opportunities for the child to express preferences and choices by looking and reaching. The feeder should encourage vocalisations during meal times, gradually pairing verbal and non-verbal communications. The child's positive and negative responses are identified and developed into yes–no responses. Pictures can be introduced to a child whose cognitive developmental level has reached 18 months. Play situations should provide the opportunity for meaningful communication. For example, through vocalising, looking at, pointing to, or directing a small light pointer placed on the forehead to a picture of shoes, the child tells the clinician or parent which clothes to put on a babydoll. The non-speech system may develop from a small number of pictures through many levels of communication boards and symbol systems, to a sophisticated computerised system.

Effectiveness of Therapy

We believe that early identification and intervention programmes which emphasise analysis and treatment of the child's total motor functioning and coordinated team and family efforts are most effective for dysarthric children. There is good face validity for pre-speech and feeding therapy with babies and young children, but we need to research further its effectiveness. Clinically, we find that CP children's speech, while improved over time, remains dysarthric. Unless they are severely mentally retarded and motorically involved, children with the spastic type of CP often become fairly intelligible speakers. Children with the athetoid type of CP, whose motor involvement is greater in the head, trunk and upper extremities, are those generally more impaired in speech. The more intelligent children learn to control their fluctuating muscle tone, incoordination and extreme movement patterns. Some never attain adequate verbal communication and are good candidates for sophisticated computerised augmentative communication systems. These usually require interfaces to input the systems by scanning or encoding techniques because their poor hand control may preclude a direct selection technique.

Conclusion

With articulatory disorders of neurogenic origin, normal speech may not be a feasible goal and additional communication modalities should be considered. The primary goal should be to help the child reach his highest potential for communication. Because apraxic and dysarthric children present such complex problems and because of the many areas that assessment and treatment touch, the clinician will find these children and the communication problems they present, extremely challenging and hopefully, rewarding.

References

ARAM, D.M. and NATION, J.E. (1982) *Child Language Disorders.* St. Louis, MO: C.V. Mosby Co.

BASHIR, A.S., GRAHAMJONES, F. and BOSTWICK, R.Y. (1984) A touch-cue method of therapy for developmental verbal apraxia. *Seminars in Speech and Language,* 5, 2, 127–38.

BLACKSTONE, S.W. (1987) *Augmentative Communication: An Introduction.* Rockville, MD: American Speech-Language-Hearing Association.

BLAKELEY, S.W. (1980) *Screening Test for Developmental Apraxia of Speech.* Tigard, OR: C.C. Publications.

BOBATH, K. and BOBATH, B. (1972) Cerebral palsy. Part 1. Diagnosis and assessment of cerebral palsy. Part 2. The neurodevelopmental approach to treatment. In P.H. Pearson and C.E. Williams (Eds), *Physical Therapy Service in the Developmental Disabilities.* Springfield, IL: Charles C. Thomas.

BOWMAN, S.N., PARSONS, C.L. and MORRIS, D.A. (1984) Inconsistency of phonological errors in developmental verbal dyspraxic children as a factor of linguistic task and performance load. *Australian Journal of Human Communication Disorders,* 12, 2, 109–19.

CAMPBELL, P.H. (1982) *Problem-Oriented Approaches to Feeding the Handicapped Child.* Akron, OH: The Children's Hospital Medical Center of Akron.

CAPOZZI, M. and MINEO, B. (1986) Nonspeech language and communication systems. In J.M. Costello and A.L. Holland (Eds), *Handbook of Speech and Language Disorders.* San Diego, CA: College-Hill.

CHAPPELI, G.E. (1973) Childhood verbal apraxia and its treatment. *Journal of Speech and Hearing Disorders,* 16, 362–8.

CHUMPELIK, D. (1984) The PROMPT system of therapy: Theoretical framework and applications for developmental apraxia of speech. *Seminars in Speech and Language,* 5, 2, 139–56.

CRARY, M.A. (1984) Phonological characteristics of developmental verbal dyspraxia. *Seminars in Speech and Language,* 5, 2, 71–83.

CRARY, M.A. and TOWNE, R.L. (1984) The asynergistic nature of developmental verbal dyspraxia. *Australian Journal of Human Communication Disorders,* 12, 2, 27–37.

DAVIS, L. (1978) Pre-speech. In F.P. Connor *et al.* (Eds), *Program Guide for Infants and Toddlers with Neuromotor and Other Developmental Disabilities.* New York: Teachers College Press.

DEPUTY, P.N. (1984) The need for description in the study of developmental verbal dyspraxia. *Australian Journal of Human Communication Disorders,* 12, 2, 3–13.

EKELMAN, B.L. and ARAM, D.M. (1983) Syntactic findings in developmental verbal apraxia. *Journal of Communication Disorders,* 16, 237–50.

FISHMAN, I. (1987) *Electronic Communication Aids: Selection and Use.* Phila., PA: College Hill/Little, Brown.

GALLENDER, D. (1979) *Eating Handicaps.* Springfield, IL: Charles C. Thomas.

GUYETTE, T.W. and DIEDRICH, W.R. (1981) A critical review of developmental apraxia of speech. In N. Lass (Ed.), *Speech and Language: Advances in Basic Research and Practice,* 5. New York: Academic Press.

GUYETTE, T.W. and DIEDRICH, W.R. (1983) A review of the Screening Test for Developmental Apraxia of Speech. *Language, Speech and Hearing Services in Schools,* 14, 202–9.

HAYNES, D. (1985) Developmental apraxia of speech: Symptoms and treatment. In D.F. Johns (Ed.) *Clinical Management of Neurogenic Communicative Disorders* (2nd ed.). Boston: Little, Brown.

JAFFE, M.B. (1986) Neurological impairment of speech production: Assessment and treatment. In J.M. Costello and A.L. Holland (Eds), *Handbook of Speech and Language Disorders.* San Diego: College Hill.

LOGUE, R.D. (1976) *Assessing speech motor behaviour: An examination Protocol.* Paper presented at the American Speech-Language-Hearing Association Convention, Houston, TX.

LOGUE, R.D. (1978) Disorders of motor-speech planning in children: Evaluation and treatment. *Communicative Disorders: An Audio Journal for Continuing Education, Vol. 3.* New York, NY: Grune and Stratton.

McGINNIS, M.A. (1963) *Aphasic Children: Identification and Education by the Association Method.* Washington, DC: Alexander Graham Bell Association for the Deaf, Inc.

MORLEY, M., COURT, D., MILLER, H. and GARSIDE, R. (1955) Delayed speech and developmental aphasia. *British Medical Journal,* 2, 463–7.

MORRIS, S.E. (1982) *Pre-Speech Assessment Scale,* Clifton, NJ: J.A. Preston.

MORRIS, S.E. and KLEIN, M.D. (1987) *Pre-Feeding Skills.* Tucson, AR: Therapy Skill Builders.

MUELLER, H.A. (1972) Facilitating feeding and pre-speech. In P.H. Pearson and C.E. Williams (Eds), *Physical Therapy Services in the Developmental Disabilities.* Springfield, IL: Charles C. Thomas, 283–310.

MUSSELWHITE, C. and ST. LOUIS, K.W. (1982) *Communication Programming for the Severely Handicapped: Vocal and Non-Vocal Strategies.* San Diego: College Hill.

MYSAK, E.D. (1980) *Neurospeech Therapy for the Cerebral Palsied* (3rd ed.), New York: Teachers College Press.

PARSONS, D.L. (1984) A comparison of phonological processes used by developmentally verbal dyspraxic children and non-dyspraxic phonologically impaired children. *Australian Journal of Human Communication Disorders,* 12, 2, 93–107.

ROSENBEK, J.C., HANSEN, R., BAUGHMAN, C.H. and LEMME, M. (1974) Treatment of developmental apraxia of speech: A case study. *Language, Speech and Hearing Services in Schools,* 5, 13–22.

ROSENBEK, J.C. and WERTZ, R.T. (1972) A review of fifty cases of developmental apraxia of speech. *Language, Speech and Hearing Services in Schools,* 3, 23–33.

ROSENTHAL, J., WILLIAMS, R. and INGHAM, R.J. (1978) *An experimental therapy programme for developmental articulatory dyspraxia.* Paper presented at the Annual Convention of the Australian Association of Speech and Hearing, Launceston, Tasmania.

SCHMIDT, P. (1976) Feeding assessment and therapy for the neurologically impaired. *American Association for Education of the Severely and Profoundly Handicapped,* 1, 8, 19–28.

SHELTON, I.S. and GARVES, M.M. (1985) Use of visual techniques in therapy for developmental apraxia of speech. *Language, Speech and Hearing Services in Schools,* 16, 3, 129–31.

SILVERMAN, F.H. (1980) *Communication for the Speechless*, Englewood Cliffs, NJ: Prentice Hall.

SMITH, P.K. and ENGEL, B.J. (1984) *Melodic Intonation Training: Stop Consonants.* Tucson, AZ: Communication Skill Builders.

YOSS, K.A. and DARLEY, F.L. (1974) Therapy in developmental apraxia of speech. *Language, Speech and Hearing in Schools,* 1, 23–31.

9   Childhood Voice Disorders

Pauline Sloane

The accurate identification, description and subsequent treatment of children with voice disorders has long been a dilemma facing speech and language clinicians. Any attempt to define voice normality represents clinical opinion, rather than objectively derived statements having professional agreement. Difficulties are therefore encountered when attempting to describe subjectively the complex acoustical pattern called voice. A valid working definition of the term voice could be considered as the sound produced primarily by the vibration of the vocal folds and the interactive effects of the sub and supraglottal structures.

There is a disparity among reports as to the prevalence of voice disorders in children. Following a review of the major studies on prevalence (Senturia and Wilson, 1968; Gillespie and Cooper, 1973; Yari, Currin, Bulian and Yari, 1974; Silverman and Zimmer, 1975; Wilson, 1987; and Sloane, 1982), one notes that estimates of the occurrence of vocal dysfunction vary from 1 per cent to 23.4 per cent. Most surveys present 6 to 9 per cent as a realistic estimate of voice deviations in children (Deal, McClain and Sudderth, 1976; Warr-Leeper, McShea and Leeper, 1979; Wilson, 1987). Regardless of whether these estimates are accurate, the speech and language clinician's typical childhood voice therapy case load does not seem to reflect the expected incidence of such disorders. There are several reasons for this: poor identification procedures; lack of recognition of voice disorder as a serious or potentially serious communication handicap; lenient sociological responses; uncertainty on the clinician's part about management; and, finally, a treatment priority system which places these children low in the therapy schedule.

Causative Factors

Laryngeal disabilities that affect children are not as varied or as plentiful as in adults (see Chapter 15). Many different organic and psychogenic conditions result in abnormal approximation and asymmetrical vibration of the vocal cords, resulting in the vocal quality deviation called hoarseness.

According to Wilson (1987), there are five primary sites of voice disorders in children: the larynx; the velopharyngeal area; the oral cavity; the nose and the ear. The normal production of voice in the child may be altered by:

1 structural anomalies
2 neurological conditions, including paralysis
3 tumours
4 trauma
5 psychological dysfunction
6 physiological dysfunction

The importance of these factors in causing voice disorders is in the way they modify the basic functional pattern of voice production and each of these will be discussed briefly to provide an overview of etiological factors.

Structural anomalies

Structural anomalies of the larynx may be present on a congenital or a developmental basis. Voice therapy is rarely the intervention of choice for congenital problems of the larynx but the clinician should be aware of such malformations and engage in close follow-up of the child as the voice develops. Structural anomalies that are earlier regarded as relatively insignificant may become important later as causes for voice disorders. Laryngeal disorders, such as webbing and stenosis, which give rise to a weak and/or hoarse cry are also likely to give rise to the more serious problem of airway obstruction. Laryngeal webs, which account for 5 per cent of congenital anomalies (Smith and Catlin, 1984) generally involve the anterior portion of the glottis and consist of thin connective tissue. Surgery is the primary form of management. Congenital supraglottic and subglottic stenosis of the laryngeal airway and larynx is generally managed conservatively. Dilation and review by the surgeon until the larynx has matured is recommended. In a few cases surgical intervention is required. Relief of the obstructed airway is usually achieved initially by endotracheal intubation but for more long term relief a tracheostomy — an artificial opening created between the cervical trachea and the neck to provide ventilatory assistance — is required. The clinician must take an active role in the management of children with tracheostomies as they are generally placed before verbal language skills are developed and consequently communicative maturation can be significantly impaired.

Another congenital condition which gives rise to a lesser degree of airway obstruction is laryngeal stridor or laryngomalacia which is caused by failure of the cartilages of the larynx to develop normally. As this condition ordinarily disappears in early childhood it may not be called to the attention of the speech and language clinician.

Neurological conditions including vocal fold paralysis

Vocal quality may be affected by impaired neurological functioning, either congenital or acquired. The vocal symptoms obviously depend on the nature and severity of the condition and include resonance problems, dysphonia and reduced loudness. Generally speaking, the vocal dysfunction forms part of a larger group of symptoms affecting muscular inco-ordination and voice therapy therefore, of and by itself, is rarely the treatment of choice.

Vocal fold paralysis that results from recurrent laryngeal nerve damage may be congenital or acquired, unilateral or bilateral and of two types, adductor or abductor. It is when the muscles of adduction are paralysed that vocal dysfunction occurs. The condition is relatively common in children and represents about 10 per cent of all congenital anomalies of the larynx. The symptoms which can include respiratory and phonatory difficulties, depend on the degree of involvement and the compensations the child has made with regard to closure of the vocal folds. Cord paralysis may result from trauma, neurological, inflammatory or vascular conditions but Wilson (1987) noted that approximately one-third of the paralyses are of undetermined etiology.

Paralysis of the left vocal fold is frequently more serious than that of the right and may not be as amenable to intervention, as it is often associated with anomalies of the heart and great blood vessels (Holinger and Brown, 1969). Children with vocal fold paralysis may require direct voice therapy by way of strengthening the healthy vocal fold and encouraging it to overadduct across the midline to achieve better approximation with the paralysed fold. The most widely used and successful method, to date, of improving laryngeal valving is the pushing method, first suggested by Froeschels, Kastein and Weiss (1955). However, it is sometimes difficult to apply this method with young children. Apart from direct voice therapy, these children may require help in adapting to disturbances in respiration.

Tumours

Perhaps the most common organic change in the laryngeal structures of children is the development of glottal margin pathologies such as vocal nodules, polyps, oedema and inflammation. Such pathologies are attributed to prolonged abuse and/or misuse of the vocal mechanism and most childhood dysphonias are thus related. Misuse includes phonation at high levels of intensity and/or phonation at an inappropriate frequency level. Vocal fold abuse may refer to inappropriate coughing and affective excesses such as prolonged shouting, screaming, yelling and cheering. Some children do not experience adverse laryngeal consequences as a result of abusive practices and it is unclear why some children seem to be particularly at risk (Anderson and Newby, 1973). Adverse physiological conditions, such as the presence of allergies and chronic upper respiratory tract infections, and adverse environmental factors such as the psychological and physical living environment may predispose a child to developing significant changes in vocal cord tissues (Wilson, 1987). A constitutional tendency and personality and adjustment factors were cited by Arnold (1963) as also being important.

Vocal nodules

These are the most common benign malignant neoplasms (Miller and Madison, 1984), resulting from functional misuse and abuse of the laryngeal tissues, in the form of excessive shouting, yelling, cheering, forms of vocal play and a multitude of other abuses. The usual site of nodule formation is at the junction of the anterior and middle one-thirds of the vocal folds and these may be unilateral or bilateral. Generally speaking, an abnormal vocal quality is perceived as soon as the mass of the cord increases and with time the hoarseness becomes progressively more severe.

The majority of laryngologists consider voice therapy the treatment of choice for children presenting with vocal nodules. Others recommend surgical intervention but the nodule will tend to return if vocal hyperfunctioning practices are not eliminated.

Vocal polyps

Vocal polyps, which are rare in children, are fluid-filled sacs of tissue similar to blisters (Stemple, 1984). They may be sessile or pedunculated and may result from a single traumatic episode of vocal abuse such as violent screaming or from vocal fold irritants such as smoke, toxic fumes or allergens. The vocal characteristics are similar to those associated with other glottal margin pathologies and vary according to the size and location of the mass. Surgery is the treatment of choice for polyps, followed by voice therapy to eliminate injurious vocal habits.

Vocal fold oedema

Children who abuse their voice over a period of time may also experience an increase in the mass of the vocal cords along the glottal margins. The membraneous tissues become swollen, irritated and reddened and this oedema, which produces a temporary dysphonia, is an early warning sign of vocal hyperfunction. Voice therapy, therefore, is the preferred method of management. In untreated cases, continued abuse and misuse of the voice may lead to the development of other glottal margin pathologies. Vocal fold oedema is also a common acute physical finding in many upper respiratory tract infections. Such oedematous conditions are generally present only for a short period of time and if the voice is not abused or misused during this period of time, hoarseness will seldom persist.

Papillomas

Papillomas are wart-like growths believed to result from viral infection and the characteristic recurrences and remission are indeed compatible with the behaviour of a viral disease (Sloan Lindsey, Montague and Buffalo, 1986). Papillomatosis of the larynx has been reported in the neonate. However, it generally becomes symptomatic in children from 3 to 12 years. They are reported to undergo remission following puberty. Laryngeal papillomatosis is a serious clinical problem in children, in that the growth can occur in the larynx and obstruct the airway. The voice is often severely impaired and whispering may only be possible. The vocal symptoms cannot readily be distinguished from those produced by less threatening glottal tumours. The long term complications have yet to be determined and it is by no means certain that voice will be normal following final resolution of the papilloma. Intervention is always medical and/or surgical. Since papilloma have a tendency to recur, repeated surgery is common (De Weese and Saunders, 1973). When airway obstruction is severe, tracheotomy is necessary. Voice therapy is a questionable form of treatment, as a recent study by Sloan Lindsey *et al.* (1986) indicated little or no relationship between the occurrence of papilloma and the frequency of vocal abuse, environmental irritants, socioeconomic conditions, and total number of surgical excisions. The clinician should monitor laryngeal and respiratory performance of the child between surgeries. In the case of a child with a tracheostomy the clinician has an obvious role in ongoing management.

Trauma

Voice disorders in children may also be associated with laryngeal trauma resulting from prolonged intubation, aspiration of foreign objects, inhalation of toxic substances and direct injuries to the neck. Cartilaginous fractures, inflammation, oedema, ulceration of the vocal folds and enlarging tumours such as granulomas and hemangiomas, leading to dysphonia or aphonia are common sequels of trauma. Surgical intervention is generally the procedure of choice and voice therapy is required for various kinds of internal laryngeal trauma (Holinger, Schild and Maurizi, 1968) and may be indicated following recovery from external trauma.

Psychological dysfunction ·

Psychogenic dysphonia may be suspected in the absence of significant laryngeal or other organic findings and when there is evidence for emotional problems that can account more readily for the dysphonia (Aronson, 1985; Morrison, Rammage, Belisle, Pullan and Nichol, 1983). The terms psychogenic or functional should imply that the clinician has isolated an active etiological agent and that the agent is non-organic. This disorder, which is not common in children, may be viewed as a manifestation of psychological disequilibrium and may be related unconsciously to stress and anxiety in the child's environment. There is some dispute as to whether voice therapy is the treatment of choice for such disorders. The traditional approach to management involved the provision of psychological support as required but the emphasis was placed on direct voice remediation. Referral to a child guidance clinic was indicated if the voice failed to improve. Current thinking dictates that if the vocal disorder is psychogenic in origin, professional counselling is indicated. Direct symptom modification will be of little avail as the disorder will be maintained by the underlying emotional conflict.

Physiological dysfunction

A variety of conditions of a physiological nature may cause and in some cases maintain a voice problem. These conditions include allergies and upper respiratory tract infections, hearing loss and glandular malfunction such as hypothyroidism. Medical treatment is the management of choice and in the majority of cases, resolution of the underlying dysfunction will result in normal voice. In other cases, voice therapy is indicated in combination with medical treatment.

Nasal resonance disorders

Many children have poor vocal resonance which affects the quality of the voice.

Disorders of nasal resonance can be divided into two main categories, characterised by either excessive or insufficient nasality. Hypernasality or excessive nasality, is related primarily to excessive coupling between the nasal cavity and oral-pharyngeal tract. All vowel sounds are nasalised and when the condition is severe, the consonants may be affected by the leakage of air pressure out of the nose, commonly referred to as nasal escape. Hypernasal voice quality is generally caused by a physiological deficit in the palatopharyngeal mechanism. The causes and treatment of such a deficit are discussed in Chapter 11.

Voice Disorders of Adolescence

According to Brodnitz (1971), mutation constitutes the most important single landmark in the vocal history of the male. Disturbed mutation can be classified into three clinical forms:

1   Mutation falsetto or puberphonia which refers to the presence of persistent falsetto voice in the physically normal male
2   Incomplete mutation, i.e. the voice does not develop the full depth of adult male pitch
3   Delayed mutation, i.e. vocal changes do not take place until several years later than usual.

Puberphonia

Greene (1982) states that the predominant characteristic of the puberphonic voice is its unnaturally high pitch. Medical examination reveals normal physical development, sexual maturation and laryngeal growth. In other words, a functional avoidance of vocal mutation has taken place. Aronson (1973) stated that in some instances the falsetto voice may be due to a structurally small larynx and Wilson (1987) comments that mutational or structural causes cannot be distinguished on the sound of the voice alone. Indirect laryngoscopic examination may reveal a slight redness of the vocal cords but this is the result of strain and not the cause of the quality deviation. The vocal quality associated with puberphonia is characterised by high pitch, mild dysphonia and low intensity.

Incomplete mutation

The voice of incomplete mutation occurs more frequently than that of puberphonia. The patient reports normal vocal changes initially but the vocal pitch levels off before reaching the full depth of adult male pitch. The folds are of normal adult length and function but reddening and thickening of the folds due to vocal strain may be present.

Delayed mutation

Aronson (1980) comments that psychological immaturity may not be the only cause of mutational voice problems. He cites such factors as:

1   delayed maturation due to endocrine disorders
2   severe hearing loss
3   general debilitating illness during puberty
4   weakness or incoordination of the vocal folds or of respiration because of neurological disease during puberty.

It is possible then, that delayed mutation may have an organic basis but both incomplete mutation and puberphonia are primarily the result of psychological influences.

Commonly, there may be a certain amount of resistance to normal voice change but in puberphonia the resistance is extreme. Authorities do not agree with the reasons for such a resistance to voice change. Some believe its presence to be related to a conflicted response to sexual maturity (Van Riper, 1972) or to problems in a relationship with the parent of the same sex (Andrews, 1986). Other reasons put forward include, a strong feminine self-identification and a wish to maintain a childhood soprano singing voice (Aronson, 1985).

Voice therapy is the procedure of choice for these disorders and the majority of these cases yield well to direct voice therapy aimed at lowering the pitch to the optimal pitch level. Counselling may be synchronised with voice therapy when necessary as psychologically the patient may resist the new pitch level. It is imperative that the clinician has an appreciation of the underlying psychological influences in this disorder. Such an understanding, combined with a series of programmed exercises, will result in a normal speaking voice (Cooper, 1973).

Assessment Considerations

Traditionally, the voice clinician has followed the medical model with regard to diagnosis and this model is based on the assumption that intervention procedures are much more successful if the etiological correlates have been identified. A number of clinicians regard treatment of vocal dysfunction as behavioural management and do not feel the necessity for pursuing etiology.

The initial step in the management of children presenting with voice disorder is to refer them for a laryngological examination. Parental support of the referral process is important. Evaluation of the voice should not be postponed if such an examination has not yet been performed as referral following the initial consultation with the speech and language clinician allows both better appreciation of the presenting problem and suggestion of certain diagnostic entities which may aid a more accurate diagnosis.

Voice evaluation involves the assembly of pertinent data such as the results of previous investigations by medical personnel, records of previous intervention and case history information directly related to the disorder. Attempts to increase objectivity and accountability in the assessment of voice disorders has led to the present emphasis on acoustic analysis of the voice, which involves an increased use of technical hardware. Although it is seen as an advance, it has also served to re-emphasise the importance of the clinician's perceptual analysis.

Indirect laryngoscopy

In the absence of objective assessment procedures the voice clinician has relied on medical evaluation, chiefly that of indirect laryngoscopy. This allows observations regarding vocal fold colour, thickness, presence or absence of pathology and symmetry of vocal fold vibration during phonation and symmetry of the folds at rest. Despite certain limitations, laryngological examination must precede any attempt at clinical intervention as the clinician's chief concern is to rule out the presence of an underlying serious medical condition in the laryngeal structures, which would require surgical or medical intervention rather than voice therapy.

Clinical evaluation

The laryngologist provides the essential information about the structures of the larynx, pharynx, oral cavity, nose, ears and neck but the clinician must identify the contributing behavioural vocal parameters. A pure tone hearing test should also be completed in order to rule out hearing impairment. Clinical evaluation consists of interview and examination, and has three main goals:

1 to determine specific characteristics of the faulty voice
2 to determine predisposing, precipitating and perpetuating factors
3 to identify specifically how the voice and related conditions can be modified or eliminated.

During the interview the clinician collects information concerning the nature of the presenting problem, its possible causes, the nature of the onset, variations in severity, possible family and environmental influences on the problem, history of voice use and related medical problems. More detailed information is available in Andrews (1986); Wilson (1987); Leith and Johnson (1986). As voice disorders are often the result of the interplay of anatomical, physiological, psychological, social and environmental factors, the voice disorder cannot be considered in isolation. The second part of the voice evaluation is the direct clinical assessment. This is usually a relatively brief procedure in the child. Laryngeal function must be analysed in relation to the antecedent conditions, present conditions and the child's future vocal usage. Evaluation of vocal quality is approached subjectively and objectively. Although there is little agreement regarding the meaning of perceptual terms such as hoarseness, harshness and breathiness, auditorily classifying the child's voice may help focus other aspects of the assessment. In addition to the clinician's subjective evaluation, the results of voice assessments should, if possible, be stated in quantitative terms. There are a number of different rating scales available, such as those devised by Wilson and Rice (1977) with which the clinician can attempt to quantify subjective judgements of the vocal parameters, pitch, intensity, range and degree of vocal fold closure on a seven point scale. Such profiles provide the clinician with an overall index of severity and generally describe the contribution of the different parameters to the child's disordered voice. Audio tape recording is necessary. A variety of more elaborate auditory analyses of the voice signal have been proposed, including spectrographic and laryngographic procedures but they are not commonly used in the voice assessment of the child and yield little clinically useful information.

The following factors should be evaluated and rated: respiratory patterns; vocal fold approximation and mode of vibration; pitch; intensity; prosody resonance and overall voice efficiency. Vocal abuses should also be identified at this time. The clinician must remember that the context in which communication takes place has at least four dimensions (De Vito, 1980; Andrews, 1986). These are physical, social, psychological and temporal and it is imperative that the clinician evaluate the child's vocal behaviour in the light of the interaction of these contexts.

Following collection of the relevant data, the clinician is in a position to form hypotheses concerning the etiology of the disorder which must be checked against medical and laryngological data. Individualised management procedures can then be determined.

Mainstream Treatment Practices

Traditionally, voice therapy programmes for children were based on a holistic approach (i.e., all the component parts of the voice production system were treated sequentially, with little emphasis placed on the underlying etiology or the presenting symptoms). This approach is not successful with children who generally lack motivation and fail to see the underlying principles involved. Specific approaches to remediation which focus on the symptoms exhibited and identifying the underlying etiological factors and vocal behaviours to be changed are generally quite successful with young children both in individual and group therapy situations. Commonalities exist between both approaches, in the form of modification and/or elimination of incorrect vocal behaviours, environmental management and counselling. Not all clinicians will have a similar procedural approach to voice modification and much depends on their philosophy, training and experience. Some authorities believe that the only logical approach to voice therapy is the behavioural approach (Leith and Johnson, 1986). This poses problems for those clinicians who adopt the more traditional physiological orientation to the presenting disorder. The behaviourists' view reflects the idea that it is the child's inability to perform certain vocal behaviours that results in his voice disorder with secondary importance being given to the question of whether this is or is not due to an underlying medical or structural problem. Behaviourists base their intervention programme on performance data to identify the behaviour change goal and on learning theory to teach a new, or modify an existing, vocal behaviour (Leith and Johnson, 1986; Wilson, 1986).

The philosophy of intervention advocated here could be considered primarily a physiological approach (i.e., efforts are made to alter or influence underlying physiological processes which are deemed responsible for the existing laryngeal pathological conditions). As the child's vocal quality is an audible manifestation of the underlying dysfunction of the phonatory and/or the resonatory mechanisms, it is this dysfunction that is the clinician's chief consideration and not the presenting perceptual vocal attributes. Regardless of the procedural approach, voice must be rehabilitated in relation to the needs of the child in context.

The majority of voice disorders in children are due to abuse and misuse of the voice and result in glottal margin pathologies. Such pathologies are treated conservatively and the management of choice is voice therapy. In discussing the voice therapy programme for children who engage in vocal hyperfunction with the concomitants of vocal fold inflammation, oedema and nodules, there is little need to make a clinical distinction in treatment as one is dealing with a common etiology. The goal of voice therapy for vocal hyperfunction is to reduce vocal fold trauma through re-education and to modify or eliminate environmental stress.

Andrews (1987) stated that there are four distinct phases that are important in a voice therapy programme for children. These are:

1 general awareness
2 specific awareness
3 production
4 carryover

These phases are interdependent and interrelated and the differenes should merely be one of emphasis.

General awareness

The initial part of the voice therapy programme should concentrate on developing an awareness of the problem and outlining the possible benefits of therapy. Explanation regarding the causative factors of the child's voice problem helps both child and parents to understand the importance of their role in vocal rehabilitation. The role of the parents and significant others in the child's environment cannot be underestimated and it may be that the ultimate success of the voice therapy programme will depend on the success achieved in gaining parental understanding and co-operation at this early stage.

Specific awareness

Once the child has developed an understanding of the presenting problem, work on specific awareness can commence. During this phase the child learns to isolate appropriate and inappropriate vocal behaviours and to discriminate between them. Successful elimination of faulty vocal habits is predicted on their accurate identification. In order to pinpoint such behaviours many clinicians opt to use the data based on vocal abuse reduction programme (VARP) introduced by Johnson (1985). This programme reports a success rate in clinical settings of greater than 95 per cent. In general childhood vocal abuses are not difficult to identify. Substitute vocal behaviours need to be introduced to compensate partly for what the child is relinquishing.

Clinicians must not fool themselves into believing that either weekly sessions or more intensive scheduling, allows sufficient time for the efficient monitoring and modification of vocal behaviour patterns. It is inappropriate to engage in vocal retraining procedures until the elimination and modification of faulty vocal behaviours has been accomplished and the vocal folds have returned to normal. Following this, and assuming continued motivation, techniques such as those recommended by Wilson (1986) and Andrews (1987) to improve vocal production may be undertaken.

Production

This phase includes the production of target behaviours, stabilising control in the immediate environment and early attempts at stabilising control in the extended environment. The child's use of abusive vocal production is often a reaction to environmental factors. With many children definite progress in the vocal abuse reduction programme results in a definite reduction in glottal margin pathology and an improvement in vocal quality. Consequently, it is rarely necessary to work directly with the child to influence or modify this phonatory behaviour.

The use of instrumentation to control the child's vocal behaviour can make voice therapy an interesting and more effective process as this allows objective assessment of habitual vocal characteristics, awareness of inappropriate vocal parameters by means of auditory and visual feedback and ease of acquisition of new vocal behaviour patterns. The use of instrumentation in vocal rehabilitation programmes continues to accelerate and professionals will find new and interesting applications for the voice disordered child.

Carryover

During this phase the child is encouraged to habituate the target vocal behaviours for increasing periods of time in his own speaking environment. Carryover and habituation is particularly difficult for children as they are more concerned with day to day issues of living than directing their energies towards changing patterns of vocal behaviour. It is difficult for any child to see the value of vocal hygiene. To ignore this reality will result in the clinician's failure to effect change. The amount and nature of responsibility placed on a child will depend on his age and on the cooperation of significant others. Unless vocal behaviours are habitually traumatic, time may be more profitably spent in controlling environmental conditions that give rise to vocally abusive patterns. Such control is considerably more certain than control of the child's vocal performance once he is in those conditions.

Children undergoing regular voice therapy should have indirect laryngoscopic examination every three months. Laryngeal changes will be apparent at this stage if voice therapy is effective. In addition, to ensure long-term carryover of new vocal behaviours, periodic reviews should be scheduled following completion of the intervention programme.

Effectiveness of Therapy

Factors which are influential in determining prognosis include history, duration and severity of the disorder, etiological correlates, intrinsic and extrinsic motivational factors and immediate and extended environmental characteristics.

The clinician should also consider the question of remission of the presenting symptoms. Many childhood voice disorders lessen in degree and frequently resolve with increase in age. This is possibly due to the stabilisation of laryngeal size and the acquisition of adult vocal behaviours during which vocal abuse is less likely to occur.

This discussion has not so far emphasised emotional factors of the dysphonia. That is not to suggest that such factors are trivial and should not be of concern during the intervention programme. If a trial period of voice therapy produces no improvement in vocal quality and the child seems to hold on to his symptoms, it may well be that the emotional problems are intractable and require referral for the appropriate expert management.

References

ANDERSON, V.A. and NEWBY, H.A. (1973) *Improving the Child's Speech* (2nd ed.). New York: Oxford University Press.

ANDREWS, M.L. (1986) *Voice Therapy for Children*. London: Longman.

ARNOLD, G.E. (1963) Vocal Nodules. In J.F. Daly (Moderator), Voice problems and laryngeal pathology. *New York State Journal of Medicine*, 63, 3096–110.

ARONSON, A.E. (1973) *Psychogenic Voice Disorders: An Interdisciplinary Approach to Detection, Diagnosis and Therapy: Audio Seminars in Speech Pathology*. Philadelphia. W.B. Saunders Co.

ARONSON, A.E. (1985) *Clinical Voice Disorders* (2nd ed.). New York: Thieme Stratton.

BRODNITZ, F.S. (1971) *Vocal Rehabilitation* (4th ed.). Rochester, New York: American Academy of Ophthalmology and Otolaryngology.

COOPER, M. (1973) *Modern Techniques of Vocal Rehabilitation*. Springfield, IL: Charles C. Thomas.

DEAL, R.E., McCLAIN, B. and SUDDERTH, J.F. (1976) Identification, evaluation therapy and follow-up for children with vocal nodules in a public school setting. *Journal of Speech and Hearing Disorders*, 41, 14–20.

DEVITO, J.A. (1980) *The Interpersonal Communication Book* (2nd ed.). New York: Harper and Row.

DEWEESE, D.D. and SAUNDERS, W.H. (1973) *Textbook of Otolaryngology* (4th ed.). St. Louis, MO: C.V. Mosby.

FROESCHELS, E., KASTEIN, S. and WEISS, D.A. (1955) A method of therapy for paralytic conditions of the mechanisms of phonation, respiration and glutination. *Journal of Speech and Hearing Disorders*, 20, 365–70.

GILLESPIE, S.K. and COOPER, E.B. (1973) Prevalence of speech problems in junior and senior high schools. *Journal of Speech and Hearing Research*, 16, 739–43.

GREENE, M.C.L. (1982) *The Voice and its Disorders* (4th ed.). New York: Pitman.

HOLINGER, P.H. and BROWN, W.T. (1967) Congenital webs, cysts, laryngoceles and other anomalies of the larynx. *Annals of Otolaryngology, Rhinology and Laryngology*, 76, 744–52.

HOLINGER, P.H., SCHILD, J.A. and MAURIZI, D.G. (1968) Internal and external trauma to the larynx. *Laryngoscope*, 78, 944–54.

JOHNSON, T.S. (1985) *Vocal Abuse Reduction Programme.* San Diego: College Hill.

LEITH, W. and JOHNSON, R. (1986) *Handbook of Voice Therapy for the School Clinician.* London: Taylor and Francis.

MILLER, S.Q. and MADISON, C.L. (1984) Public school voice clinics, Part 1:A working model. *Language Speech and Hearing Services in the Schools*, 15, 51–7.

MOORE, G.P. (1971) Voice disorders organically based. In L.E. Travis (Ed.), *Handbook of Speech Pathology and Audiology.* New York: Appleton Century Crofts.

MORRISON, M.D., RAMMAGE, L.A., BELISLE, G.M., PULLAN, C.B. and NICHOL, H. (1983) Muscular tension dysphonia. *Journal Otolaryngology*, 12, 302–6.

SAUNDERS, W.H. (1964) The Larynx. *Clinical Symposia*, 16, 67–99.

SENTURIA, B.H. and WILSON, F.B. (1968) Otorhinolaryngic findings in children with voice deviations. *Annals of Otology, Rhinology and Laryngology*, 77, 1027–42.

SILVERMAN, E.M. and ZIMMER, C.H. (1975) Incidence of chronic hoarseness among school-aged children. *Journal of Speech and Hearing Disorders*, 40, 211–5.

SLOAN, L.P., MONTAGE, J.E. and BUFFALO, M.D. (1986) A preliminary survey on the relationship of exogenous factors to laryngeal papilloma. *Language, Speech and Hearing Services in the Schools*, 17, 292–9.

SLOANE, P.M. (1982) *The Prevalence of Voice Quality Deviations in the Irish School Age Population in the Light of Laryngological Examinations.* Unpublished Masters Thesis, University of Dublin, Trinity College.

SMITH, R.J.H. and CATLIN, F.L. (1984) Congenital anomalies of the larynx. *American Journal of Diseases of Children*, 138, 35–9.

STEMPLE, J.C. (1984) *Clinical Voice Pathology: Theory and Management.* Columbus, OH: Charles C. Merrill.

VAN RIPER, C. (1972) *Speech Correction, Principles and Methods* (6th ed.). Englewood Cliffs, NJ: Prentice Hall.

WARR-LEEPER, Y.A., McSHEA, R.S. and LEEPER, H.A. (1979) The incidence of voice and speech deviations in a middle school population. *Language, Speech and Hearing Services in the Schools*, 10, 14–20.

WILSON, D.K. (1987) *Voice Problems of Children* (3rd ed.). Baltimore: Williams and Wilkins.

WILSON, F.B. and RICE, M. (1977) *A Programmed Approach to Voice Therapy.* Allen, TX: DLM Teaching Resources.

WYNTER, H. (1974) An investigation into the analysis and terminology of voice quality and its correlation with the assessment reliability of speech therapists. *British Journal of Disorders of Communication*, 9, 102–9.

YARI, E., CURRIN, L.H., BULIAN, N. and YARI, J. (1974) Incidence of hoarseness in school children over a 1-year period. *Journal of Communication Disorders*, 7, 321–8.

10   Childhood Stuttering

Irmgarde Horsley

Dysfluency, in its various forms such as hesitations, pauses, repetitions, revisions, interjections and prolongations, is a natural aspect of speaking. It reflects various cognitive, affective and linguistic processes that occur when both children and adults are speaking, and, by and large, these dysfluencies are either ignored by the listener or are used as clues to meaning (Kowal, O'Connell and Sabin, 1975; Sabin, Clemmer, O'Connell and Kowal, 1979; Brotherton, 1979). Clinically, the problem is to decide whether or not a child displaying dysfluencies is likely to develop chronic stuttering. The term *dysfluency* is often contrasted with normal non-fluency.

Stuttering may be defined as an involuntary disruption in the flow of speech which may take the form of repetitions, prolongations, or stoppages which interfere with the speaker's intended utterance. A child's speech is likely to attract the label 'stuttering' when either an excess of dysfluencies or less common forms of dysfluency, such as part-word repetitions and prolongations are present and perceived by a listener. Stuttering usually appears initially between the ages of 2 and 5 years (Andrews and Harris, 1964) at a time when a child's language is in a state of rapid growth. Delayed speech and language development is more often reported in the case histories of stutterers than non-stutterers (Wingate, 1983). Boys are more likely to stutter than are girls at an estimated ratio of three to one (Bloodstein, 1981) and possibly higher (Wingate, 1983). The familial risk is also increased if at least one parent ever stuttered and is related to the sex of the relative (Kidd, 1985).

Causative Factors

Past theoretical positions as to the causes of stuttering have included either organic or neurologically disposing factors or environmental and emotional factors to be the source. Current thinking, however, supports a combination of both organic predisposing factors and environmental aspects in the causation of stuttering.

A seminal paper by Andrews, Craig, Feyer, Hoddinott, Howie and Neilson (1983) comprehensively reviewed only replicated findings about various aspects of stuttering. They concluded that there are two aspects to the disorder of stuttering. The first is a genetically determined reduction in central capacity for efficient sensory motor integration, a conclusion mirrored by a number of other recent individual reports on various aspects of sensory motor functioning in stutterers. The second aspect is that of psychosocial factors which contribute to and maintain learned aspects of stuttering. These include communicative and general stresses which have been demonstrated to be of importance because their removal or reduction may result in stuttering being removed or reduced. In other words, some, but not all, children who stutter have a familial history of stuttering but there are various factors as a child is acquiring speech and language and maturing which may determine whether or not stuttering behaviour emerges. However, a consideration of environmental factors must also include such aspects as pre- and peri-natal conditions, and accidents and illnesses which may result in a detrimental effect on a child's capacity for fluent speech organisation. Stuttering is also reported to be more prevalent amongst those who have suffered some form of cerebral damage (Bloodstein, 1981; Van Riper, 1982). Whether or not a child without any pre-disposing factors but subject to various environmental stresses would develop a chronic stutter is not clear.

Assessment Considerations

The speech of any child referred to a clinician because of dysfluency noted by someone in the child's environment needs to be evaluated because, if for no other reason, concern about some aspect of the child's speech development has been expressed. The extent of the evaluation may vary depending on the information gained from the interview with the parents and initial contact with the child. Not only must the clinician satisfy herself about various components of the child's development which will include more than actual speech, she also needs to decide to what extent environmental factors may be contributing to the difficulty. Only then can the level of intervention be decided.

The case history, usually through parental interview, is the beginning of the compilation of information and should take place without the child being present. The clinician, through sensitive and informed discussion, will hope to obtain information about familial speech and language development and the stage and course of the child's development of speech and language. Of equal importance is information about general and motor development, behaviour, health, and parental attitudes towards these. In essence, what is being built up is a picture of the child's communication environment together with a description of the dysfluent behaviours, as well as when and how often they occur. As childhood dysfluency is very often cyclical, one needs to discover the presence and length of such cycles.

One is attempting to discover both overt and covert contributions to the child's dysfluency; in other words, those aspects over various situations which may be important. However, not every case interview will be ideal and yield the desired information on the first occasion, and perhaps not even on subsequent ones. Often, the informant may be one parent only, who is unaware of specific aspects of family history and/or may find it difficult to be informative. In that event even more emphasis will be placed on the second aspect of evaluation.

Here, one needs, insofar as possible, an environment that fits the child. This second aspect will include an assessment by the clinician of the child's speech, language and possibly hearing. This should include a recording of the child's spontaneous conversation both with parents and with the clinician as well as more structured evaluations where necessary.

Wherever possible though, multiple evaluations of the child's speech should be made in naturalistic settings (e.g., in the home, at nursery or school). Traditionally, the age of the child has been a major factor in evaluating stuttering symptoms and deciding on the course of therapy (i.e., the dysfluent pre-school child has usually been treated differently from the school-age child). However, as each child needs individual evaluation, the age of the child can only serve as a rough guide at best. Excellent detailed models for evaluation may be found in Wall and Myers (1984), Gregory (1973, 1985), Riley and Riley (1983), Cooper (1978, 1984), Curlee (1980, 1984) and Adams (1984a,b) as well as in many other current texts (Rustin *et al.,* 1987).

One aim is to decide to what extent the child's dysfluency is within normal limits, commensurate with both general and speech development and chronological age and, therefore less likely to be a matter of future concern. There is reasonable agreement over a number of studies as to what are normal and less usual nonfluencies, although there can also be an overlap in that both types have been found to be present in the speech samples of young children labelled as stutterers and non-stuttering controls (Johnson and Associates, 1959; Floyd and Perkins, 1974; Bjerkan, 1980; Bloodstein and Grossman, 1981; Wexler and Mysak, 1982; Horsley, Bills, Eason and Kilford, 1988). The important ones to note as abnormal dysfluencies are part-word sound and syllable repetitions (broken works) and sound prolongations. Normal dysfluencies include silent and filled pauses such as interjections of sounds and syllables, revisions and incomplete phrases and whole-word repetition.

As Gregory (1986) points out, dysfluencies are best viewed on a continuum from the more usual to the more unusual as a guide to evaluation. Several warning signs include the presence of the *schwa* vowel, air-flow disruptions, irregular temper and/or breathing patterns, and signs of excess tension in articulation. However, dysfluencies of any kind may interact with how frequently they occur in the child's speech. Even so-called normal dysfluencies may lead to a diagnosis of stuttering if they are a substantial portion of the child's speech. Not surprisingly, dysfluent speech often interacts with the acquisition and use of more complex syntactic and semantic structures (Bloodstein, 1981). A child's awareness of difficulty in speaking takes on different degrees of importance, depending on the extent of this awareness, behavioural reaction to this awareness, and the age of the child.

Theoretical Basis of Intervention

Andrews *et al.* (1982), among many experts, have pointed out that stuttering onset most often appears at a time when a child is experiencing an explosive growth in language ability, but has an immature speech motor apparatus (usually between 3 and 6 years of age). It is estimated that 60 per cent of children who have stuttered for less than one year will spontaneously recover without direct intervention (Andrews, 1985) and that the recovery rate in school-age children by 16 years of age is 78 per cent (Andrews *et al.*, 1983). Kent (1976), reviewing acoustic data on various aspects of speech production, concludes that the accuracy of motor control improves with age until about 11–12 years of age, depending upon the child's individual pattern of motor development, until adult-like performance is reached. As Curlee (1980) points out, it is tempting to speculate about the possible relationship between these high recovery rates and maturational processes. Also, Palermo and Molfese (1972) indicate that various aspects of language development continue until adolescence with periods of instability. It is possible that cyclical dysfluency in young children is a reflection of both these periods of linguistic instability combined with variability in motor control. However, it is by no means clear which children will recover and which will go on to develop chronic stuttering. Given the interactive effects of environment and individual predisposition, the primary aim of intervention with the young dysfluent child is one of *prevention*. As Prins (1983) points out whether or not to intervene is not simply a matter of decision about the presence of stuttering versus normal non-fluency.

Indirect Therapy

Indirect approaches to treatment have been the most common line adopted for young children, particularly for those just beginning to stutter. The provision of clear and simple information at the appropriate level so that parents may understand the nature of a child's speech and language development is the first essential step. The second stage involves the identification and modification of environmental factors which may be affecting the child's fluency. This is achieved through parental counselling and guidance. The assumption of the indirect approach is that a reduction in communicative pressures and environmental stress will have a positive effect on a child's fluency.

Van Riper (1973) and Irwin (1988) clearly described the kinds of difficulties that can arise in the verbal behaviour between parent and child and the importance of introducing positive behaviours and perceptions into the relationship. The type of verbal behaviours identified as potential fluency disruptors include excessive interruptions, finishing the child's statements, filling in words, asking multiple questions at once, constant correction of a child's verbal and non-verbal behaviour, a very rapid speech and conversation rate and topic switching. More general disruptive communicative behaviours may involve such things as listener loss, competition and time pressure over speaking, display and demand speech. There are also emotionally disruptive factors such as inconsistent family routines or severe family problems.

There are often subtle aspects of the parent/child relationship, particularly expectations or negative perceptions of the child, which need to be uncovered and discussed. These are often based on ordinary and understandable anxieties caused by comparisons with other children or by negative comments made by other people in the family environment. Parental expectations about children's speech and general behaviour may be uninformed or unrealistic. It is essential to avoid imparting a sense of blame to the parents who are already concerned. Those individual factors that need to be dealt with will be obtained from the case history and from observation and analysis of the communicative and general relationship of parents and child. Wherever possible, the counselling process needs to involve all those individuals in the environment likely to have an effect on the child's fluency (e.g., siblings, grandparents and teachers). However, despite the widespread use of this indirect approach and the many claims for its efficacy, the absence of matched control groups which would indicate the degree of spontaneous recovery means that its real value is not known.

Direct therapy

Whether or not some degree of direct therapy with the child is also indicated will depend on the presence and degree of borderline stuttering behaviours previously described, the length of time they have been present, and the child's reactions to his speech disruptions. Direct treatment approaches are therefore employed when the clinician has reason to believe that the child's symptoms indicate the likelihood of a chronic stutter developing and that direct work will not be harmful in the sense of exacerbating the dysfluency or by introducing awareness of speech difficulty where none previously existed. Adams (1984a,b) succinctly summarises the guidelines arising out of differential diagnosis. When a child displays little or infrequent awareness of speech difficulty and therefore no serious reactions, when there are no other developmental problems, behavioural or speech and language related and where the environment presents no apparent difficulties, then the indirect method would be the most likely approach to management.

The combination of indirect treatment including environmental manipulation and parental counselling together with direct modification of the child's speech is the form of treatment followed by most experts today: e.g., Wall and Myers (1984), Gregory (1986), Rustin and Cook (1983), Cooper (1984), and Riley and Riley (1984) to name only a few.

Mainstream Treatment Practices

During the last ten years, an enormous amount of information on stuttering has been published. More is currently known about childhood dysfluency at a descriptive level, and various steps and aspects of treatment have been systematically described, some in the form of comprehensive treatment packages. Increasingly, attempts at follow-up and evaluation of therapy are also being undertaken. The importance of this latter factor cannot be underestimated. Despite the fact that the vast majority of childhood dysfluency disorders will, for one reason or another, resolve themselves, we remain desperately short of information as to the course this resolution follows. Even if some of the children treated might have recovered with no intervention, without information as to the progression to normal fluency, we remain working in the dark.

Currently, there are many important and interesting models for treating childhood dysfluency, many of which share similar principles in both differential diagnosis and therapy but use different terminology. Consideration will be given to those which make more than a token effort to assess the effectiveness of their approach or which are considered to represent a significant trend in the management of childhood stuttering. While some of them, however, may still fail to demonstrate the basic requirements needed to indicate the efficacy of the therapy used (Bloodstein, 1981; Ingham, 1983), their clarity of approach recommends them as a starting point for the newly qualified clinician.

Differential diagnosis and therapy

The first model to be considered is that of Gregory (1985) and Gregory and Hill (1980) because it covers the whole range of possible approaches. By its very nature, it is the least controversial and perhaps the most helpful to the clinician, beginning or experienced. The determination of treatment is systematically explored through the evaluation of the individual child. This model identifies four possible results of differential diagnosis with corresponding treatment approaches. The treatment strategy followed when identifying the 'typically' dysfluent child is preventive parent counselling only. What is important here is that even when the child's non-fluency is clinically considered to be within acceptable ordinary limits, parents who have been concerned about a child's fluency should receive some counselling. The form of the counselling will initially always involve attention to parental concerns and observations about the child.

As 'preventive' counselling the process will focus on providing the parents with information. Such information would include a description of speech development and of normal non-fluency. An exploration of, rather than a lecture on, environmental factors conducive to fluency and those related to increased dysfluency will help the parents understand and manage their child's fluency. An important part of their understanding would also include the concepts of time and other communication competence. An important aspect is to maintain contact with the parents over a subsequent period of time and ensure that they will feel comfortable about contacting the clinician should they become concerned about the child's speech.

Where the child is displaying borderline type dysfluencies, e.g., more unusual dysfluencies, more definite stuttering behaviours but no other difficulties with speech and language development, and, the problem has been noted for less than a year, Gregory's approach is to again counsel the parents and see the child for brief therapy. The general principles of preventive counselling are followed but additional procedures which come under the heading of prescriptive counselling are added. These are based on involving the parents more deeply, by providing information in regard to the clinician's judgements about the child's general skills and training the parents to be aware of various types of dysfluency.

With the child, the clinician models a slower, easier and relaxed speaking method with pauses between shorter phrases. This modelling behaviour extends to and includes the parents who will view the sessions and gradually take them over from the clinician.

When the child is, in addition, showing complicating speech, language, or behavioural problems or, when the dysfluencies are largely composed of speech behaviours judged as typical of stuttering behaviours, usually compounded by reports of long-term parental concern, then the approach involves a comprehensive therapy programme. This third strategy obviously includes the elements of the first two approaches as well as a highly individualised and intensive treatment programme involving both child and parents. The main aim is to enhance fluency by the use of direct speech modification procedures, depending on the needs of the individual child. These methods enhance fluency, and though often called by different names, are central to the remediation of dysfluency. These will be mentioned when considering Cooper's (1978, 1984) approach to treatment, but they are also well described in Costello (1983), Adams (1984b), and Gregory and Hill (1980).

Gregory and Hill (1980) reported that, of the children in the comprehensive therapy programme, 70 per cent developed and maintained fluency as evaluated in a follow-up of 9 to 18 months. The remaining 30 per cent were referred to other disciplines after interfering factors were identified. Subsequently, this figure was raised to 75 per cent, and reports about preventive parental counselling with and without limited treatment for the child simply state success after 4 to 8 weekly sessions (Gregory, 1986).

Personalized Fluency Control Therapy

Cooper and Cooper (1976, 1985), over an extended period, have developed a programme called Personalized Fluency Control Therapy which integrates both cognitive and behaviour therapy for stutterers of all ages. The therapeutic activities are highly individualised and depend on the client's abilities, type of dysfluency problems and environmental factors. Obviously, the age level of the child is important. There are several useful graphic representations of various aspects of the therapeutic process which would certainly be appealing to the young child. These include the 'stuttering apple' which visually incorporates individual stuttering behaviours. 'My monkeys' help identify negative feelings and attitudes, and the 'FIG' tree aims to identify fluency-initiating gestures in pictorial form.

Considerable emphasis is placed on the need for a positive relationship between clinician and child. The aim, for any age group, is the feeling of fluency control, which is achieved by working through a well-defined series of stages, with specified short-term and long-term goals. The first stage is *identification* and *structuring,* which enables the individual to identify the feelings, attitudes and actual behaviours which are all part of the problem of stuttering and to understand the direction and goals of therapy. It is at this stage that the structure of the therapeutic relationship is established.

The second stage is *examination* and *confrontation.* In this stage, the modification of various behaviours related to dysfluency both within and outside the clinical setting are introduced. Both resistance and success are verbally identified by the clinician and reinforcement of the client's expressions and opinions about the therapeutic process is provided. The emphasis and method in this stage will depend on the individual client's needs. There is, however, a clear marriage between consideration of the stutterer's feelings and attitudes and the modification of stuttering behaviours. The third stage of *cognition* and *behaviour orientation* continues the process of reinforcement and facilitation of both self-evaluation and commitment.

The use of fluency-initiating gestures introduce behaviours which promote increased fluency and are methods which form a part of most therapeutic approaches. These are reduction of speech rate, easy voice onset combined with a consciously controlled inhalation. Control of loudness together with light articulatory contact during speech as well as manipulation of stress patterns are other concepts introduced to the child, usually together with the parents. Transfer to specific situations outside the clinic is the next procedure followed.

Cooper emphasises that therapeutic success or failure should be judged on changes in the client's fluency, attitudes, and feelings. He advises that evaluation follow-ups after therapy is terminated, should continue for at least three years. His own status report of evaluation insofar as children are concerned is couched in very general terms: i.e., four out of every five abnormally dysfluent pre-school children can be helped to achieve normal fluency by the time they complete the primary school years (approximately 80 per cent) (Cooper, 1984). Assessment and therapy procedures are well described in both the therapy package (Cooper and Cooper, 1976, 1985) and in a status report (Cooper, 1984).

Operant conditioning approaches

The issue of whether the young stutterer should be treated directly has often been considered in relation to the age of the child, i.e. treatment for the pre-school child should be indirect or preventive and treatment for the school-age child should most likely be a combination of indirect and direct work on stuttering symptoms. Several proponents of direct amelioration of stuttering, even in the very young child, include Costello (1983, 1984, 1985), Shine (1984a, 1984b), Ryan (1974, 1986) and Riley and Riley (1983, 1984). These authors take the view that the earlier the direct intervention in any communication disorder, the more likely the chance of success. They reject the idea that calling the young child's attention to stuttering will increase his/her awareness and exacerbate the problem. Some recent opinions offer support for this view (Cooper, 1984; Ingham, 1983). Both point out that at least some of the spontaneous remission reported may in fact be due to parental intervention of this nature.

Differential diagnosis ranges from the quite complex (Riley and Riley, 1983, 1984) to simpler forms prior to therapeutic intervention. Therapy is based on the principles of operant conditioning which in essence involves the manipulation of consequences to increase or decrease a behaviour; in this case to increase fluency and decrease stuttering. This feedback may be either positive (a reward) or negative (punishment). Costello (1981, 1983, 1985) succinctly states the rationale for this approach by pointing out several assumptions in the use of the indirect or parental counselling method which may be unwarranted. She points out that no valid empirical evidence exists to indicate that family and environmental variables are functionally related to stuttering and asks whether the clinician has the right to ask families to rearrange their lives when it cannot be said with any confidence which of any aspects in the child's environments are contributing to and maintaining stuttering. The second issue she raises is that attempting to change familial behaviour over which one has no control is at best a difficult process and certainly not one amenable to observation or measurement. The clinician is reliant on parental reports of unverifiable accuracy.

Instead, her approach is to directly teach the young child how to produce fluent speech, irrespective of environmental aspects. The treatment strategy is simple and structured, moving from short and simple fluent utterances to longer and more complex ones, termed the Extended Length of Utterances (ELU) programme which is similar to the Graduated Increase in Length and Complexity of Utterance (GILCU) of the Monterey Programme (Ryan, 1974, 1986). During each stage of the treatment programme, the child's behaviour is systematically rewarded or punished and in this way guided on to the next stage. Positive reinforcement for non-stuttered utterances is by means of a token system together with social reinforcement, i.e., positive verbal comments of a general nature.

Punishment contingencies for stuttering may take the form of the clinician saying 'stop' (time-out procedure) as soon as a stuttered utterance occurs so that the child does not continue speaking until the next trial begins. Reinforcers are gradually faded out as the programme progresses so as to prevent the child's becoming dependent on external feedback. In this approach, explanations of the rationale underlying therapy are not given to the child nor are they considered advisable.

Other components may be added to the treatment programme if deemed necessary (i.e., if adequate change in fluency is not attained and if evaluation indicates that certain aspects of the child's speech need attention). For example, rate control might be introduced by either instruction or modelling or a combination of both. Easy voice onset and the reduction of linguistic complexity in utterances are other possible additions, depending again on assessment data. Parents are involved as much as possible, observing every session and being taught to recognise fluent utterances and give positive reinforcers, but not to use punishment procedures. The latter is avoided because of the danger of inappropriate or excessive use of punishment and is controlled for by not having the parent perform a step in the programme until the child has satisfactorily performed at that level in the clinic.

Several questions arise when considering this approach. For one thing, how does the clinician ensure that parents do not use the punishment procedures they have observed in the clinic at home. Also, the therapy programme depends on the child performing various speaking tasks of increasing complexity in the clinic. Costello (1985) considers that any child speaking in connected utterances who has been labelled a stutterer may be a candidate for direct work on stuttering. However, some young children who stutter are not very verbal or are more interested in play activities which although capable of eliciting speech do not invariably lend themselves to structuring of speech situations. Young children who are engrossed in play situations may not attend to reinforcers. Childhood stuttering is very often cyclical, both in severity and occurrence and there may be too few examples of dysfluency in the clinic.

The force and simplicity of the approach is obvious but not its general applicability. In many cases, the clinician has no choice but to work with the family and the environment. Also, as Prins (1983) points out, there are many reported clinical observations that manipulating patterns of listening to and responding to the young stuttering child result in fluency changes. Evaluation data is sparse.

Wall and Myers (1984) present a model for the assessment and treatment of stuttering children which comprises the three factors known to be of interactive importance, namely, psycholinguistic, physiological and psycho-social factors. In their model, variables under each heading are examined and their contribution to the problem evaluated. Basically, theirs is an eclectic and broad-based view which considers the child's overall communicative functioning at every level and so provides the clinician with guidelines which will ensure that no possible contributing factor will be inadvertently ignored.

Effectiveness of Therapy

For most approaches, published evaluation data in general is at best incomplete and at worst vague and anecdotal. There is little data on recovery as a direct result of treatment available for scrutiny. Consequently, it is not really possible to exclude reported success rates from spontaneous recovery rates (i.e., an estimated 78 per cent based on the results of several studies, Andrews *et al.*, 1983). This observation is not meant to suggest that treatment approaches for children are of no or little benefit but rather to highlight the need to continue to obtain and publish information about the characteristics and progress of young stuttering children as they are treated. This means designing and implementing carefully-controlled longitudinal studies together with the appropriate control groups (see St. Louis and Westbrook, 1987 and Purser, 1987). Andrews (1985), however, puts this view more strongly by saying that no study purporting to benefit pre-school stutterers should be accepted unless it compares a randomised controlled trial of treatment with a placebo condition.

Conclusion

What is clear is that there is not, nor probably ever can be, a blanket approach to the treatment of childhood dysfluency. Obviously, a child who exhibits dysfluent speech behaviours sufficient to cause concern at any level needs to be considered in relation to all aspects of development and environment. Given the current state of our knowledge, it would seem wise to use a therapy programme that is concerned with all areas of language as suggested by Homzie and Lindsay (1984) rather than a purely symptomatic approach. But that is a matter for future research.

References

ADAMS, M.R. (1984a) The differential assessment and direct treatment of stuttering. In J. Costello (Ed.), *Speech Disorders in Children: Recent Advances*. San Diego: College Hill.

ADAMS, M.R. (1984b) The young stutterer: Diagnosis, treatment and assessment of progress. In W.H. Perkins (Ed.) *Stuttering Disorders*. New York: Thieme Stratton.

ANDREWS, G. (1985) Epidemiology of stuttering. In R.F. Curlee and W.H. Perkins (Eds), *Nature and Treatment of Stuttering: New Directions*. London: Taylor and Francis.

ANDREWS, G., CRAIG, A., FEYERS, A.M., HODDINOTT, S., HOWIE, P. and NEILSON, M. (1983) Stuttering: A review of research findings and theories circa 1982. *Journal of Speech and Hearing Disorders*, 48, 226–46.

ANDREWS, G. and HARRIS, M. (1964) *The Syndrome of Stuttering. Clinics in Developmental Medicine* (No. 17). London: Heinemann.

BJERKAN, B. (1980) Word fragmentations and repetitions in the spontaneous speech of 2–6 year-old children. *Journal of Fluency Disorders*, 5, 137–48.

BLOODSTEIN, O. (1981) *A Handbook of Stuttering* (3rd ed.) Chicago, IL: National Easter Seal Society.

BLOODSTEIN, O. and GROSSMAN, M. (1981) Early stutterings; Some aspects of their form and distribution. *Journal of Speech and Hearing Research*, 24, 298–302.

BROTHERTON, P. (1979) Speaking and not speaking: processes for translating ideas into speech. In A.W. Siegman and S. Feldstein (Eds), *Of Speech and Time*. Hillsdale, NJ: Lawrence Erlbaum.

COOPER, E.B. and COOPER, C.S. (1976) *Personalized Fluency Control Therapy Kit*. Hingham, MA: Teaching Resources.

COOPER, E.B. (1978) Facilitating parental participation in preparing the therapy component of the stutterer's individualised education program. *Journal of Fluency Disorders*, 3, 221–8.

COOPER, E.B. (1984) Personalized fluency control therapy; a status report. In M. Peins (Ed.), *Contemporary Approaches in Stuttering Therapy*. Boston: Little Brown.

COOPER, E.B. and COOPER, C.S. (1985) *Personalized Fluency Control Therapy*. Leicester: (Developmental Learning Materials) Taskmaster, Ltd.

COSTELLO, J. (1985) Treatment of the young chronic stutterer: Managing fluency. In

R.F. Curlee and W.H. Perkins (Eds), *Nature and Treatment of Stuttering: New Directions*. London: Taylor and Francis.

COSTELLO, J. (1984) Operant conditioning and the treatment of stuttering. In W.H. Perkins (Ed.), *Stuttering Disorders*. New York: Thieme Stratton.

COSTELLO, J. (1983) Current behavioral treatments for children. In D. Prins and R.J. Ingham (Eds), *Treatment of Stuttering in Early Childhood: Methods and Issues*. San Diego: College-Hill.

CURLEE, R.F. (1980) A case selection strategy for young disfluent children. *Seminars in Speech, Language and Hearing*, 1, 4, 277–87.

CURLEE, R.F. (1984) A case selection strategy for young disfluent children. In W.H. Perkins (Ed.) *Stuttering Disorders*. New York: Thieme Stratton.

FLOYD, S. and PERKINS, W.H. (1974) Early syllable dysfluency in stutterers and non-stutterers: A preliminary report. *Journal of Communication Disorders*, 7, 279–82.

GREGORY, H. (1973) *Stuttering: Differential Evaluation and Therapy*. Indianapolis: Bobbs-Merrill.

GREGORY, H. and HILL, D. (1980) Stuttering therapy for children. In W.H. Perkins (Ed.), *Strategies in Stuttering Therapy*. New York: Thieme Stratton.

GREGORY, H. (1985) Prevention of stuttering: Management of early stages. In R.F. Curlee and W.H. Perkins (Eds), *Nature and Treatment of Stuttering*. London: Taylor and Francis.

GREGORY, H. (1986) Environmental manipulation and family counselling. In G.H. Shames and H. Rubins (Eds), *Stuttering Then and Now*. Columbus, OH: Merrill.

GREGORY, H. and HILL, D. (1984) Stuttering therapy for children. In W.H. Perkins (Ed.), *Stuttering Disorders*. New York: Thieme Stratton.

HOMZIE, M.J. and LINDSAY, J.S. (1984) Language and the young stutterer: A new look at old theories and findings. *Brain and Language*, 2, 232–52.

HORSLEY, I. Linguistic characteristics of early dysfluency and normal non-fluency, in prep.

INGHAM, R.J. (1983) *Stuttering and Behavior Therapy: Current Status and Experimental Foundations*. San Diego: College Hill.

IRWIN, A. (1988) *Stammering in Young Children*. Wellingborough: Thorsons.

JOHNSON, W. AND ASSOCIATES (1959) *The Onset of Stuttering*. Minneapolis: University of Minnesota Press.

KENT, R.D. (1976) Anatomical and neuromuscular maturation of the speech mechanism; evidence from acoustic studies. *Journal of Speech and Hearing Research*, 19, 421–47.

KIDD, K.K. (1985) Stuttering as a genetic disorder. In R.F. Curlee and W.H. Perkins (Eds), *Nature and Treatment of Stuttering: New Directions*. San Diego: College Hill.

KOWAL, S., O'CONNELL, D.C. and SABIN, E.J. (1975) Development of temporal patterning and vocal hesitations in spontaneous narratives. *Journal of Psycholinguistic Research*, 4, 195–207.

PALERMO, D.S. and MOLFESE, D.L. (1972) Language acquisition from age five onward. *Psychological Bulletin*, 78, 409–28.

PRINS, D. (1983) Continuity, fragmentation, and tensions: Hypotheses applied to evaluation and intervention with preschool disfluent children. In D. Prins and R.J. Ingham (Eds), *Treatment of Stuttering in Early Childhood: Methods and Issues*. San Diego: College Hill.

PURSER, H. (1987) The psychology of treatment evaluation. In L. Rustin, D. Rowley and H. Purser (Eds), *Progress in the Treatment of Fluency Disorders*. London: Taylor and Francis.

RILEY, D.G. and RILEY, J. (1983) Evaluation as a basis for intervention. In D. Prins and R.J. Ingham (Eds), *Treatment of Stuttering in Early Childhood: Methods and Issues*. San Diego: College Hill.

RILEY, D.G. and RILEY, J. (1984) A component model for treating stuttering in children. In M. Peins (Ed.), *Contemporary Approaches in Stuttering Therapy*. Boston: Little Brown.

RUSTIN, L., ROWLEY, D. and PURSER, H. (Eds) (1987) *Progress in the Treatment of Fluency Disorders*. London: Taylor and Francis.

RUSTIN, L. and COOK, E. (1983) Intervention procedures for the disfluent child. In P. Dalton (Ed.), *Approaches to the Treatment of Stuttering*. Beckenham, Kent: Croom Helm.

RYAN, B. (1974) *Programmed Therapy for Stuttering in Children and Adults*. Springfield, IL: Charles C. Thomas.

RYAN, B. (1986) Operant procedures applied to stuttering therapy for children. In G.H. Shames and H. Rubin (Eds), *Stuttering Then and Now*. Columbus, OH: Merrill.

SABIN, E.J., CLEMMER, E.J., O'CONNELL, D.C. and KOWAL, S. (1979) A pausological approach to speech development. In A.W. Siegman and S. Feldstein (Eds), *Of Speech and Time*. Hilsdale, NJ: Lawrence Erlbaum.

SHINE, R.E. (1984a) Direct management of the beginning stutterer. In W.H. Perkins (Ed.), *Stuttering Disorders*. New York: Thieme Stratton.

SHINE, R.E. (1984b) Assessment and fluency training with the young stutterer. In M. Peins (Ed.), *Contemporary Approaches in Stuttering Therapy*. Boston: Little Brown.

ST. LOUIS, K. and WESTBROOK, J. (1987) The effectiveness of treatment for stuttering. In L. Rustin, D. Rowley and H. Purser (Eds), *Progress in the Treatment of Fluency Disorders*. London: Taylor and Francis.

VAN RIPER, C. (1973) *The Treatment of Stuttering*. Englewood Cliffs, NJ: Prentice-Hall.

VAN RIPER, C. (1982) *The Nature of Stuttering*. Englewood Cliffs, NJ: Prentice-Hall.

WALL, M.J. and MYERS, F.L. (1984) *Clinical Management of Childhood Stuttering*. Baltimore, MD: University Park Press.

WEXLER, K. and MYSAK, E. (1982) Disfluency characteristics of 2-, 4-, and 6-year-old males. *Journal of Fluency Disorders*, 7, 37–46.

WINGATE, M.E. (1983) Speaking unassisted: Comments on a paper by Andrews *et al. Journal of Speech and Hearing Research*, 48, 255–63.

YAIRI, E. (1982) Longitudinal studies of disfluencies in 2-year-old children. *Journal of Speech and Hearing Research*, 25, 155–60.

11 Cleft Palate and other Craniofacial Anomalies in Children

Jane Russell

The speech and language clinician now has a recognised and significant role in the management of children born with cleft lip and palate, from the identification of the abnormality and throughout the whole process of medical treatment into adulthood. Because of the physical defect, these children are known to be at risk for factors which adversely influence the development of normal communication skills. Although many will achieve normal speech and language with little or no direct intervention, their progress needs to be carefully monitored by a speech and language clinician so that any potential problems are detected and managed appropriately at an early stage. In addition, following recent advances in the medical treatment of the rarer and more complex craniofacial anomalies, such cases are beginning to be encountered in speech pathology clinics and may present with communication disorders associated with the physical defect or particular syndrome. These can be further complicated by associated conditions such as hearing loss, learning difficulties and psychosocial factors. These cases, therefore, also require careful assessment, monitoring and treatment by the speech and language clinician.

The aim of this chapter is to describe briefly cleft lip and palate and other craniofacial anomalies and to discuss the potential effects of a physical defect on speech and language development. In addition the ongoing role of the speech and language clinician in the management of such conditions is outlined. In the space available here it is only possible to present an overview of this subject. Reference is made to other texts where more detailed information can be found.

Cleft Lip and Palate

Cleft lip and cleft palate are the most common types of congenital orofacial defects. It is difficult to obtain exact figures but the incidence is estimated to be in the region of 1 in 750 live births (McWilliams, Morris and Shelton, 1984). This estimate is based on overt clefts which are diagnosed at birth and on a Caucasian population. There are some racial differences, for example, a higher incidence is reported for Chinese/Oriental people and American Indians and the lowest incidence for Afro-Caribbean people (McWilliams *et al.,* 1984). There are two genetically distinct groups, that is cleft lip with or without cleft palate CL(P) and isolated cleft palate (CP). Sparks (1984) describes how clefts can occur with other malformations (see further below) as part of a syndrome. 'Nonsyndromic' clefts (not symptoms of a syndrome) in both CL(P) and CP 'can be caused by familial etiology or be an isolated event' (Sparks, 1984, p. 76).

Facial clefts originate in the first three months in utero when the anatomical processes which will ultimately form the face, fail to fuse at the appropriate stage in embryological development (Bzoch and Williams, 1979; Watson, 1980; McWilliams *et al.,* 1984). The resultant defect ranges from slight to severe and can affect the lip, alveolus, hard palate and soft palate. Clefts may be unilateral, bilateral, or median and can occur in different combinations as described by McWilliams *et al.* (1984). Submucous clefts of the palate in which there are muscle and bone defects underlying what appears to be an intact palate, often remain undiagnosed unless they give rise to associated speech disorders. Similarly, other congenital defects resulting in 'palatopharyngeal incompetence' and hypernasal speech, in the absence of a cleft palate, are diagnosed from the resulting speech characteristics (McWilliams *et al.* 1984).

Surgery

In advanced countries, clefts of the lip and palate are routinely repaired surgically, usually in early childhood. There is considerable variation in the timing and type of surgical procedures and a continuing debate concerning the resultant effects on facial growth and speech development (Watson, 1980; McWilliams *et al.,* 1984; Pigott, 1986; Harding, 1988). In some centres orthodontists undertake pre-surgical orthopaedics prior to lip repair. This involves the use of an intra-oral appliance and lip strapping of the pre-maxilla in order to protect exposed nasal mucosa during feeding and to influence the alignment of the cleft segments of the lip and alveolus (Foster, 1980; Hathorn, 1986).

Craniofacial Anomalies

Craniofacial anomalies are anatomical deviations which may or may not include cleft palate. They are rare but as McWilliams (1984, p. 187) comments they 'constitute a major group of handicaps in children'. Such abnormalities can affect the oral and facial structures, the cranium or both. They are often complex and, as indicated above, may occur with cleft palate as features of a particular syndrome. Although it is possible for similar physical abnormalities to occur as a result of trauma, they are usually congenital and often of genetic origin (Sparks, 1984). McWilliams *et al.* (1984) provide a useful introduction to this subject. They describe the primary features, incidence, embryology, etiology, major hazards and communication problems associated with the syndromes such as Apert syndrome[1] and Crouzon disease.[2] Major hazards are factors such as poor life expectancy, severe disfigurement, physical limitations, hearing loss and psychosocial problems.

Craniofacial surgery

Until recently, congenital craniofacial abnormalities were generally considered to be untreatable. Witzel (1983) describes the development of craniofacial surgery and comments that 'the surgery is often drastic, detailed and dangerous'. She describes operative procedures (see also McWilliams *et al.* 1984) and the effects of craniofacial surgery on articulation and velopharyngeal function. Both Witzel (1983) and McWilliams *et al.* (1984) stress the need for a multi-disciplinary team approach to the management of patients with craniofacial anomalies. The speech and language clinician should be an integral member of such a team in order to document communication difficulties associated with craniofacial anomalies and to record changes in speech patterns following any operative procedures, even when there are no obvious speech problems initially.

Articulation problems associated with orofacial and craniofacial anomalies are described by Peterson-Falzone (1982), Witzel (1983) and McWilliams (1984). Although more severe structural defects are likely to result in greater articulation problems, both Peterson-Falzone and McWilliams comment on the lack of correlation between structure and articulatory function, and the ability of some patients to compensate for severe physical defects. In addition, McWilliams (1984) comments that speech therapy may not be effective in the presence of 'massive oral deformities'. Spontaneous improvement often occurs following surgery, without the need for speech therapy. It should be noted, however, that this does not apply in cases of late cleft palate repair, from about six years upwards, when almost all patients will need some speech therapy (Sell and Grunwell, personal communication).

However, it is often the conditions associated with craniofacial anomalies which give rise to the types of speech and language difficulties that require intervention. Language delay, for example, may result from mental retardation, hearing loss or psychosocial factors (McWilliams, 1984). It is, therefore, important for patients with craniofacial anomalies to receive a comprehensive assessment covering all aspects of communication development. The results of such an assessment must then be carefully evaluated in the context of any associated conditions and with regard to the overall team management of the child.

Cleft Palate and Communication Development

In this section the discussion focuses on the cleft palate anomalies but the reader will appreciate that many of the implications for communication development may also apply to other craniofacial anomalies. From birth the physical defect influences behaviours such as feeding and parent-child interaction, which in turn can subsequently influence normal communication development (Russell, 1989).

Feeding

One of the initial consequences of cleft lip and palate, except the most minor kind, is a disruption of feeding (Campbell and Watson, 1980). Because of the abnormal physical structures the infant is unable to establish normal sucking patterns. Abnormal feeding patterns and the physical defect can also affect oral motor and oro-sensory development (Edwards, 1980; Russell, 1989). Bzoch (1979, p. 73) suggests that abnormal neuromotor patterns may develop because 'auditory decoding and neuromotor encoding skills are learned when the vast majority of infants with a palatal defect have an abnormal mechanism'. Both the abnormal physical structures and neuromotor patterns may result in delayed, or deviant phonetic development.

A further effect of feeding difficulties is the potential disruption of normal mother-child interaction which is vitally important for pragmatic development (Carpenter, Mastergeorge and Coggins, 1983). If feeding is a slow, arduous process and causes anxiety, a pattern of negative interaction may develop. Mother and child may not have the time or inclination to participate in normal communicative interaction because of the pressures of the feeding situation (Russell, 1989).

Hearing

Otitis media is frequently present from birth in children with cleft palate and is thought to be due to Eustachian tube malfunction (Heller, 1979; Lencione, 1980; McWilliams *et al.,* 1984; Maw, 1986). This results in a conductive hearing loss which may fluctuate and which can seriously affect auditory skills and communication development (Bamford and Saunders, 1985). Sensori-neural hearing losses may also occur but much less frequently than conductive problems. In craniofacial anomalies there are often associated ear deformities and these can also result in conductive or sensori-neural hearing losses (McWilliams, 1984).

Parent/child communication

The effect of feeding on mother-child interaction and subsequent pragmatic development is indicated above. It is also possible that the presence of a physical defect will affect the parents' attitude to the child and thus their response to and initiation of communication. As Edwards (1980, p. 84) points out; 'it has been shown that parents of a child with a congenital handicap tend to regard them as being different long after they have in fact moved towards normality.' This may mean that parental expectations of a child's potential are underrated. Attempts by the child to communicate may not be recognised by the parents, particularly because the effects of the cleft on articulation development can cause different vocal output from that which might be expected from the normal child (Russell, 1989). From the start, therefore, the child may experience failure in communication which can result in delayed speech and language development.

Further stress can be placed on the parent-child relationship and communicative interaction by the experience of hospitalisation and the trauma of the operation itself (Russell, 1989). In addition, there is also the need to attend out-patient clinics for individual or joint consultations with a number of different professionals, such as the plastic surgeon, orthodontist, otolaryngologist and speech and language clinician. This places an additional strain on the parents, child and other members of the family, which again has the potential to affect family relationships and pragmatic development.

Language development

From the foregoing discussion it will be appreciated that the cleft palate child is at risk for delayed language development. In the many studies of the language development of cleft palate children, there is considerable variation in the aspects of language investigated and the variables taken into account (see McWilliams *et al.,* 1984 for a comprehensive survey). There is, however, general agreement that the language abilities of cleft palate children are delayed, particularly in expressive language development (Philips and Harrison, 1969; Nation, 1970; Pannbacker, 1971; Fox, Lynch and Brookshire, 1978; Bzoch, 1979; McWilliams *et al.,* 1984). The effect of cleft palate on the phonological aspects of language development is discussed below.

Studies involving younger children have shown that it is possible to detect delay in the pre-linguistic period of development (Fox *et al.,* 1978; Bzoch, 1979; Long and Dalston, 1982). Long and Dalston found that cleft palate children differed significantly from normal children in the development of 'paired gestural and vocal behaviour' at twelve months of age. The combination of gestural and vocal development is a prerequisite for early pragmatic development and is also linked to the origins of grammar (Griffiths, 1979). Fox *et al.* (1978) found that cleft palate children were performing less well than their normal peers on both linguistic and non-linguistic tasks even below the age of three years. Significant areas of difference were found on both receptive and expressive language subtests. There is, therefore, a need for close monitoring of the linguistic development of cleft palate children commencing in the prelinguistic period of development and continuing into later childhood.

Articulation and phonetic development

Recent studies of the babbling patterns of cleft palate children have confirmed delay and differences from the normal pattern of development (Mousset and Trichet, 1985; O'Gara and Logemann, 1985; Grunwell and Russell, 1987). Grunwell and Russell (1988), and O'Gara and Logemann (1985) report a predominance of glottal and 'back' articulation as well as the frequent occurrence of glides. Mousset and Trichet (1985) report a delay in the development of the voiceless plosives [p] [t] and [k] after palate repair, particularly in the group who had their operation at eighteen as opposed to six months of age. Dorf and Curtin (1982) report a higher incidence of 'compensatory articulations (mid-dorsum palatial stops, posterior nasal fricatives, velar fricatives, pharyngeal stops, pharyngeal fricatives and glottal stops)' in a group of children who had 'late' (after twelve months) as opposed to 'early' (prior to twelve months) palatal repairs.

Deviant phonetic patterns have also been reported in the speech of older cleft palate children. Bzoch (1979) and Morris (1979) both describe the predominance of glottal stop articulation, the use of pharyngeal fricatives and the lack of normal plosives and fricatives. Both authorities attribute these characteristics to velo-pharyngeal insufficiency (see further below) or abnormal learned motor patterns. Bzoch comments that the abnormal learned motor patterns can be identified 'as early as 3 years of age . . .' McWilliams *et al.* (1984) in an extensive review of the literature, illustrate the high risk of disordered articulation for cleft palate children and the occurrence of improvement with age, especially in the articulation of plosives and fricatives. They also point out the considerable variability between individual cleft palate children in the extent and nature of their speech sound errors and conclude that they are a heterogeneous population in this respect.

Phonological development

Ingram (1976) demonstrates by analysing data from previous studies that there are systematic processes in cleft palate speech. Following Ingram's lead, reports employing phonological techniques in the investigation of cleft palate children's speech have begun to appear in the literature (Hodson, Chin, Redmond and Simpson, 1983; Lynch, Fox and Brookshire, 1983; Broen, Felsenfeld and Bacon, 1986; Grunwell and Russell, 1988). Crystal (1981) highlights the need to investigate the speech of cleft palate children using phonological as well as phonetic analyses in order to determine the extent and nature of any deviance or delay and whether these result primarily from phonetic or phonological bases. McWilliams *et al.* (1984) also comment on how information about the child's phonological system helps in clinical speech therapy management. The relationship between phonetic and phonological development in the speech patterns of cleft palate children is described further in Russell (1989). It should also be stressed that a child with cleft palate may present with a phonological delay or disorder in the absence of or in addition to any phonetic deviance. This may be related to an overall expressive language delay as described above, or to other factors such as hearing problems.

Broen *et al.*, (1982) illustrate how phonological analysis helped to identify, at the age of 2.5, children requiring secondary surgery for velopharyngeal insufficiency. Lynch *et al.* (1983) report differences in the developing phonological systems of two children. For one subject, phonological analysis revealed the characteristics of developmental delay rather than deviation, whereas in the other subject deviant characteristics of 'structural inadequacy' were detected. Grunwell and Russell (1988) also studied two children and report differences in their phonological development. The results for one subject indicate the possibility of spontaneous recovery from phonetic deviance and relatively normal phonological development once palatal surgery has provided an intact intra-oral mechanism. For the second subject, however, there is evidence of persisting phonetic influence on phonological development. Both these studies bear out the observation of McWilliams *et al.*, (1984) mentioned above, that in respect of their articulatory patterns cleft palate children constitute a heterogeneous group. Each individual, therefore, requires a detailed speech assessment including both phonetic and phonological analyses.

Velopharyngeal insufficiency

Inappropriate nasal escape on non nasal consonants and vowels, and hypernasal resonance during speech may indicate velopharyngeal insufficiency (VPI). VPI occurs when the physical structures which constitute the velopharyngeal sphincter are inadequate or function inadequately. As a result the child is unable to build up sufficient intra-oral pressure for the articulation of oral phonemes, particularly plosives. The underlying cause may be a residual palatal fistula, poor soft palate function or a palate which is too short to reach the posterior pharyngeal wall. There may be associated facial movements such as 'nares constriction or facial grimacing during speech' (McWilliams *et al.,* 1984). Patients who are suspected of having VPI need careful investigation including assessment of nasal airflow during speech, radiographic and endoscopic procedures (Huskie, 1989). A comprehensive phonetic and phonological assessment of speech is also required (Russell, 1989). When there is consistent nasal escape and hypernasality as a result of structural inadequacy, rather than abnormal learned motor patterns (see phonetic development above), secondary surgery is usually indicated. Operative procedures employed in secondary surgery are described by Randall (1980).

In the space available here it has only been possible to give a brief overview of the influences of cleft palate on communication development. It has been demonstrated that such influences are potentially wide ranging and are not just concerned with the physical nature of the defect. It should also be remembered that, as well as being vulnerable to speech and language problems because of the cleft condition itself, cleft palate children are also subject to the same influences which affect the development of communication in the normal population. For example, a child with a cleft lip only may have a language disorder or delay which is unrelated to the physical condition.

The Role of the Speech and Language Clinician

Once palatal surgery has provided an intact intra-oral mechanism, many cleft palate children will achieve normal speech and language skills with little or no active speech therapy intervention. It is, however, important to monitor closely the communication development of all the children in order to identify as soon as possible those who will require specific help and/or further surgery. In some cases direct intervention may be unnecessary as a result of the ongoing advice and help which the speech and language clinician has given to the parents while monitoring the child's progress.

The clinician's involvement with the cleft palate child should commence at or soon after birth and may continue into the teenage years. The type and frequency of clinical involvement varies, however, according to the age and needs of the child and the counselling needs of the parents. The clinician, therefore, has to adopt a changing role in such cases. Management and treatment of the cleft palate child may be undertaken by the speech and language clinician who is an integral member of the cleft palate team, the clinician in the child's home locality or, in some cases, a combination of both. In the latter situation there should be close liaison between the clinician from the cleft palate team and the child's local clinician, concerning management of the child's communication development. In order to illustrate the changing role of the speech and language clinician the following discussion describes the clinical management of such children in a developmental chronology.

Before speech

Once the parents have come to terms with the cleft palate condition and have coped with initial problems such as feeding, their next major concern is often associated with speech development. The initial role of the speech and language clinician, therefore, is one of counsellor, although there may also be some involvement with regard to feeding. The aim of the clinician is to establish the foundations of a long term relationship with the parents and to provide them with accurate and comprehensible information regarding speech development. In some cases it is often helpful to supplement verbal with written information but this should be used with care (Russell, in press).

Excellent guidelines for those undertaking parent counselling are provided by MacDonald (1979). She emphasises the need to adopt a positive approach and to listen carefully in order to be guided by the parents themselves. In particular the clinician should avoid 'suggesting to the parents what they should be experiencing' by telling them what not to do, for example 'not to feel guilty . . .' (MacDonald, 1979). The counselling aspect of the speech and language clinician's role is ongoing and should continue throughout childhood and into adolescence and adulthood as required. The family's need for support will change over time and extra help may be required at times of stress, such as when children are in hospital for lip and palate operations, or in adolescence.

At the initial meeting with the parents a brief explanation of the speech and language clinician's involvement with cleft palate children is provided. It is explained that the physical defect may have implications for speech and language development, that many children will develop normal communication skills, but others may need further help from the clinician. This lays the foundation of the clinician's role in monitoring communication development (Russell, in press), which is usually carried out at subsequent clinic visits in conjunction with the cleft palate team, or with only the speech and language clinician. In some cases it is appropriate for the clinician to visit the child's home.

Most monitoring of early development is carried out through observation and discussion with the parents. Any cause for concern is then investigated in greater detail as appropriate. A knowledge of normal development is obviously essential and it can be useful to refer to developmental checklists such as the REEL scale (Bzoch and League, 1971). The speech and language clinician should monitor all aspects of communication development including parent-child interaction, the development of understanding and expression, and early phonetic development. Appropriate advice can then be offered to the parents who can be shown how to help their child progress on to the next stage of communication development.

The pre-school child

If there has been no previous concern regarding communication development a routine assessment should be carried out at about the age of 1.5 to 2.0 years, in order to ensure that the child is making satisfactory progress along normal lines. As in the pre-speech stage, all areas of communication development should be screened. The speech and language clinician needs to consider the whole child in relation to his environment. The assessment procedure, therefore, should not differ from that adopted for the speech and language assessment of any young child. Factors relating to the physical defect should obviously be taken into account but these must not prevent the clinician from being open-minded until a differential diagnosis is reached. It should be stressed that a specialist knowledge of cleft palate is not required, the speech and language clinician has the necessary expertise to assess and manage children of all ages. Applicable assessment procedures are outlined in McWilliams *et al.* (1984) and Russell (1989).

In the assessment of a child with a cleft palate or other craniofacial anomaly, there are some additional factors which need to be covered in the case history. Details of early feeding, the nature and extent of the original defect, and information about operations all need to be included. When discussing this with the parents the clinician will be able to gain some insight into their understanding of the problem and their attitudes towards the child (Russell, 1989). In addition, particular attention should be paid to the oro-facial examination (Huskie, 1989) as the child's articulatory ability may be directly related to dentition, occlusion, or the presence of a palatal fistula (residual, usually small, open cleft remaining following palatal surgery). As indicated above this may in turn influence phonetic and phonological development.

From the results of an initial assessment the clinician is able to identify areas which need further investigation and to implement appropriate action. This may involve reference to other members of the cleft palate team, as in the case of a child who appears to have hearing difficulties, and/or direct or indirect intervention from a speech and language clinician (see below). Cleft palate children should, of course, be receiving regular hearing checks and the routine developmental screening which is carried out on all children.

The school-age child

In an ideal situation the procedures of counselling, monitoring and assessment which have been outlined above will have been ongoing enabling early diagnosis and intervention and, to some extent, the prevention of secondary problems, for example reluctance to communicate because of unintelligible speech. Many cleft palate children will have achieved good communication skills by the time they reach school age but there will also be those who require continued help. This may be due to the severity of the communication problem, the lack of provision for early intervention and other factors such as poor attendance records for speech therapy.

The speech and language clinician should carry out informal and formal assessment procedures which are appropriate for the age of the child, and assess all areas of communication, including verbal comprehension, vocabulary, syntax, semantics, articulation, phonetic and phonological development and the pragmatic aspects. As highlighted above, factors relating to the physical defect and to the child's environment are taken into account in order to construct a profile of the child's communicative abilities. Appropriate intervention is based on the results of the assessment with referral to other professionals if necessary, for example, when further investigation of velopharyngeal function is indicated. When therapy is not indicated the clinician will continue to monitor the child's communicative abilities at regular intervals in order to record any changes and to identify whether help is needed at some time in the future.

With children of all ages one of the main responsibilities of the speech and language clinician is to document and report on the child's communicative development to other members of the cleft palate team. It is particularly important to include the results of the phonetic and phonological analysis, as well as other speech parameters, in the battery of procedures required to evaluate VPI (Van Demark, Bzoch, Daly, Fletcher, McWilliams, Pannbacker and Weinberg, 1985; Huskie, 1989). Some procedures such as nasal anemometry and radiography may be successfully used with pre-school children but the more invasive procedure of nasendoscopy requires a higher degree of active cooperation from the child (Pigott, 1980). The likelihood of success with this procedure increases in proportion with the age of the child. With regard to these investigations, the speech and language clinician takes an active role in the recording and interpretation of data with other members of the diagnostic team. Subsequently, the clinician may be involved in counselling the child and parents with regard to secondary surgery. Such surgery may be required to modify the results of the earlier primary lip or palate repair, for example closure of an oronasal fistula or adjustment to the shape of the lip. An operation termed a pharyngoplasty may be needed to provide a competent velopharyngeal sphincter in cases of VPI (Randall, 1980; Pigott, 1986). Further speech assessment and possibly intervention will be required following such surgery (Peterson-Falzone, 1982; McWilliams *et al.*, 1984).

Mainstream Treatment Practices

The methods of intervention employed by the speech and language clinician will vary according to the age and needs of the child and his family. With the very young child, intervention is usually implemented through the parents who, on a daily basis at home, carry out activities suggested and demonstrated by the clinician (Russell, 1989). Most intervention with young cleft palate children is carried out on an individual basis with the child and his parents. It may be appropriate however, to include children, from about three years of age, in groups. These may be made up of cleft palate or non-cleft palate children provided that the needs of the children are similar. Older children may be seen in an individual or group situation and there are considerable advantages when either of these methods are carried out on an intensive basis (Bzoch, 1979; Huskie, 1979; Albery and Enderby, 1984; Grunwell and Dive, 1988; Scanlon, personal communication).

Intervention strategies also vary according to the age of the child and his needs as indicated by the communication assessment. Strategies which can be used with the younger child are described in Hahn (1979); Philips (1979); Brookshire, Lynch and Fox (1980); McWilliams *et al.* (1984) and Russell (1989). Brookshire *et al.* (1980) provide detailed objectives for facilitating speech and language development from birth up to three years of age. These are presented in six monthly stages and this programme is a valuable resource for those lacking experience with younger children. Philips (1979) describes a programme for 'stimulating syntactic and phonological development' which she recommends is initiated when the child is between 1.5 and 2.0 years old. It is important to take advantage of what the child is doing naturally to reinforce and encourage appropriate development so that suitable activities become part of the daily routine (Russell, 1989).

With regard to the treatment of 'cleft palate speech' in older children, there is currently a trend towards a combination of articulatory and phonological strategies versus traditional articulation therapy per se (McWilliams *et al.,* 1984; Grunwell and Dive, 1988). Grunwell and Dive studied two children who attended an intensive therapy course and demonstrated that a combined articulatory and phonological strategy 'facilitates the reorganisation and expansion of previously static phonological systems, sometimes in spite of persisting articulatory disabilities, sometimes accompanied by improvements in articulatory abilities'. The strategy adopted by the clinician is obviously directly related to the results of the assessment: for example some children will need help with language and not speech development. In view, however, of the evidence provided by Grunwell and Dive (1988), a phonological approach will enhance and broaden articulation therapy.

McWilliams (1984) comments with regard to speech problems associated with craniofacial anomalies, that 'therapy for these patients does not differ in any remarkable way from speech therapy in general'. This as also applicable to children with cleft palate except perhaps in cases where VPI is a significant factor. Even then the clinician can often continue to work on different aspects of speech, such as encouraging appropriate tongue placements, while waiting for investigations of velopharyngeal function to be implemented. Albery (1986) stresses that the clinician 'should always be aware of the possibility of potential competence' of the velopharyngeal sphincter and recommends a period of diagnostic therapy for children with 'a total glottal stop pattern'. The child may therefore learn to produce some consonants, such as bilabial plosives, with the correct articulatory placement, which may improve intelligibility even when there is nasal escape resulting from VPI.

When it appears that VPI is not a result of abnormal physical structures but is due to the inadequate function of a potentially competent velopharyngeal mechanism, the use of tongue and palate training aids or biofeedback may be indicated (McWilliams *et al.,* 1984; Hardcastle, 1984; Stuffins, 1989). Prior to the use of training aids, detailed assessment is required along with close liaison with other professionals such as the orthodontist. It is also important to continue therapy while an aid is being used (Stuffins, 1989). Biofeedback devices, such as the Nasal Anemometer which visually indicates nasal airflow (Ellis, 1979) and the Electro-palatograph (Hardcastle, 1984) which visually displays tongue contacts against the hard palate, can be used to help the child learn to control the movements of the articulators.

In some cases it may be necessary for the speech and language clinician to compromise over some aspects of speech development. This may occur when accurate articulation is difficult for the child to achieve due to dental or occlusal abnormalities causing, for example, some lateral escape of air on an /s/. In such instances the decision regarding further therapy depends on the results of the oral examination, the phonetic and phonological analysis, and the motivation of the child. If the problem does not cause the child to be misunderstood and if he is unconcerned, therapy is unlikely to be effective. The clinician should continue to review the child at regular intervals and therapy may be indicated following orthodontic treatment or secondary surgery.

Conclusion

In this chapter the role of the speech and language clinician in the management of children with orofacial defects, in particular cleft palate, has been outlined. The continuing nature of this role from birth and through childhood into adolescence and adulthood has been discussed. It has been demonstrated that the same basic principles of therapeutic practice which are used routinely by the clinician are applicable to the assessment and management of children with cleft palate. The clinician should take into account relevant factors related to the physical defect but a specialist knowledge of cleft palate is not required. When necessary the clinician is able to refer to appropriate texts for further information and to seek the advice of a more experienced colleague who works routinely as a member of a cleft palate or craniofacial team.

Notes

1   *Apert Syndrome* (Peterson-Falzone, 1982; McWilliams, 1984; McWilliams *et al.,* 1984). Apert's syndrome is always characterised by craniosynostotis (premature osseous union of bones that are normally distinct) and syndactyly (webbing or union) of the hands and feet. Such children have a high steep forehead, a flattened occiput, hypertelorism and exopthalmos. Thirty per cent of cases have a cleft of the soft palate but a high arched complete palate is more common. Mental retardation may occur in as many as 50 per cent of those affected. Communication skills are affected by factors such as severe malocclusion, an abnormal nasopharyngeal airway, the anomalous shape of the palatal vault, hearing loss and psychosocial problems.

2   *Crouzon Disease* (Peterson-Falzone, 1982; McWilliams, 1984; McWilliams *et al.,* 1984). Crouzon disease is also known as craniofacial dysostosis. It is less severe than Apert syndrome and is characterised by an abnormally shaped head, maxillary hypoplasia (midfacial deficiency), prognathism (prominent mandible), hypertelorism (wide set eyes), exophthalmus (protruding eyes) and low set ears. These children are not usually mentally retarded. They may have essentially normal speech but defective speech is usually related to structural abnormalities. Airway problems can restrict respiration and conductive hearing losses are common.

References

ALBERY, E.H. (1986) Type and assessment of speech problems. In E.H. Albery, I.S. Hathorn and R.W. Pigott (Eds), *Cleft Lip and Palate: A Team Approach.* Bristol: Wright.

ALBERY, E. and ENDERBY, P. (1984) Intensive speech therapy for cleft palate children. *British Journal of Disorders of Communication,* 19, 115–24.

BAMFORD, J. and SAUNDERS, E. (1985) *Hearing Impairment, Auditory Perception and Language Disability.* London: Edward Arnold.

BROEN, P.A., FELSENFELD, S. and KITTLESON BACON, C. (1986) *Predicting from the Phonological Patterns Observed in Children with Cleft Palate.* Paper presented at the Symposium on Research in Child Language Disorders, University of Wisconsin, Madison.

BROOKSHIRE, B.L., LYNCH, J.I. and FOX, D.R. (1980) *A Parent-Child Cleft Palate Curriculum: Developing Speech and Language.* Oregon: C.C. Publications.

BZOCH, K.R. (1979) Etiological factors related to cleft palate speech. In K.R. Bzoch (Ed.), *Communicative Disorders Related to Cleft Lip and Palate.* Boston: Little, Brown.

BZOCH, K.R. and LEAGUE, R. (1971) *Assessing Language Skills in Infancy.* Baltimore: University Park Press.

BZOCH, K.R. and WILLIAMS, W.M. (1979) Introduction, rationale, principles and related basic embryology and anatomy. In K.R. Bzoch (Ed.), *Communicative Disorders Related to Cleft Lip and Palate.* Boston: Little Brown.

CAMPBELL, M.L. and WATSON, A.C.H. (1980) Management of the neonate. In M. Edwards and A.C.H. Watson (Eds), *Advances in the Management of Cleft Palate.* London: Churchill Livingstone.

CARPENTER, R.L., MASTERGEORGE, A.M. and COGGINS, T.E. (1983) The acquisition of communicative intention in infants eight to fifteen months of age. *Language and Speech,* 26, 101–16.

CRYSTAL, D. (1981) *Clinical Linguistics.* Vienna: Springer.

DORF, D.S. and CURTIN, J.W. (1982) Early cleft palate repair and speech outcome. *Plastic and Reconstructive Surgery,* 70, 74–9.

EDWARDS, M. (1980) Speech and language disability. In M. Edwards and A.C.H. Watson (Eds), *Advances in the Management of Cleft Palate.* Edinburgh: Churchill Livingstone.

ELLIS, R.E. (1979) The Exeter nasal anemometry system. In R.E. Ellis and F.C. Flack (Eds), *Diagnosis and Treatment of Palato Glossal Malfunction.* London: The College of Speech Therapists.

FOSTER, T.D. (1980) The role of orthodontic treatment. In M. Edwards and A.C.H. Watson (Eds), *Advances in the Management of Cleft Palate.* Edinburgh: Churchill Livingstone.

FOX, D., LYNCH, J. and BROOKSHIRE, B. (1978) Selected developmental factors of cleft palate children between two and thirty-three months of age. *Cleft Palate Journal,* 15, 239–46.

GRIFFITHS, P. (1979) Speech acts and early sentences. In P. Fletcher and M. Garman (Eds), *Language Acquisition.* Cambridge: Cambridge University Press.

GRUNWELL, P. and DIVE, D. (1988) Treating 'cleft palate speech': Combining phonological techniques with traditional articulation therapy. *Child Language Teaching and Therapy,* 4, 193–210.

GRUNWELL, P. and RUSSELL, J. (1987) Vocalisations before and after cleft palate surgery. *British Journal of Disorders of Communication,* 22, 1–17.

GRUNWELL, P. and RUSSELL, J. (1988) Phonological development in children with cleft lip and palate. *Clinical Linguistics and Phonetics,* 2, 75-95.

HAHN, E. (1979) Directed home training program for infants with cleft lip and palate. In Bzoch, K.R. (Ed.), *Communicative Disorders Related to Cleft Lip and Palate.* Boston: Little Brown.

HARDCASTLE, W.J. (1984) New methods of profiling normal and abnormal lingual palatal contact patterns. *Work in Progress, University of Reading Phonetics Laboratory,* 4, 1–40.

HARDING, A. (1988) A comparison of the speech results after early and delayed hard palate closure. *British Journal of Plastic Surgery.*

HATHORN, I.S. (1986a) Classification. In E.H. Albery, I.S. Hathorn and R.W. Pigott (Eds), *Cleft Lip and Palate: A Team Approach*. Bristol: Wright.

HATHORN, I.S. (1986b) Dental management. In E.H. Albery, I.S. Hathorn and R.W. Pigott (Eds), *Cleft Lip and Palate: A Team Approach*. Bristol: Wright.

HELLER, J.C. (1979) Hearing loss in patients with cleft palate. In Bzoch, K.R. (Ed.), *Communicative Disorders Related to Cleft Lip and Palate*. Boston: Little Brown.

HODSON, B.W., CHIN, L., REDMOND, B. and SIMPSON, R. (1983) Phonological evaluation and remediation of speech deviations of a child with a repaired cleft palate: A case study. *Journal of Speech and Hearing Disorders*, 48, 93–8.

HUSKIE, C.F. (1979) Intensive therapy — Glasgow experience. In R.E. Ellis and F.C.Flack (Eds), *Diagnosis and Treatment of Palato Glossal Malfunction*. London: The College of Speech Therapists.

HUSKIE, C.F. (1989) Assessment of speech and language status: Subjective and objective approaches to the appraisal of vocal tract structure and function. In J. Stengelhofen (Ed.), *Cleft Palate: The Nature and Remediation of Communication Problems*.

INGRAM, D. (1976) *Phonological Disability in Children*. London: Edward Arnold.

LENCIONE, R.M. (1980) Associated conditions. In M. Edwards and A.C.H. Watson (Eds), *Advances in the Management of Cleft Palate*. London: Churchill Livingstone.

LONG, M. and DALSTON, R.M. (1982) Paired gestural and vocal behaviour in one-year-old cleft lip and palate children. *Journal of Speech and Hearing Research*, 47, 403–6.

LYNCH, J.L., FOX, D.R. and BROOKSHIRE, B.L. (1983) Phonological proficiency of two cleft palate toddlers with school age follow up. *Journal of Speech and Hearing Disorders*, 48, 274–85.

MACDONALD, S.K. (1979) Parental needs and professional responses: A parental perspective. *Cleft Palate Journal*, 16, 118–92.

McWILLIAMS, B.J. (1984) Speech problems associated with craniofacial anomalies. In. W.H. Perkins (Ed.), *Recent Advances: Speech Disorders*. San Diego: College Hill.

McWILLIAMS, B.J., MORRIS, H.L. and SHELTON, R.L. (1984) *Cleft Palate Speech*. London: B.C. Decker.

MAW, A.R. (1986) Ear disease. In E.H. Albery, I.S. Hathorn and R.W. Pigott (Eds), *Cleft Lip and Palate: A Team Approach*. Bristol: Wright.

MORRIS, H.L. (1979) Evaluation of abnormal articulation patterns. In K.R. Bzoch, (Ed.), *Communicative Disorders Related to Cleft Lip and Palate*. Boston: Little Brown.

MOUSSET, M.R. and TRICHET, C. (1985) *Babbling and Phonetic Acquisitions After Early Complete Surgical Repair of Cleft Lip and Palate*. Paper presented at the Fifth International Congress on Cleft Palate and Related Craniofacial Abnormalities, Monte Carlo.

NATION, J.E. (1970) Vocabulary comprehension and usage of preschool cleft palate and normal children. *Cleft Palate Journal*, 7, 639–44.

O'GARA, M.M. and LOGEMANN, J.A. (1985) *Phonetic Analysis Pre and Post Palatoplasty*. Paper presented at ASHA convention.

PANNBACKER, N. (1971) Language skills of cleft palate children: A review. *British Journal of Disorders of Communication*, 6, 37–44.

PETERSON-FALZONE, S.J. (1982) Articulation disorders in orofacial anomalies. In N.J. Lass, Yoder and McReynolds (Eds), *Speech, Language and Hearing.*

PIGOTT, R. (1980) Assessment of velopharyngeal function. In M. Edwards and A.C.H. Watson (Eds), *Advances in the Management of Cleft Palate.* London: Churchill Livingstone.

PIGOTT, R. (1986) Primary repair of the cleft lip and palate. In E.H. Albery, I.S. Hathorn and R.W. Pigott (Eds), *Cleft Lip and Palate: A Team Approach.* Bristol: Wright.

PHILIPS, B.J.W. (1979) Stimulating syntactic and phonological development in infants with cleft palate. In K.R. Bzoch (Ed.), *Communicative Disorder Related to Cleft Lip and Palate.* Boston: Little Brown.

PHILIPS, B.J. and HARRISON, R.J. (1969) Language skills of preschool cleft palate children. *Cleft Palate Journal,* 6, 108–19.

RANDALL, P. (1980) Secondary surgery. In M. Edwards and A.C.H. Watson (Eds), *Advances in the Management of Cleft Palate.* London: Churchill Livingstone.

RUSSELL, J. (1988) Early intervention. In J. Stengelhofen (Ed.), *Cleft Palate: The Nature and Remediation of Communication Problems.* London: Churchill Livingstone.

SCANLON, E. (1987) Personal communication.

SELL, D. and GRUNWELL, P. (1988) Personal Communication (Sri Lanka Project).

SPARKS, S.N. (1984) *Birth Defects and Speech-Language Disorders.* San Diego: College Hill.

STUFFINS, G. (1989) The use of tongue and palate training aids in the treatment of speech problems. In J. Stengelhofen (Ed.), *Cleft Palate: The Nature and Remediation of Communication Problems.* London: Churchill Livingstone.

VAN DEMARK, D., BZOCH, K., DALY, D., FLETCHER, S., McWILLIAMS, B.J., PANNBACKER, M. and WEINBERG, B. (1985) Methods of assessing speech in relation to velopharyngeal function. *Cleft Palate Journal,* 22, 281–5.

WATSON, A.C.H. (1980) Embryology of cleft lip and palate. In M. Edwards and A.C.H. Watson (Eds), *Advances in the Management of Cleft Palate.* London: Churchill Livingstone.

WITZEL, M.A. (1983) Speech problems in craniofacial anomalies. *Communicative Disorders,* 8, 4, 45 59.

II COMMUNICATION DISORDERS IN ADULTS

12   Aphasia: Theory-based Intervention

Ruth Lesser

Like many other definitions, the definition of aphasia (here used as synonymous with acquired dysphasia) has fuzzy boundaries. Classically it is described as a language disorder resulting from the sudden onset (or relatively sudden onset) of focal brain damage. The delimitation of what language is, however, has been shifting, and with it the delimitation of what constitutes a language disorder. For example, the inclusion of pragmatics and paralinguistics within the proper study of linguistics has extended our awareness of the communication difficulties experienced by people who have right brain damage but who would be excluded from the classical definition of aphasia. Similarly major developments in aphasiology have occurred through the involvement of cognitive psychologists, whose interest in aphasic language is as a variety of normal language; for them the fact, location and extent of damage to the brain is of subsidiary interest to how some speakers may be used to show fractionation of normal language processing.

The classical definition has also become blurred on another front, beside the linguistic and the psychological, and this is in respect of the focal nature of the brain damage. Developments in brain imaging have shown that anatomical location of a site of lesion, as established through transmission computerised tomography, is not necessarily the same as the 'functional' lesion, as established through the various types of investigations of cerebral blood flow. The damage may extend beyond a focal area. Particularly in some types of aphasia the expected damage is extensive rather than focal (for example, as in 'isolation of the speech area'). There is also, therefore, some controversy as to whether other patients with language disorders accompanied by widespread and scattered cerebral damage, as in multi-infarct dementia, should properly be described as aphasic, when the language disorder is but one facet of a generalised cognitive impairment.

Fortunately for the purpose of this chapter we can step delicately out of this minefield by using an empirical definition. Aphasia is the language disorder experienced by individuals who are referred to the speech therapist after observation and/or some screening procedure has indicated the relatively sudden development of some difficulty in understanding and/or producing speech and/or writing where there has been no such previous difficulty. Although in the great majority of cases referred to the speech therapist, the 'ands' will apply rather than the 'ors', this will allow us to include within the speech therapist's province the rare cases of single modality impairment. More importantly it allows us to be flexible as to the nature of aphasia, while insight into the nature of language develops and, in parallel, let us hope, the skills of the observers and screeners (patient, relative, nurse, doctor) who seek the therapist's help.

Causative Factors

The event which precipitates a referral to the speech therapist for investigation for or of aphasia is most likely to be a stroke. According to Vignolo (1988) up to 70 per cent of referrals for rehabilitation of language have this aetiology of cerebrovascular lesion. Such an interference with the blood supply of the brain can result from some form of blockage of an artery, or from a haemorrhage. Both cut off the supply to the areas fed by the artery and its branches, but the haemorrhage has the additional complication of leaving a build up of fluid and clot which may have pressure effects on a more extensive area of brain. Haemorrhage is therefore sometimes followed by surgery to remove the clot or to prevent further bursts by clipping of a weak place on an artery. Aphasia may also arise after surgery when a life-threatening tumour or arterio-venous malformation has been removed. Slow-growing tumours which affect only the glial cells of the brain (gliomas) rather than the neurones themselves may produce very little effect on language, until surgery is undertaken which removes the whole brain tissue involved.

Another cause of aphasia is head-injury (either open or closed) from road traffic accidents (particularly to unprotected pedestrians), street violence, domestic battering and dangerous sports. The damage in closed head injuries tends to affect the surface of both cerebral hemispheres, and often the brain stem as well, resulting in forms of dysarthria with aphasia which are different from those caused by stroke, in which unilateral subcortical structures may be involved as well as cortical. Aphasia can also result from a variety of other causes: infections resulting in encephalitis, deprivation of oxygen supply (as in carbon monoxide poisoning, or arterial spasm during an operation), other kinds of toxicity, inflammatory diseases, abscesses and degenerative or psychiatric conditions.

Assessment and Treatment

In what follows these two aspects of the speech therapist's involvement with aphasia have not been separated. This is not only because treatment cannot be planned without assessment, but because both are continuing and interactive commitments for the therapist. In our present state of knowledge (and the field is so complex that this is likely to remain valid for many decades to come), assessment is a matter of forming hypotheses which responses to intervention will test and modify. Aphasia therapy is therefore of a very different order from the dominant medical model, in which a patient's symptoms lead to a diagnostic category which has a recommended prescriptive treatment. Speech therapists working with aphasic adults have, in fact, for a long time been seeking theories of aphasia which could explain why what they have been doing intuitively with their patients sometimes seems to work and sometimes does not.

Theoretical Bases of Intervention

Neurological theory

The first elaborated theory of aphasia was the neurological one — initially proposed in the nineteenth century by Wernicke, popularised more recently by Geschwind in the form of connectionist theory. This theory proposes that there are zones in the brain which control particular language functions, and tracts which connect them. Damage to these zones and tracts can account for the various phenomena of apraxia, alexia without agraphia and varieties of aphasia. The theory unfortunately brings with it few implications for aphasia therapy. From it an influential battery of tests has been developed, the *Boston Diagnostic Examination of Aphasia* (Goodglass and Kaplan, 1983), which claims to provide a 'comprehensive assessment of the assets and liabilities of the patient in all language areas as a guide to therapy'. These implications for therapy have never been spelled out in detail — possibly because the authors of the Examination are not speech and language therapists. The implications drawn from the test in practice seem to be that, having found that the patient has problems with particular tasks on the Examination, the therapist should work on that particular difficulty. For example, if the patient fails on Complex Ideational Material in the Auditory Comprehension Section, the inference is often drawn that the therapist should devise practices to improve that skill. As a theory of language, this only skims the surface.

We fare a little better with the neurological theory in respect of the syndromes which it has specified (Broca's aphasia, Wernicke's aphasia, anomia, etc). Therapy programmes have been devised which are targeted at such specific syndromes: e.g.,

Helm-Estabrooks' (1981) HELPSS, or Helm Elicited Language Program for Syntax Stimulation, for the agrammatic component of Broca's aphasia, and SLAC, Sentence Level Auditory Comprehension treatment, Naeser, Haas, Mazurski and Laughlin's (1986) programme for comprehension difficulties in Wernicke's aphasia. A further addition to the therapist's repertoire from the neurological theory has been the notion of right hemisphere stimulation to assist in language recovery by the left hemisphere or to develop latent language in the right hemisphere. The best known application of this is Melodic Intonation Therapy (Sparks and Holland, 1976), which draws on the prosodic abilities of the right hemisphere. None of these, however, helps us into a deep understanding of the nature of the language deficit in aphasia. The whole notion of syndromes as applied to aphasia has been severely criticised on the grounds that they are polythetic, with heterogeneous elements combined (see, for example, Ellis, 1987). As a theory basis for therapy, therefore, what they can offer provides little advance beyond what clinicians already get from intuition.

Unitary theory

A second theory of aphasia has been the unitary theory, in its various forms of asymbolia, specific language disorder and reduction of efficiency. For the aphasia therapist its dominant influence has been through the ideas of Schuell (Schuell, Jenkins and Jiminez-Pabon, 1964), herself a speech pathologist. She proposed a model of language which required concerted action from the whole of the brain, subcortical structures as well as cortical. She accounted for the superficial differences amongst types of aphasia in terms of different kinds of non-aphasic deficits being added to simple aphasia — for example, sensorimotor deficits adding articulation difficulties, and visual deficits adding particular problems with reading. She advocated and described a range of techniques for coping with essential aphasia and these additional difficulties, which are still widely used in many clinics today. Unitary theory as Schuell propounded it has fallen out of fashion, however, largely due to the advent of a more powerfully explanatory and testable theory, which I shall discuss shortly. Nonetheless there are still elements of unitary theory which provide a valuable complement to more modern ideas. We see these in Luria's (1966) theory, which reconciles neurological and unitary theory. Neurologically localisable syndromes are proposed (afferent motor, semantic, sensory, etc.), but as well there is explanation in terms of disruption in neurophysiological activities which concern the whole brain such as excitation, inhibition, perseveration, retention of traces, inertia. The current expressions of such a modified unitary theory are in terms of control systems (see Butterworth and Howard, 1987, for an example applied to jargonaphasia), accounts of the disparity between willed and automatic processing (Schacter, McAndrews and Moscovitch, 1988), and a new 'connectionism' which has nothing to do with Wernicke-Geschwind theory but is derived from computer modelling. This employs processors connected in parallel and engages in interactive parallel activity rather than serial activity referred back to a central memory store (see Schneider, 1987, for an introduction, and Allport, 1985, for an application to anomia). The unitary theory of aphasia is not therefore to be dismissed as entirely superceded, although, in the form in which Schuell expressed it, it comes nowhere near to accounting for the complex phenomena of aphasia.

Linguistic theories

I have mentioned theories devised by neurologists (and supported by psychologists working with them) and by a speech pathologist. What about the other major discipline to which aphasiology looks for help, linguistics? Linguistics has in fact been extremely helpful to aphasiology, but it has primarily been through providing frameworks for description and analysis (notably the framework which distinguishes the language domains of phonology, syntax, semantics and pragmatics). For clinical practice it has provided theory-based notions of rank order of complexity in language, for example in terms of distinctive features in phonology, of phrase structure trees in syntax and of sense relations in semantics. It has also provided empirically derived rank orders associated with order of acquisition by children. There have been attempts to apply to aphasia specific linguistic theories as these have emerged. Examples are Jakobson's (1964) interpretation of Luria's syndromes, applying the linguistic notion of paradigmatic and syntagmatic dimensions of language, the attempts of Meyerson and Goodglass (1972) to account for aphasic difficulties in terms of transformational complexity, essays of my colleagues and myself at applying Bresnan's lexical functional grammar (Lesser, 1985), and the current interpretations of aphasia by Caplan and his colleagues (Hildebrandt, Caplan and Evans, 1987) in terms of government and binding theory. In as much as they make a contribution to aphasia therapy, these efforts have so far added depth to our knowledge of what makes language complex, but they have not yet led to direct applications to remediation.

Sociolinguistic description

There is one aspect of linguistics which is rather further ahead in its implications for therapy, and that is the study of conversational analysis by sociolinguistics. Of particular concern to sociolinguists is the study of the varieties of spoken language (and a reminder that spoken language is very different from written language). The message has well and truly been got across in aphasia therapy that the therapist is concerned in restoring, not some abstract norm of language, but the colloquial spoken language of individual patients in their particular speech communities and social networks. As distinct from central language as a medium for the user's thoughts, spoken language had a dual function. It serves to give and receive information and control the behaviour of others, but it also serves a solidarity function. It establishes the individual in a social context through the style and accent in which he or she speaks and in the content of what is said, including social small talk. The aphasia therapist has to be sensitive to this second dimension of the patient's needs as well as to disruptions in the central use of language and the more obvious information-giving use of language. Hence there is a burgeoning interest for aphasia therapists in conversational analysis.

Detailed work is now being undertaken into the behaviour of aphasic individuals and their partners during conversational exchanges (see, for example, de Bleser and Weisman, 1986). To what extent do aphasic speakers retain turn-taking abilities, use cohesive devices for linking sections of discourse, achieve clarifications and repairs, for example? Although there are now a number of protocols for measuring this aspect of language (Skinner, Wirz, Thompson and Davidson, 1984; Penn, 1985; Prutting and Kirchner, 1987), they have the limitation of assessing only the aphasic speaker rather than the dynamic exchange between both partners in the conversational dyad, and more sensitive protocols are needed which analyse the exchange itself. To cater for this dimension of language use, the aphasia therapist needs to think of the patient not as an isolated individual but as a member of a community. Very often this may be a shrunken community due to the physical and communication handicaps. The therapist may seek to extend this where possible, for example by introducing the patient to a Speech after Stroke Club or by arranging for visiting volunteers where this is appropriate; but much of the therapist's efforts will be directed at improving the patient's spouse's understanding of the aphasic's conversational limitations, so that joint communication can be enhanced. Examples of the application of this aspect of sociolinguistic theory can be found in Green (1984).

Psycholinguistics models

I want to turn now to a different approach to aphasia therapy, which is also derived from theory, and which stems from another discipline, psycholinguistics as developed by cognitive psychologists. Its application to aphasia has become known as the cognitive neuropsychological approach. A key notion in this approach is that mental processes are organised in modules. These modules are essentially distinct from each other in their functions although they work interactively and cooperatively. This is not a neurological model, and there is no implication that these modules are specifically localised in any centres in the brain, nor indeed that they have to be physically real in terms of having a specific brain substrate. They use essentially abstract notions such as 'logogens', 'buffers', 'phonemes', 'graphemes'. They do, however, seem to be psychologically and neuropsychologically real, in that brain damage seems to show that the language system can fractionate in such a way as to disturb modules selectively.

Since early psycholinguistic studies focused on single words, the best developed cognitive neuropsychological models concern the processing of single words. Fig. 12.1 shows a simple cross-modal model of the processes which intervene between hearing or reading single words and repeating them or writing them. Much of the evidence in support of such a model comes from psychologists' experiments with normal subjects (mostly students), but the models have been refined from observations of brain damaged adults. For example, the notion that there may be two lexical routes in writing to dictation, one which bypasses the semantic/cognitive system as well as one which uses that system, is based on observations from brain-damaged individuals (Patterson, 1986). For the aphasia therapist to apply such a model to the remediation of reading or spelling difficulties in a patient, it is necessary first to be able to identify which of these hypothetical modules or processes may be malfunctioning.

Reading

To take reading aloud as an example, the therapist needs to test whether the patient's reading aloud shows the influence of variables which can be linked back to different modules. If the disorder is in the visual word analysis system, there will be effects of the length of the word, and possibly of the visual form of presentation (though note that the absence of an effect may be significant also, e.g., if the individual is using a letter-by-letter strategy, the presence of crosses between each letter may not reduce speed of reading, as it does with normal subjects). If the reader is predominantly using the subword route to phonological assembly rather than the visual input lexicon, there will be effects of whether or not the word has an irregular print-to-sound correspondence. For example, a word like COLONEL may be read as /kolonɛl/ rather than /kɜnal/. On the other hand non-words or unfamiliar words should be read correctly, since the subword route is the normal way for coping with such novelties. If the patient cannot read non-words, this suggests malfunction of the subword route and reliance on the visual input lexicon. There should therefore be a significant effect of word frequency, since word frequency norms are based specifically on counts of the number of times whole words have appeared in print. If processing draws on the semantic/cognitive system there are likely to be effects of

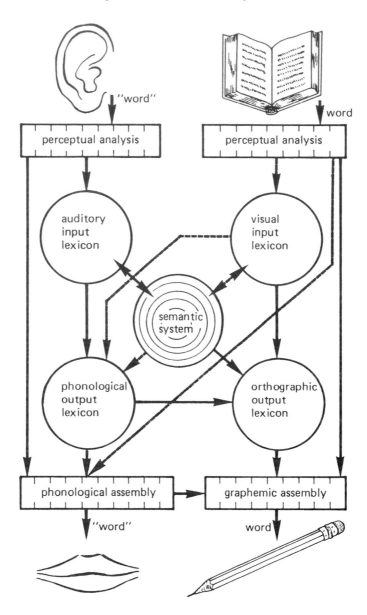

Figure 12.1

the imageability ratings of the words, with high imagery words producing fewer errors than low imagery words. There may also be effects which show the influence of other language processes, in that grammatical words result in more errors than nouns, and that inflected and derived words cause more mistakes.

From such measurements, different types of alexia (or dyslexia) syndromes have been described (e.g., surface, phonological, deep and visual dyslexias). In surface dyslexia the lexical route is impaired, and reading shows the effects of use of the subword route. In phonological dyslexia, the subword route is impaired. Deep dyslexia is like phonological dyslexia with added complications implicating the semantic and grammatical systems. Visual dyslexia shows significant effects of word length, and implicates the visual word analysis system. There are many differences of behaviour within these and other dyslexia syndromes, and the same criticism of heterogeneity has been applied to them as to the aphasia syndromes. Nevertheless, as a working framework, they have been applied productively in therapy. For example, de Partz (1986) diagnosed a patient of hers as a deep dyslexic, with malfunctioning subword route, and devised methods of re-establishing this route with such success that the patient then showed signs similar to those of surface dyslexia during his recovery to functional reading.

Naming

Another related model expands the part of this model which relates to the production of names of words in speech, in order to account for different kinds of anomic difficulties on confrontation naming (i.e., looking at a picture of an object and saying what it is). It is proposed that different types of difficulties can be related to the different processes involved (i.e., semantic), accessing the item in the phonological lexicon, assembling the accessed item and planning of phonetic realisation (for a more detailed justification of this model, see Lesser, in press). All of these can lead to a failure to produce the correct name, although different kinds of behaviours will be observed. A patient with a semantic disorder may produce semantic paraphasias for the target words, though this in itself is not definitive of a central semantic disorder — since normal speakers are not immune from such errors. Such a patient is likely, however, to have difficulty on semantic comprehension tests, where fine semantic discriminations have to be made. Such tests may be given in picture form with the stimulus a spoken or written word. Tests can also be given in reading or auditory versions where the response is to select a written or spoken word rather than a picture. With a central semantic deficit, all these measures should reveal impairment. When trying to name a picture unsuccessfully, a patient with a central semantic disorder will also accept phonemic cues for associates of the target word as correct for the target word.

Other patients appear to have intact semantic representations for the target word they cannot find, but their main difficulty seems to be in accessing the item in the phonological lexicon — a 'tip-of-the-tongue' condition. They often show partial awareness of some indexing information for the word — its initial sound, the number of syllables, sometimes the number of letters in the visual lexicon — although the item in the phonological lexicon can only be accessed after considerable delay, if at all. During the searching behaviour the patients experiment with attempts at the word which result in phonemic paraphasias. When the word is finally accessed, however, or if it is given to them to repeat, they have no difficulty in recognising it as correct and in producing it. In respect of the latter behaviour, they can be distinguished from patients whose naming disorder can be attributed to a difficulty in phonemic assembly.

Like these 'phonological lexicon' patients, 'phonemic assembly' patients produce phonemic paraphasias in their searching for a word, but they are phonemic paraphasias which are more closely related to a target word, and the patient shows the same type of behaviour when given the whole word to repeat. This seems, therefore, to be essentially a different disorder, one of organising retrieved lexical information phonemically so as to output it as the correct phonemic assembly. Beyond this, difficulties can arise at the stage of planning the phonetic realisation. This corresponds to one definition of apraxia of speech (or verbal dyspraxia). This patient has difficulty, not only in organising a seriation of phonemes but in organising each phoneme; hence phonetically deviant sounds may be produced, with difficulty in transition from one phoneme to another. It differs from a phoneme assembly disorder as such in that speech is often facilitated by being given a model to imitate. It is a planning disruption, not an articulatory executive disruption, however, empirically distinguishable from dysarthria, because the patient has no difficulty in articulating some overlearned, affective, spontaneous utterances. Table 12.1 summarises the diagnostic distinctions proposed in this model.

Table 12.1: Diagnostic Behaviours in Naming Difficulties

Level of Disorder	Behaviour
Semantic	Semantic paraphasias Errors on semantic discrimination tests Accepts cued semantic associates as correct
Phonological lexicon	'Tip-of-the-tongue' or partial indexing Circumlocutions and exploratory phonemic paraphasias Good recognition and imitation of target word
Phoneme assembly	Target-oriented phonemic paraphasias with little circumlocution Difficulty in imitating multisyllabic target word
Verbal praxis	Search for phoneme shape Well-articulated 'asides'
Articulation	Consistent articulatory difficulties

As a working theory for remediation, such a model has direct implications. Different kinds of naming disorders need different kinds of treatment. The 'semantic' patient needs therapy aimed at clarifying word meaning, and producing sharper distinctions between words and associates. There is essentially no need for the patient to be asked to produce any speech during such therapy, since the assumption is that if the semantic system is improved the rest will follow. The 'phonological lexicon' patient needs repeated practice at linking items in the semantic lexicon with those in the phonological lexicon. He or she is likely to show an effect of word frequency, for the reasons given before. Making words more frequently retrieved for this patient should therefore improve the available phonological lexicon. For the 'phonemic assembly' patient the best strategy may be to reduce the complexity of the assembly required by breaking the words down into component syllables, which are processed singly and then combined; classically, seeing the words in written form helps to facilitate this. There are many well known techniques for the other types of patients with more peripheral difficulties in the naming process, which I do not need to rehearse here, as they are discussed in chapters 13 and 14 on dysarthria and apraxia of speech.

We do not yet know how accurate this model is. Consistent with modular theory it implies that there can be a disorder at any one stage without consequences for other stages, at least for those higher up the system. The model is certainly oversimplified; retrieving items from a phonological lexicon, for example, may well be influenced both by their semantic import for the individual and by their ease of phonemic assembly. But one subsidiary function of therapy is that it can be used to test the validity of such a model.

Sentence production

Another expansion of the model has been proposed, in respect of an aspect of its central component — specifically how intentions to speak are converted into producible sentences. This draws particularly on inferences made about the nature of sentence production from observations of the errors made by normal speakers, in collections made particularly in American English in UCLA, MIT and Cornell University, by Fromkin (1973), Garrett (1982), Shattuck-Hufnagel (1979), and others.

The model of sentence production proposed from this by Garrett has been applied to aphasia by Schwartz (1987), though in what follows I have added my own interpretation.

Table 12.2 shows the representation Garrett has included in his model of how individual speakers move from the thought of what they want to say to saying it. Word exchanges and word substitution errors are evidence for the Functional Level. They occur only on content words, the only kind of words which are specified at

Table 12.2: Levels of Representation in Sentence Production (after Garrett, 1982)

Message level representation
(Logical processes and verb arguments)
Functional level representation
(Syntactic frame and frame element processes)
Positional level representation
(Phonological processes)
Phonetic level representation
(Motor coding processes)
Articulatory level representation

this level. In contrast sound exchange errors occur as content words are inserted into syntactic frames at the Positional Level. Inflections and grammatical words can remain stranded when content words are exchanged (e.g., 'He is schooling to go' for 'He is going to school') and this is adduced as evidence that these sentence elements are attached to the syntactic frame before the content items are inserted. That the Phonetic Level occurs at a later stage than this is evident because the inflections and grammatical words are adjusted to accommodate the content words (e.g., the indefinite article 'a' becomes 'an' if appropriate, or syllabic or non-syllabic plural inflections are formed according to the new context).

Fig. 12.2 illustrates the processes which are hypothesised to occur in producing a specific sentence.

In applying this to disorders of grammar in aphasia, it seems sensible to see if we can distinguish between disorders which affect the achieving of the different Levels of Representation. If the problem lies in moving from the Message to the Functional Level, it may be suspected that patients would have difficulty in retrieving the appropriate content words from the semantic lexicon to express their meaning and/or in establishing the thematic roles of the sentence (e.g., who does what to whom, and with what). If the semantic item has been correctly accessed these thematic roles will be to some extent specified by the notion which has been retrieved which will take the form of the main verb of the sentence. A transitive verb, for example will specify that there must be an object for the sentence as well as a subject. Some verbs, such as 'pub' and 'set' have arguments which specify location slots which must be filled; others such as 'give' and 'offer' have slots for recipients which generally must be filled. Problems at this level of representation, therefore, have sometimes been considered to be specifically related to difficulty with verbs. Disturbances in the transition from the Functional to the Positional Level may be of different kinds. They may affect the ability to construct a syntactic frame, or they may affect the ability to select and insert the appropriate inflections and

"A man's giving money to a girl"

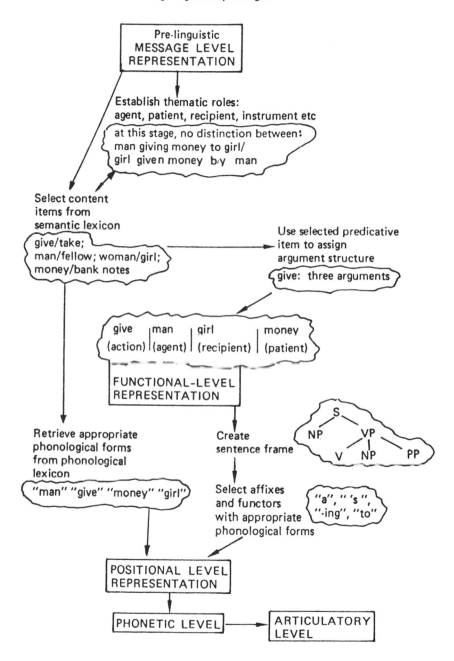

Figure 12.2

grammatical words (indeed there are linguistically principled reasons, as well as some actual evidence, that subcategories of these may be selectively impaired).

Analysing aphasic speech in terms of such a model is still new. In principle it should be possible to establish from a speech sample whether a patient shows features of restriction of number of verb arguments, problems of sentence construction or specific problems with inflections or grammatical words. Saffran, Berndt and Schwartz (1986) suggest asking the patient to tell the story of Cinderella and have devised a method of analysis.

A working assumption is also made that at least the central stage of these processes will apply in the comprehension of sentences as well as in their production. Comprehension tests can therefore be used to supplement the information from the patient's spoken language. Difficulty in interpreting reversible sentences has been taken as indicative of problems in extracting thematic roles (Schwartz, Saffran and Marin, 1980), since it is assumed that comprehension does not necessarily impose a need to reconstruct a syntactic frame as such, though this is somewhat controversial (see Caplan, 1987, pp. 316–7). A set of non-reversible sentences can also provide information on a patient's ability to extract thematic roles, which is not dependent on the ability to process word order in working memory. These are sentences with unfilled gaps such as 'John's demonstrating what to do' which can be contrasted with sentences such as 'John's asking what to do' where the unfilled referent for the verb complement differs according to the semantics of the verb.

Having assessed the patient along these parameters, the therapist then at least has some basis on which to justify selection of a particular method to assist in the improvement of sentence production. It may be specific work on the insertion of grammatical words, on the production of syntactic frames, on the identification of thematic roles or on lexical retrieval particularly of verbs. The important point is that the practice is related to a particular theoretical model and that the patient has been identified in terms of that model. This model is being applied in therapy by an increasing number of therapists (see for example Jones, 1986; Byng, 1988).

Effectiveness of Intervention

A final aspect of this discussion of the relationship between theory and practice in aphasia therapy is the question of evaluation of the effectiveness of therapy. This is important in any kind of intervention, and applies to pragmatic intervention with spouses using a sociolinguistic perspective as much as to the cognitive neuro-psychological approach. With the latter approach it has an additional value in that the results of therapy (i.e., whether it was effective or not) can feed back into the models and justify them, or show how they require further elaborations. This in turn feeds back into clinical practice. Evaluation requires accurate and replicable measurement, and the means for achieving this in terms of the models decribed are becoming available (see, for example, Kay, Lesser and Coltheart, in preparation). There have been several expositions in the literature recently of designs which can be used in single case studies of the effectiveness of therapy, in particular, AB designs which contrast treatment and non-treatment periods of two different tasks, multiple baseline designs where treatment is expected to be item-specific and extended baseline designs. The latter can be used where the treatment might be expected to have generalised effects but where the effects of a non-treatment period can be subtracted from the effects of treatment (for reviews see McReynolds and Thompson, 1986; Pring, 1986; Howard and Hatfield, 1987).

All these are beginning to make evaluation of therapy a practical proposition in the working clinic, provided that reliable instruments are available to measure changes in the processes or situations which are being treated. Great advances have been made in linking theory and the practice of aphasia therapy over the last few years; students are now graduating from their degree courses better equipped than ever before to push both theory and practice forward together, and an increasing number of clinicians are recognising that making time to apply the newer theories to therapy promises to benefit their patients.

References

ALLPORT, D.A. (1985) Distributed memory, modular subsystems and dysphasia. In S. Newman and R. Epstein (Eds), *Current Perspectives in Dysphasia.* Edinburgh: Churchill Livingstone.

BUTTERWORTH, B. and HOWARD, D. (1987) Paragrammatisms. *Cognition,* 26, 1–37.

BYNG, S. (1988) Sentence processing deficits: theory and therapy. *Cognitive Neuropsychology,* 5, 629–76.

CAPLAN, D. (1987) *Neurolinguistics and Linguistic Aphasiology: An Introduction.* New York: Cambridge University Press.

DE BLESER, R. and WEISMAN, H. (1986) The communicative impact of non-fluent aphasia on the dialogue behavior of linguistically impaired partners. In F. Lowenthal and F. Vandamme (Eds), *Pragmatics and Education.* New York: Plenum Press.

DE PARTZ, M.P. (1986) Reeducation of a deep dyslexic patient: rationale of the method and the results. *Cognitive Neuropsychology,* 3, 149–77.

ELLIS, A.A. (1987) Intimations of modularity, or, the modelarity of mind: Doing cognitive neuropsychology without syndromes. In M. Coltheart, G. Sartori and R. Job (Eds), *The Cognitive Neuropsychology of Language.* London: Lawrence Erlbaum.

FROMKIN, V.A. (1973) *Speech Errors as Linguistic Evidence.* The Hague: Mouton.

GARRETT, M.A. (1982) Production of speech: Observations from normal and pathological language use. In A.W. Ellis (Ed.), *Normality and Pathology in Cognitive Functions.* London: Academic Press.

GOODGLASS, H. and CAPLAN, E. (1983) *Assessment of Aphasia and Related Disorders.* Philadelphia: Lea and Febiger.

GREEN, G. (1984) Communication in aphasia therapy: Some of the procedures and issues involved. *British Journal of Disorders of Communication,* 20, 35–46.

HELM-ESTABROOKS, N. (1981) *Helm Elicited Language Program for Syntax Stimulation.* Austin, TX: Exceptional Resources Inc.

HILDEBRANDT, N., CAPLAN, D. and EVANS, K. (1987) The Man$_i$ left t$_i$ without a trace: A case study of aphasic processing of empty categories. *Cognitive Neuropsychology,* 4, 257–302.

HOWARD, D. and HATFIELD, F.M. (1987) *Aphasia Therapy: Historical and Contemporary Issues.* London: Lawrence Erlbaum.

JAKOBSON, R. (1964) Towards a linguistic typology of aphasic impairments. In A.V.S. deReuck and M. O'Connor (Eds), *Disorders of Language.* Edinburgh: Churchill.

JONES, E.V. (1986) Building the foundations for sentence production in a non-fluent aphasic. *British Journal of Disorders of Communication,* 21, 63–82.

KAY, J. LESSER, R. and COLTHEART, M. (in preparation) *The Psycholinguistic Assessment of Language Processing in Aphasia.* London: Lawrence Erlbaum.

LESSER, R. (1985) Sentence comprehension and production: an application of lexical grammar. In F.C. Rose (Ed.), *Recent Advances in Neurology, 42: Progress in Aphasiology.* New York: Raven.

LESSER, R. (in press) Some issues in the neuropsychological rehabilitation of anomia. In: X. Seron and G. Deloche (Eds), *Cognitive Approaches in Neuropsychological Rehabilitation.* London: Lawrence Erlbaum.

LURIA, A.R. (1966) *Higher Cortical Functions in Man.* London: Tavistock.

McREYNOLDS, L.V. and THOMPSON, C.K. (1986) Flexibility of single-subject experimental designs, Part 1: review of the basics of single-subject designs. *Journal of Speech and Hearing Disorders,* 51, 194–203.

MEYERSON, R. and GOODGLASS, H. (1972) Transformational grammars of three agrammatic patients. *Language and Speech,* 15, 40–50.

NAESER, M.A., HAAS, G., MAZURSKI, P. and LAUGHLIN, S. (1986) Sentence level auditory comprehension treatment program for aphasic adults. *Archives of Physical Medicine and Rehabilitation,* 67, 393–6.

PATTERSON, K.E. (1986) Lexical but non-semantic spelling? *Cognitive Neuropsychology,* 3, 341–67.

PENN, C. (1985) The profile of communicative appropriateness: a clinical tool for the assessment of pragmatics. *The South African Journal of Communication Disorders,* 32, 18–23.

PRING, T. (1986) Evaluating the effects of speech therapy for aphasics: developing the single case methodology. *British Journal of Disorders of Communication,* 21, 103–15.

PRUTTING, C.A. and KIRCHNER, D.M. (1987) A clinical appraisal of the pragmatic aspects of language. *Journal of Speech and Hearing Disorders,* 52, 105–19.

SAFFRAN, E., BERNDT, R. and SCHWARTZ, M. (1986) *A System for Quantifying Sentence Production Deficits in Aphasia.* Academy of Aphasia.

SCHACTER, D.L., McANDREWS, M.P. and MOSCOVITCH, M. (1988) Access to consciousness: dissociations between implicitn and explicit knowledge in neuropsychological syndromes. In L. Weiskrantz (Ed.), *Thought Without Language.* London: Oxford University Press.

SCHNEIDER, W. (1987) Connectionism: Is it a paradigm shift for psychology? *Behavior Research and Methods,* 19, 73–83.

SCHUELL, H.M., JENKINS, J.J. and JIMINEZ-PABON, E. (1964) *Aphasia in Adults: Diagnosis, Prognosis and Treatment.* New York: Harper and Row.

SCHWARTZ, M.F. (1987) Patterns of speech production deficit within and across aphasia syndromes: application of a psycholinguistic model. In M. Coltheart, G. Sartori and R. Job (Eds), *The Cognitive Neuropsychology of Language.* London: Lawrence Erlbaum.

SCHWARTZ, M.F., SAFFRAN, E. and MARIN, O. (1980) The word order problem in agrammatism: 1. *Comprehension. Brain and Language,* 10, 249–62.

SHATTUCK-HUFNAGEL, S. (1979) Speech errors as evidence for a serial-ordering mechanism in sentence production. In W.E.Cooper and E.C.T. Walker (Eds), *Sentence Processing.* New York: Lawrence Erlbaum.

SKINNER, C., WIRZ, S., THOMPSON, I. and DAVIDSON, J. (1984) *Edinburgh Functional Communication Profile.* Buckinghamshire: Winslow Press.

SPARKS, R. and HOLLAND, A. (1976) Method: Melodic Intonation Therapy for Aphasia. *Journal of Speech and Hearing Disorders,* 41, 287–97.

VIGNOLO, L.A. (1988) The anatomical and pathological basis of aphasia. In F.C. Rose, R. Whurr and M.A. Wyke (Eds), *Aphasia.* London: Whurr.

13 Assessment of Dysarthria: The Critical Prerequisite to Treatment

James H. Abbs and Roxanne De Paul

(In the following chapter, the authors examine the growing data that exists regarding the neuromotor speech disorders grouped under the term dysarthria. In Chapter 8, Jaffe describes dysarthria in childhood; here, the manifestation of the acquired disorder in adults is the main focus of attention. Dysarthria is the term given to a group of related neuromotor speech disorders where paralysis, weakness or incoordination of the speech musculature is caused by damage in the central or peripheral nervous systems. The clinical presentation may include impairments in the movement and synchrony of speech components in terms of range, timing, force, speed or direction. These result in a range of problems that may include difficulty in respiration, phonation, articulation and prosody. Non-speech activity involving the vocal organs may also be affected. Dysarthria may occur as a single disorder or it may be accompanied by other speech and/or language disorders such as apraxia of speech or aphasia. It is necessary to distinguish which condition contributes most and the way in which it contributes to the overall disability of the individual patient. *Editor's note*).

The last two decades have been witness to an unprecedented increase in clinical research on the disorders of speech associated with brain impairments. A new era of theory, description, and diagnosis of dysarthria was begun with the pioneering efforts of James Hardy at the University of Iowa and Ronald Netsell then at the University of Wisconsin, in describing these disorders using techniques previously reserved for physiology studies. In parallel and of equal significance were the extensive and landmark nosological analyses of Frederic Darley and his colleagues at Mayo Clinic, including a comprehensive attempt at providing a complete set of categories of these inflictions. In this context, the present chapter is an attempt to update and extend that earlier work, as well as correct some misconceptions that appear to reflect overinterpretation or misunderstandings in its subsequent application.

The quality of clinical treatment generally is related to the degree of knowledge of the pathophysiology and the extent to which reliable assessment procedures can be devised to exploit that knowledge. Dysarthria treatment is not an exception to this principle. Based upon a recent orientation towards the assessment of the underlying pathophysiology, treatment of dysarthria increasingly has involved focused physical intervention, including biofeedback, palatal lifts, posturing, abdominal binding, respiratory exercise, bite-block prostheses, etc. (cf. Bless, Rubow and Braun, 1983; Hixon, 1975; Lybolt, Netsell and Farrage, 1982; McNamara, 1983; Netsell and Daniel, 1979; Rosenbek and LaPointe, 1978; Rubow, 1981; Rubow and Netsell, 1979). In contrast to more global approaches (e.g., behavioural modification techniques aimed at general behavioural variables such as 'correct articulation') the prescription of such focused, physically oriented intervention, requires detailed information concerning the speech mechanism pathophysiology (Netsell and Daniel, 1979). For example, it would not be justified to undertake biofeedback as a means to reduce muscle tone if information was not available on (a) the severity and distribution of that increased muscle activity and (b) whether or not it causes problems in speech performance.

It is obvious that the long-term advancement of intervention in dysarthria depends upon the reliability and validity of assessment in revealing the underlying motor pathophysiology. New rehabilitation techniques are difficult to develop, apply or refine without concrete information concerning these characteristics. Unfortunately, the effectiveness and validity of current dysarthria assessment procedures have not been evaluated quantitatively in their relative sensitivity to the underlying pathophysiology. Indeed, many assessments for dysarthria have been developed in isolation and hence are idiosyncratic to particular clinicians or particular clinics, making global evaluation difficult. Despite these problems it is worthwhile to examine dysarthria assessment with a view toward the strengths and weaknesses of the different approaches currently being utilised.

Effectiveness of Current Dysarthria Assessment

Generally, there appear to be two general avenues in dysarthria assessment: (1) the listener judgement-inferential approach and (2) the multiple component approach (cf. Abbs, Hunker and Barlow, 1983 for a further description of these two approaches). Within a broader perspective, these two avenues have increasingly merged in the last ten years (as reflected in Rosenbek and LaPointe, 1978), although this may not be uniformly manifest in most clinical settings. In any case, at present there is not a widely accepted or standardised set of approaches to this problem. These issues not withstanding, a brief review of these two major assessments highlights a number of key issues in clinical management of dysarthria.

Evaluation of assumptions underlying assessment

The listener judgment-inferential approach, as it was originally advocated for use in many clinical settings, involves several serial steps in determining the speech system neuropathophysiology. Initially, a speech pathologist listens to and evaluates the dysarthric speech with attempts, via speech task manipulations, to identify the nature of impairments in the three 'major' components of the speech production system (i.e., respiratory, phonatory, and articulatory). In most clinical settings this evaluation is augmented by a routine, but usually unstandardised examination (the oral peripheral exam) and sometimes a test of articulation (cf. Logemann, Fisher, Boses, and Blonsky, 1978). The second stage of this particular assessment process involves differential categorisation of the apparent dysarthric subgroup based upon the auditory-perceptual classification of the speech patterns (cf. Darley, Aronson and Brown, 1969a; 1969b; 1975). The final step in 'determining' the underlying pathophysiology is based upon inferences from the dysarthric subgroup categorisation. These critical inferences commonly are drawn from (1) parallel neurological examinations of limb impairments, and (2) classical profiles of the nonspeech symptoms and signs as provided in traditional neurological descriptions. For example, if the differential diagnosis (step 2) results in the categorisation of hypokinetic dysarthria (namely, dysarthria associated with Parkinson's disease), the speech motor problem has been suggested to be due to hypo- or bradykinesia, rigidity, and tremor in the muscles and movements of the speech production system. This profile of signs and symptoms is, of course, the classical one found in descriptions of limb impairments in this population (DeLong and Georgopoulos, 1981; Marsden, 1982).

There is no question that a number of experienced speech and language clinicians can categorise a given speech motor disorder by listening to the associated speech patterns. However, the question is whether such identification provides optimal or useful directions for treatment. In particular, it is apparent that there is not a common profile of symptoms and signs for all patients with a given neurological disease. The further presumption that inferences from limb signs and symptoms to orofacial motor impairments are clinically valid is also unsupported. In evaluating the viability of these inferences, interestingly, one must in turn address the multiple speech component approach, as reflected in the physiological perspectives of Hardy (1967) and the representation of the speech production system offered by Netsell and Daniel (1979). This multicomponent orientation evolved from the concept that assessment of individual speech motor subsystems (e.g., lips, jaw, tongue, velum, larynx, etc.) is necessary to develop optimal programmes of focused, physically-oriented rehabilitation. This approach is particularly appealing in evaluating potential lower motoneuron disorders where differences in subsystem impairments might be present due to select damage in some cranial nerves.

However, it also appears valuable to conduct multiple subsystem assessment in dysarthrias of suprabulbar origin. Earlier data from articulation tests in patients with dysarthrias due to supranuclear lesions indicate non-uniform patterns of impairment (cf. Logemann *et al.*, 1978). Further, most neurologists and speech and language clinicians are acutely aware of the fact that individuals with Parkinson's disease, congenital or acquired spasticity, etc. do not have equivalent degrees of impairment across all orofacial or limb motor systems. Obviously, if supranuclear lesions yield differential impairments among orofacial and limb muscle groups, it would be difficult to make inferences from limb motor impairments to determine the pathophysiology in the orofacial system (cf. Darley *et al.*, 1975).

By way of direct physiological measures, several recent observations in hypokinetic, ataxic, spastic, and flaccid dysarthrics indicate that differential impairment among the motor subsystems of the speech production mechanism is the rule rather than the exception. These studies indicate differential degrees of:

1   rigidity and hypokinesia in the upper vs. lower lips of Parkinson subjects (Hunker, Abbs and Barlow, 1982)

2   hypertonicity, fine force control, fine position control impairment in the lips, tongue, jaw and upper limbs of congenital spastic subjects (Barlow and Abbs, 1984; 1986)

3   multimovement decomposition in the orofacial vs. respiratory motor systems in ataxic patients (Abbs *et al.*, 1983; Abbs, 1985)

4   variations in bradykinesia of speech movements of the upper lip, lower lip, and jaw of Parkinson patients (Connor, Forrest, Cole, Gracco and Abbs, 1987)

5   motoneuron loss for the tongue, lip, jaw and laryngeal muscles in patients with amyotrophic lateral sclerosis (DePaul, Abbs, Caligiuri, Cracco and Brooks, 1988), and

6   fine force control impairment among the lips, tongue, and jaw of Parkinson patients (Abbs, Hartman and Vishwanat, 1987).

Given these data, one major issue concerns the nature of impairment differences among different orofacial and limb motor systems. If these differential impairment profiles are systematic, one would be able to utilise that information clinically. For example, it appears that there are subgroups of patients within the Parkinsonian population with different sub-clusters of motor signs and deficits (cf. Hunker and Abbs, 1984; Mortimer, Perozzolo, Hansch, and Webster, 1982). Different treatments for these two groups of Parkinson patients might be indicated.

A second major issue is related to the underlying reason for a differential distribution of impairment manifestations across orofacial, laryngeal, respiratory, and limb muscle groups. Obviously, multiple factors are involved, at least in some disorders. Focal dysfunctions of portions of the primary motor or premotor cortex, the basal ganglia or the cerebellum could selectively impair parts of the orofacial system, or the upper or lower limbs, especially given the consistent somatotopy manifest throughout the nervous system. Variation due to differential loss of neural tissue is most probable with lacunar insults such as those associated with cerebral vascular accident or trauma. However, it appears that consistent patterns of differential impairment are manifest in systemic diseases as well, including amyotrophic lateral schlerosis and Parkinson's disease. In individual patients, progressive neuromotor diseases commonly are first observed in a single part of the body and then in other parts over the time course of the disease. Recent studies with the differential impairment profiles associated with amyotrophic lateral sclerosis (ALS) address this point quite well.

Even retrospective clinical studies of ALS support differential orofacial muscle group impairment. For example, Carpenter, McDonald and Howard (1978), studying twelve bulbar ALS patients, observed that weakness and fasciculations were most common in the tongue (66 per cent, 54 per cent respectively) and much less prominent in the facial (23 per cent, 8 per cent), velopharyngeal (8 per cent, 2 per cent) or jaw muscles (10 per cent). Predictably, these patients also reported greater difficulties in tongue muscles (68 per cent) than in laryngeal (14 per cent), pharyngeal (13 per cent) or jaw muscles (1 per cent). These kinds of differential impairments have important implications for the progression of functional deterioration, especially with regard to manifestations of dysphagia, aspiration and dysarthria.

More recent quantative work with ALS patients, along with neuropathological data further addressed the consistency of this differential pattern and the neuropathological origins. In one recent study, maximum strength was measured for the lips, tongue, and jaw of ALS patients using special force transducers. (DePaul *et al.*, 1988). Fig. 13.1 shows force signals for multiple MVC (Maximum Voluntary Contraction) trials. As shown, tongue MVC signals in the ALS patient are substantially more reduced (in relation to the normal subject) and the lip or jaw MVC signals. Quantitatively, the normal MVC values of the tongue, lips and jaw vary substantially from one another (reflected in the calibration bars in Figure 13.1); as such it is not meaningful to compare absolute ALS decrements in lip, jaw and tongue strength directly. To permit such comparisons, MVC values for ALS patients were expressed as a percentage of normal (i.e., one-half normal equals a 50 per cent decrement). Figure 13.2 illustrates the percentage of strength loss for the lip, jaw and tongue of two subgroups of these ALS patients — (1) bulbar ALS patients, and (2) those manifesting the earliest signs of ALS in the extremities (nonbulbar).

Clearly, in both subgroups, the tongue is significantly weaker than either the lips or the jaw. However, it also is worthy to note (Fig. 13.2) that the nonbulbar subgroup does not have normal lip, jaw or tongue strength. These data thus not

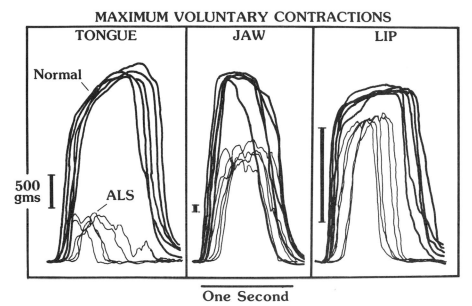

Figure 13.1: MVC signals showing differential involvement of facial, trigeminal and hypoglossal motoneurons for one ALS subject relative to a normal control.

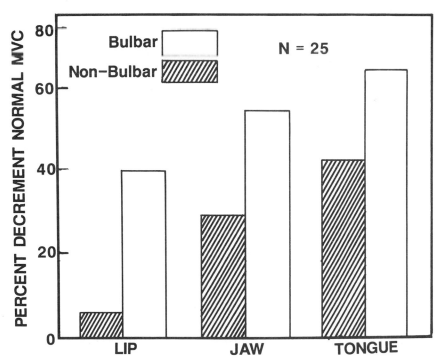

Figure 13.2: Differential involvement of facial, trigeminal and hypoglossal motoneurons for bulbar and non-bulbar ALS subjects relative to normal controls.

only support the clinical observations of Carpenter *et al.,* 1978), indicating a disproportionate degree of tongue muscle group involvement in ALS, but are consistent with Gubbay, Kahana, Zilber, Cooper, Pintov and Liebowitz (1985) finding that even patients with initial ALS symptoms in the extremities manifest bulbar signs. Obviously separating ALS patients into bulbar and nonbulbar subgroups is tenuous.

Obtaining instrumental measures of this kind in most clinical settings is difficult. Of additional concern is whether maximum strength measures lack sensitivity in some stages of ALS during which MN collateral reinnervation minimises actual muscle strength changes. As such, it is useful to consider other techniques which reflect other manifestations of motor neuron disease, including fasciculations, muscle wasting and mobility. Such data, while largely unpublished (see, however, DePaul and Abbs, 1987), were obtained using a standardised dysarthria examination, the Frenchay Test (Enderby, 1980; 1983a; 1983b). The data obtained from the Frenchay examination corroborate the findings of differential ALS symptoms in the orofacial muscles. Fig. 13.3 illustrates results from the Frenchay evaluations for fifteen of the patients studied above; a high positive correlation was found between degree of MVC decrement and the degree of Frenchay test impairment. Overall, with clinical observation and two sets of measures, it is clear that there is a consistent pattern of differential tongue, larynx, lip, and jaw muscle impairments in ALS. These results have important clinical implications with regard to assessment and management, as well as providing better prognostic indicators for the influence of this insidious disease upon speech. However, such consistent patterns of differential motor impairment should also have neuropathological correlates.

The predominant neuropathologic changes in ALS patients are degeneration and depletion of neurons in cranial motor nuclei, degeneration of the corticospinal pathways (Hughes, 1982; Hirano, 1982), and loss primary of motor cortex pyramidal cells. While limited data are available, neuropathological studies in ALS patients support the MVC and Frenchay profiles shown in Figs. 13.1–3. Specifically, all available studies indicate differential degrees of involvement in cranial motor nuclei V, VII, X and XII. For example, Lawyer and Netsky (1953) reported hypoglossal nucleus alterations in 50 of 53 patients, with only 4 of the 50 brains manifesting trigeminal motor nucleus changes; facial nucleus involvement was not mentioned. These observations directly support the data reported above. Notably, only 14 of Lawyer and Netsky's 53 patients initially manifested cranial motor signs. Comparable observations have been made by other authors (Bonduelle, 1975; Brain, Croft and Wilkinson, 1969; Shiraki and Yase, 1975). Specifically, Bonduelle (1975) noted common alterations of motorneuron cells in hypoglossal nucleus, while motor trigeminal nucleus was much less impaired and there was only limited isolated groups of MN loss in the facial nucleus. Shawker and Sonies (1984) also argued for

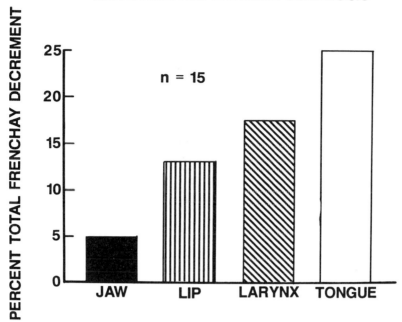

Figure 13.3: Differential orofacial impairment of mandibular, labial, laryngeal and lingual subsystems for ALS subjects using the Frenchay Dysarthria Assessment (1983b).

differential impairment of extrinsic and intrinsic tongue muscles; however, a paucity of information on the organisation of the hypoglossal nucleus makes evaluation of potential neuropathological correlates difficult.

In addition to XIIth and Vth cranial MN changes, Lawyer and Netsky (1953) also observed changes in the nucleus ambiguus in 43 of their 53 patients and in the dorsal motor nucleus of 35 of these patients. Although frequencies of MN alteration were not given, Bonduelle (1975) made comparable observations regarding nucleus ambiguus and dorsal motor nucleus involvement. Some authors assert that the intrinsic laryngeal muscles do not manifest involvement in ALS (Kushner, Parrish, Burke, Behrens, Hays, Frame and Rowland, 1984). However, change in phonation typically is an early ALS symptom, and given the obvious alteration of nucleus ambiguus MNs, this assertion may simply be due to limitations in objective measures of these muscles in ALS patients. Interestingly, the observations of the Frenchay evaluation (Fig. 13.3) indicate laryngeal involvement was second only to that of the tongue muscles. Further, the very common observation of ALS aspiration argues for some impairments in the laryngeal muscles. Potential loss of nucleus ambiguus innervation to the pharyngeal constrictor and velopharyngeal muscles may relate to 'nasality' in the speech of ALS patients and with dysphagia.

While the motor contributions of dorsal motor nucleus are controversial (cf. Carpenter and Sutin, 1983), if MNs innervate the pharyngeal constrictors and some extrinsic laryngeal muscles (Alba, Pilkington, Kaplan, Baum, Schultheiss, Ruggieri and Lee, 1976; Davis and Nail, 1985), their degeneration could also contribute to ALS swallowing problems. Overall, these data illustrate that the differential impairment of the tongue, larynx, lip, and jaw MNs is consistent across the ALS population and because this is a systemic disease, these differences must be due to variation in susceptibility of different cranial motoneuron pools to the underlying disease process.

In the same way, one could argue that differences in Parkinson upper lip, lower lip, tongue and jaw impairments relate to differences in the way that these muscle groups are influenced by this systemic metabolic disease. The recent work by Abbs *et al.* (1987) indicates that within an isometric fine force control task the tongue was much more impaired than the lips or jaw. In terms of underlying pathophysiology, these data would support the position that the movement impairments associated with Parkinson's disease (PD) are related to aberrant basal ganglia (BG) inputs to the motor or somatic sensory cortices (Mortimer and Webster, 1978; Tatton and Lee, 1975). That is, the tongue muscles, without spindle afferent projections to MNs or the cerebellum (Bowman and Combs, 1969), should be particularly reliant upon sensorimotor actions at the motor cortex (Neilson, Andrews, Guitar and Quinn, 1979) and hence, as observed, would be disproportionately impaired in PD. Interestingly, however, the lip muscles, devoid of muscle spindles, manifest PD rigidity similar to that observed in the extremities (Hunker *et al.,* 1982).

The disproportionate tongue impairment observed in Parkinson's disease is also subject to an alternative interpretation. While major BG outputs project to cortical sites (DeLong and Georgopoulos, 1981), there are also descending pathways directly to the brain stem. Several studies (Lidsky, Robinson, Denaro and Weinhold, 1978; Labuszewski and Lidsky, 1979; Welzl, Schwarting and Huston, 1984) indicate that BG lesions yield particular orofacial dysfunctions consistent with swallowing in Parkinson's disease (Palmer, 1974; Logemann, Blonsky and Boshes, 1975; Robbins, Logemann and Kirshner, 1986), and upper airway respiratory (Vincken, Gauthier, Dollfus, Hanson, Darauay and Cosio, 1984) problems. Inasmuch as the motor cortex is not primarily involved in the functions of swallowing or respiration, these latter disorders are difficult to reconcile with the concept that PD impairments are due to aberrant BG influences upon the motor cortex. However, reported orofacial reflex aberrations in PD (Gracco and Abbs, 1984; Kimura, 1973) are consistent with swallowing and upper airway breathing problems and with the Abbs *et al.* data.

In view of the special anatomical and physiological characteristics of the orofacial system, and apparently unique interrelationship with the basal ganglia, orofacial motor impairments in PD are likely to be different from those manifest in the extremities. As such, orofacial movement disorders with PD may not respond to drug manipulation in the same way as the muscle groups of the extremities. Thus, Abbs *et al.* (1987) data in PD suggest that efficacy of treatment in the limb and the orofacial muscles should be evaluated separately. These considerations in Parkinson's disease also indicate that the possible basis for differential impairments may be due not only to variable susceptibility of different neural centres to a disease process, but possible also to the particular central representation of a given muscle group. Apparently the somatic sensory aspects of the tongue are not represented at the levels of the cerebellum and cerebrum in the same manner as the lips and jaw, hence a possible basis for their being impaired to differing degrees.

While a comprehensive review of the multiple neurophysiological and neuroanatomical factors that might predict differential impairments would be prohibitive in the present chapter, other reviews in earlier papers (cf. Abbs, 1985; Abbs *et al.,* 1983) provide sufficient documentation that these differences are commonplace. Indeed, in an earlier paper it was noted that the major and unquestionable neurophysiological and neuroanatomical differences among different speech system muscle groups was almost irrefutable evidence that the CNS does not control the spinal and cranial systems nor their respective subsystems in the same manner ... and hence, if there is damage to the nervous system at a suprabulbar/supraspinal level, the result will be impairments in movements and muscle contractions that are different among the speech production systems and the limbs. For example, hypo- and hyper-gamma drive to muscle spindles, loss or aberrations in recurrent inhibition, and impairment of selective influences on motoneuron recruitment patterns all have enjoyed some popularity as partial pathogenic explanations for spasticity, rigidity, tremor, ataxia, hypotonia, dysmetria, and asthenia. If some of these explanations are even partially correct, and the implicated physiological processes (e.g., presence of spindles, operation of recurrent inhibition) differ from one motor system to another, then the pathophysiology must vary as well (Abbs *et al.,* 1983, p. 30).

The implications of this nonuniformity of speech motor subsystem impairments are several. Initially, because global measures of the speech motor system are generally unlikely to reveal such impairments, determination of speech motor subsystem pathophysiology may need to be enhanced by use of direct observations using voluntary, nonspeech tasks. In this manner, it may be possible to identify those speech motor subsystems manifesting the greatest degree of impairment and focus treatment for maximum effectiveness.

Improvements in speech motor function could possibly be enhanced by initial emphasis upon those subsystems that are either most severely impaired or allow for the most direct and effective intervention.

Diagnostic Signs, Neural Control Aberrations
and Performance Deficits

Table 13.1 provides an overview of the signs and movement aberrations classically associated with different classes of movement disorders. This is a catalogue of some value in distinguishing among these disorders. However, it has become increasingly apparent in the last decade that it is not satisfactory to describe or list the various speech motor system aberrations associated with a given neuromotor disorder. That is, describing the presence or absence of particular pathophysiological signs across the speech motor subsystems and the limbs is of limited value unless it is possible to determine whether the salient aberrations are primary or causal factors in the speech motor performance deficit, or simply tertiary manifestations that accompany the syndrome. More specifically in relation to Table 13.1, the relations among the major and minor signs and the movement aberrations are uncertain. As such, the effort must be made to ensure that each particular aberration has a causal relation to the performance deficits prior to the expenditure of energy, time and money on treatment programmes to eliminate or minimise it. Neurological signs or motor manifestations that are simply different from normal do not necessarily play a causal or important role in a patient's clinical disability.

Aberrant manifestations that are tertiary were recognised by Hughlings Jackson over 100 years ago, and labelled *positive signs* (e.g., due to 'release' of certain nervous system functions or simply irritations to nervous system tissue). Negative signs, according to Jackson, are aberrant disease characteristics that are causally associated with the performance deficit or the clinical disability, *per se*. Clearly the white lock of hair (a positive sign) associated with Waardenberg's syndrome is not a causal factor in the hearing disability (a negative sign) also manifest in this population. In this vein, one also must be very careful in interpreting abnormal patterns that might be compensatory in nature. For example, the ubiquitous slowing of speech in many dysarthric subjects may be primarily a compensation for certain general aberrations of control that are deleterious at a more rapid rate. No one would undertake to treat the Waardenberg white hair lock with an expectation of improving the patient's hearing. Attempting to treat such compensatory patterns as speech slowing also could be counterproductive unless the complex factors associated with this behaviour are also understood.

In this context, it is enlightening to consider some of the assessment procedures utilised in dysarthria and evaluate the extent to which it is possible to discriminate positive signs and compensations from factors causally intertwined with actual performance deficits. By using customary diagnostic procedures, it has been common to distinguish the different neuromotor pathologies of speech via contrastive profiles of descriptive behaviours. As highlighted above, a common assumption has been that diagnostic indicators of a particular neuropathological

Table 13.1 Lists neurological signs and movement aberrations associated with different classes of movement disorders

	Major signs	*Other signs*	*Movement aberrations*
HYPERKINETIC CLUSTER	– fluctuating tone – shortening reaction	– reflex reinforcement absent – stretch reflexes variable	– athetosis – chorea – dystonia – ballismus
FLACCID CLUSTER	– hypotonia – weakness – muscle atrophy	– reduced or absent reflexes – fasciculations	– reduced velocity and extent of movement
SPASTIC CLUSTER	– spastic hypertonicity – clasp-knife reflex (lengthening reaction) – clonus	– hyper-brisk stretch reflexes – babinski sign	– restricted or weak movement – loss of fine adjustments
CEREBELLAR CLUSTER	– ataxia – tremor: postural and intention – hypotonia	– reduced stretch reflex – pendular reflexes – rebound phenomenon	– asynergia – decomposition of multi-joint movement – dysmetria
HYPOKINETIC CLUSTER	– rigidity: plastic/lead-pipe and cogwheel	– shortening reaction – reflex reinforcement absent	– hypo-, brady- and akinesia – kinesia paradoxica

syndrome are coincident with or underlie the debilitating performance deficits associated with the disease. An assumption of this kind is found with the so-called spastic dysarthric. In this group, it has been indicated that several of the distinct speech motor symptoms can be related to increased muscle tone or muscle spasms. Such a phenomenon as the feature of strain-strangled voice observed in these patients has been argued to be caused by co-contraction of antagonistic intrinsic laryngeal muscles or spasms in the same. This example presents several problems clinically. First, the term spasticity is ill-defined, even in neurology. Secondly, assumptions have been made that (1) the antagonistic co-contraction thought to be manifest in the limbs is also operating in the larynx, and (2) this spastic hypertonicity is a causative factor underlying the speech motor disability.

Unfortunately, muscle activity in the intrinsic laryngeal muscles is difficult to record and thus has not been evaluated in a patient with spastic dysarthria; as such, the argument for antagonistic co-contraction or laryngeal muscle hypertonicity is without documentation. Further, the clinical neurology literature is ambiguous as to the definition of spasticity or its quantification (Lance, 1980; Landau, 1980). Controversy continues as to whether spasticity is primarily a velocity of stretch-related activation of stretch reflexes yielding a pathological resistance to a clinical examiner's passive displacement, or rather is descriptive of an entire syndrome which includes increased reflex excitability, muscle weakness, clumsiness, greater than normal stiffness, and flexion reflexes that are hyperactive. Aside from this controversy, obviously spasticity is not unidimensional. Of greatest importance is the fact that clinical neurologists realise that spasticity (narrowly defined) is primarily a clear diagnostic sign, but largely unrelated to the actual motor performance deficits manifest in this population. Perhaps no author has been more clear in stating these points than William Landau (1980), who in reviewing several sets of corroborative studies of evidence (Denny-Brown, 1980; Duncan, Shahani and Young, 1976; Landau, 1974, 1980; Sahrman and North, 1977) commented directly regarding the hypertonicity and motor disability in individuals with spasticity:

> However useful to clinical diagnosis may be the increase of excitability at anterior horn cells and to some extent muscle spindles, these phenomena have little more relation to the patient's disability than does the insertion of the rectal thermometer in pneumonia. (Landau, 1980, p. 20).

Obviously in this context, one must seriously question the assertion that so-called strain-strangled voice is the result of antagonistic muscle/spastic hypertonus in the larynx.

These observations point very clearly to the need for distinguishing between diagnosis and assessment! That is, while it often appears logical to infer that diagnostic signs are a major underlying cause of motor disabilities in individuals with neuromuscular disease, even the most 'apparent' of these inferences need to be tested empirically. That is, it is likely that some of the most striking distinguishing features for differential dysarthria classification may not be related causally to the speech deficits. One must examine the extent to which certain features of speech abnormality are related causally to deficits in functional communication or speech movement coordination and control. In the example of spasticity discussed above, reducing or eliminating flexor spasms or hyperactive stretch reflexes through various treatments is not of particular benefit in improving motor function. Treating certain superficial speech aberrations may be similarly futile unless such aberrations have been demonstrated to be related to deficits of speech performance. Apparent compelling causal relations among symptoms and signs one might observe in clinical populations may not be valid; the nervous system usually functions in ways not intuitively obvious, and the requirement for testing of unquantified assertions, no matter how appealing they may be, cannot be compromised.

Can Motor Speech Impairment be Predicted from Nonspeech Measures?

If one accepts the arguments that (1) the various speech motor subsystems are differentially impaired and (2) many aberrations or signs accompanying a particular disorder do not have a causal relation to deficits in speech movement performance, then measures obtained during ongoing speech behaviour may be very difficult to interpret as a basis for determining the critical elements of the underlying pathophysiology. For example, if one observes alterations in the temporal properties of speech, it may be very difficult to discern whether those aberrations are due to a uniform impairment in all speech system muscle groups, or primarily disproportionate aberrations in one or two components. For example, analyses of the infleunce of disproportionate aberrations in jaw control (DePaul and Abbs, 1984) suggested that such aberrations were manifest during speech in structures that are mechanically isolated from the jaw (e.g., the upper lip), possibly reflecting attempts at compensation for the jaw control aberrations. These and other related data indicate that experimental and clinical assessment of motor speech disorders could be enhanced through the utilisation of measures obtained during nonspeech tasks.

Many measures currently utilised either experimentally or in clinical settings with instrumental capabilities indicate that measures of speech motor subsystem performance simplify assessment substantially by dealing with one subsystem at a time. Differential impairment is clearly manifest as in the work described previously with cases of amyotrophic lateral sclerosis (DePaul *et al.,* 1988) and Parkinson's disease (Abbs *et al.,* 1987; Connor *et al.,* 1987). Presumably with such information one can consider focusing rehabilitation or clinicial management at those more specific, less global motor malfunctions. In general, this seemingly logical approach is dependent upon the assumption that nonspeech motor impairments are of value in assessing and managing motor speech disorders. This assumption raises the classical issue of whether speech and nonspeech motor functions are dependent upon a sufficiently common neural substrate so that impairments in speech can be predicted from nonspeech measures and further that enhancements in nonspeech performance will lead to parallel improvements for speech tasks.

It has been a long-standing question in the assessment and treatment of motor speech disorders as to whether (1) impairments in the motor control of nonspeech activities such as chewing and swallowing, or volitional nonspeech manoeuvres (as observed in the oral peripheral examination) correlate with or are indicative of parallel impairments in speech motor function, and further, whether (2) rehabilitation focused upon either feeding or nonspeech voluntary control of speech motor systems will effectively carry over to speech control. This issue has been debated most intensely regarding speech motor problems resulting from supranuclear damage, either of a congenital or acquired nature.

There are several lines of evidence that appear particularly relevent. It is, however, important that speech and nonspeech motor tasks be defined from a current neurophysiological perspective. Chewing, swallowing and other orofacial vegetative functions are known to be neurophysiologically distinct from nonspeech tasks performed voluntarily. That is, these vegetative functions appear, to a large extent, to be controlled via certain subcortical pattern generators and/or networks of brainstem reflexes (cf. Dubner, Sessle and Storey, 1978; Wyke, 1974). For example, Hoffman and Luschei (1980) demonstrated that primary motor cortex activity was not related to movements during chewing in rhesus monkeys. However, operantly conditioned biting (a 'more voluntary' task using the same jaw muscles) was clearly under motor cortex influence. Hoffman and Luschei noted, 'a likely explanation for this observation is that the reciprocal action of the jaw-closing and opening muscles during chewing is patterned elsewhere in the brain' (1980, p. 345). Other recent work suggests a parallel dichotomy for the muscles of the respiratory system (Phillips and Porter, 1977) and the facial muscles (Denny-Brown, 1960). As noted by Evarts:

> It might at first seem odd that corticospinal neurons controlling precise skilled movements terminate on motoneurons controlling intercostal muscles that participate in an act as automatic and primitive as respiration, but Phillips and Porter point out that these terminations are probably related to the use of respiratory muscles in speech and song rather than in breathing ... Destroying the corticospinal projection to thoracic motoneurons does not impair the use of respiratory muscles for respiration, though these same muscles may be useless for speech. (Evarts, 1981, p. 1113).

These considerations offer a different perspective on the long-standing speech-nonspeech controversy. That is, these recent neurophysiological observations indicate that this issue is not one of speech versus nonspeech motor control. The critical distinction may be whether the nonspeech movements are controlled in a conscious, voluntary manner as in speech, or, by contrast, represent vegetative movements that are more automatic. This interpretation is compatible with earlier and more recent data that address this issue. As was noted recently in a re-evaluation of this issue:

These data and the previously considered neurophysiological/neuroanato-mical findings suggest that nonspeech control of precise, *voluntary* activities is likely to be impaired in the same manner and to the same degree as speech motor behaviour. (Abbs and Rosenbek, 1985, p. 39).

The implications for assessment and for rehabilitation based upon this working hypothesis are several. Recent data indicate that assessment of impairments solely on the basis of spontaneous speech behaviour, whether one uses movement observations, acoustic analyses or simply a sage clinical ear, may not permit discrimination of a jaw control impairment from a lip or tongue impairment. Spastic and hypokinetic dysarthric data in particular address an important point made previously regarding the relative insensitivity of more global indices provided by acoustic or aerodynamic analyses. For example, changes in the speech of a congenital spastic subject by inserting a bite-block was not discernible from such measures as perceptual judgments (DePaul and Abbs, 1984). Similarly, conventional global measures are not likely to be sensitive to the differential degree of upper and lower lip rigidity in the Parkinsonian dysarthrics. Hence, observations of voluntary nonspeech control tasks apparently are useful for disambiguating potential subsystem motor impairments. This line of reasoning applies to treatment as well. If impairments in voluntary nonspeech control are parallel to those for speech, improvements on selected, voluntary nonspeech tasks should enhance speech control as well, depending on the site of the lesion and neural tissue remaining to support less automatic behaviours.

These interpretations have interesting implications for other forms of rehabilitation as well. For example, some schools of cerebral palsy treatment have emphasised that facilitation of chewing and swallowing is a means for improving speech function. Despite the enthusiasm for these particular programmes, direct evidence to support their value for speech improvement is lacking. Indeed, difference in neural control between chewing and speech/nonspeech voluntary behaviour argues against the utility of these therapies for speech. This argument is supported by the recent observations of Love, Hagerman and Taimi, (1980) who found no consistent relation between severity of speech impairment in sixty cerebral palsied children and the presence of dysphagia. Other data to this point are those of Schliesser (1982), who reported that in the cerebral palsy population certain non-speech alternate motion rate tasks predicted dysarthria severity quite well.

While these considerations offer a suporting basis for assessment and treatment of dysarthria via nonspeech voluntary control tasks, the details of this approach need to be considered in light of current state-of-the-art assessment procedures and their underlying neurophysiological rationale. Obviously, it is of particular value to test the above distinctions empirically in studies designed to offer more direct evidence for predicting speech motor impairment from nonspeech measures.

What are the Implications for Treatment?

At the outset of this chapter it was noted that the most promising new approaches for treatment of speech motor disorders lay with physically-oriented techniques such as prostheses, biofeedback to reduce increased muscle tone, muscle strengthening exercises, and so on. Obviously, the ultimate objective of dysarthria assessment in this context must be to provide empirical indications of the pathophysiology in each of the speech motor subsystems (Abbs *et al.,*1983; Netsell and Daniel, 1979). However, to date many of these efforts have involved instrumentally-based techniques; one is faced with the question as to the practical clinical utility of measures that largely have been confined to research laboratories. Based upon some efforts in the last five years, we have been increasingly convinced that some measures of this kind provide information of potential clinical value to the patient's physicians and speech and language clinicians. However, the issue is whether technically complex and instrumentally intensive procedures can be readily adopted for routine clinical evaluation. Certainly most speech and language clinics will not be able to exploit these measures in the foreseeable future without some assistance from engineering and computer experts as well as an influx of monies with which to purchase electronic and computer systems. To this end however, one may be able to rely upon non-instrumental measures. In two circumstances, we have been able to replicate the results of instrumental analyses utilising non-instrumental measures. Specifically, as described, utilising the Frenchay Dysarthria test it has been possible to replicate the results of Abbs *et al.* (1987) with Parkinson patients and the findings of DePaul *et al.* (1988) with ALS patients. Given the relatively high reliability of this examination (cf. Enderby, 1980; 1983a; 1983b), it would appear reasonable to include a standardised orofacial exam to clinical assessment procedures. From the foregoing considerations it appears that the optimal success of treatment is conditioned not only by the degree to which the distribution of motor impairments across muscle groups is identified, but also if determinations are made as to which of the identified aberrations are contributing factors to the patient's speech motor disability. Treatment of so-called positive signs is unlikely to be useful. However, even if these important conditions are satisfied, the directions of treatment must also be conditioned by other factors. One of these is the careful consideration of the disease process and awareness of what influences treatment might have on that process. For example, in diseases influencing motoneurons (e.g., ALS), strengthening exercises appear to be of questionable value and may even be contraindicated. Specifically, it appears, based upon preliminary evidence in the limb musculature that exercise may stress motoneurons and accelerate their death and exacerbate consequent muscle weakness. The data on post-polio syndrome clearly point in this direction. Additionally, such exercise does not appear to provide even transient plateaus of muscle strength in those patients so tested. In these cases, say for example one wishes to minimise the influence of substantially weakened ALS tongue muscle group function, the alternate approach may be to begin working toward enhancing a patient's ability to use compensatory jaw or extrinsic tongue muscles in anticipation of failure of primary muscles. This approach to treatment thus implies that all differential impairment profiles must be individually evaluated with an understanding of disease prognosis and pathophysiology to determine the optimal course.

Conclusion

Finally, as reflected in this chapter, irrespective of the specific treatment or management programme undertaken, the current emphasis in motor speech disorders is on improved objective measures of system performance. With such measures subtle alterations in performances can be documented in relation to various therapeutic endeavours, or to the progression of the disease condition. Improved measures limit speculation and assumptions; medical colleagues can be provided with clearly defined observations rather than subjective impressions of symptoms and signs. In this manner, handling of patients with motor speech disorders is certain to improve.

References

ABBS, J.H., HUNKER, C.J. and BARLOW, S.M. (1983) Differential speech motor subsystem impairments with suprabulbar lesions: Neurophysiological framework and supporting data. In W.R. Berry (Ed.), *Clinical Dysarthria*. San Diego: College Hill.

ABBS, J.H. (1985) Motor impairment differences in orofacial and respiratory speech control with cerebellar disorders: A response to Hixon and Holt. *Journal of Speech and Hearing Disorders*, 50, 3, 306–12.

ABBS, J.H. and ROSENBEK, J.C. (1985) Some motor control perspectives on Apraxia of Speech and Dysarthria. In J.M. Costello (Ed.), *Recent Advances Speech Disorders in Adults*. California: College Hill.

ABBS, J.H., HARTMAN, D.E. and VISHWANAT, B. (1987) Orofacial motor control impairment in Parkinson's disease. *Neurology*, 37, 394–8.

ALBA, A., PILKINGTON, L.A., KAPLAN, E., BAUM, J., SCHULTHEISS, M., RUGGIERI, A. and LEE, M.H.M. (1976) Long-term pulmonary care in amyotrophic lateral sclerosis. *Respiratory Therapy*, Nov-Dec, 1–11.

BARLOW, S.M. and ABBS, J.H. (1984) Orofacial fine motor control impairment in congenital spastics: Evidence against muscle spindle-related performance deficits. *Neurology*, 34, 145–50.

BARLOW, S.M. and ABBS, J.H. (1986) Fine force and position control of select orofacial structures in the upper motor neuron syndrome. *Experimental Neurology*, 94, 699–713.

BLESS, D.M., RUBOW, R.T. and BRAUN, S. (1983) Speech breathing patterns in cerebral palsied adults. *Folia Phoniatrica*, 24, 107.

BONDUELLE, M. (1975) Amyotrophic lateral sclerosis. In P.J. Vincken, G.W. Bruyn and J.M. DeJong (Eds), *Handbook of Clinical Neurology*. New York: Elsevier Publishing Company.

BOWMAN, J.P. and COMBS, C.M. (1969) Discharge patterns of lingual spindle afferent fibers in the hypoglossal nerve of the Rhesus monkey. *Experimental Neurology*, 21, 105–19.

BRAIN, LORD, CROFT, P. and WILKINSON, M. (1969) The course and outcome of motor neuron disease. In F.H. Norris and L.T. Kurland (Eds), *Motor Neuron Disease: Research on ALS and Related Disorders*. New York: Grune and Stratton.

CARPENTER, R.J., MCDONALD, T.J. and HOWARD, F.M. (1978) The otolaryngologic presentation of amyotrophic lateral sclerosis. *Otolaryngology*, 36, 479–84.

CARPENTER, R.J. and SUTIN, J. (1983) *Human Neuroanatomy*. Baltimore, Williams and Wilkins.

CONNOR, N.P., FORREST, K., COLE, K.J., GRACCO, V.L. and ABBS, J.H. (1987) *Kinematic Analyses of Parkinsonian Dysarthria*. Paper presented at the American Speech–Language–Hearing Association Convention, New Orleans, Louisiana.

DARLEY, F.L., ARONSON, A.E. and BROWN, J.R. (1969a) Differential diagnostic patterns of dysarthria. *Journal of Speech and Hearing Research*, 12, 246–69.

DARLEY, F.L., ARONSON, A.E. and BROWN, J.R. (1969b) Clusters of deviant speech dimensions in the dysarthrias. *Journal of Speech and Hearing Research*, 12, 462–69.

DARLEY, F.L., ARONSON, A.E. and BROWN, J.R. (1975) *Motor Speech Disorders*. Philadelphia, PA: W.B. Saunders.

DAVIS, P.J. and NAIL, B.S. (1984) On the location and size of laryngeal motoneurons in the cat and rabbit. *Journal of Comparative Neurology*, 230, 13–32.

DELONG, M. and GEORGOPOULOS, A.O. (1981) Motor functions of the basal ganglia. In V.B. Brooks (Ed.), *Handbook of Physiology, Section 1, Vol 2: Motor Control, Part 2*. Maryland: American Physiological Society.

DENNY-BROWN, D. (1960) Motor mechanisms — introduction: The general principles of motor integration. In H.W. Magoun (Ed.), *Handbook of Physiology*. Washington, DC: American Physiological Society.

DENNY-BROWN, D. (1980) Preface: Historical aspects of the relation of spasticity to movement. In R.G. Feldman, R.R. Young, and W.P. Koella, (Eds), *Spasticity: Disordered Motor Control*. Chicago: Year Book Medical Publishers.

DEPAUL, R. and ABBS, J.H. (1984) *Physiologic and Acoustic Analyses of the Effect of a Bite-Block Prosthesis in a Spastic Dysarthric*. Paper presented at the Clinical Dysarthria Conference, Tucson, Arizona.

DEPAUL, R. and ABBS, J.H. (1987) Manifestations of ALS in the cranial motor nerves: Dynametric, Neuropathologic, and speech motor data. In B.R. Brooks (Ed.), *Neurologic Clinics of North America: Amyotrophic Lateral Sclerosis, Vol 5*. Philadelphia: W.B. Saunders Co.

DEPAUL, R., ABBS J.H., CALIGIURI, M.P., GRACCO, V.L. and BROOKS, B.R. (1988) Hypoglossal, trigeminal and facial motoneuron involvement in amyotrophic lateral sclerosis. *Neurology*, 38, 2, 281–3.

DUBNER, R., SESSLE, B.J. and STOREY, A.T. (1978) *The Neural Basis of Oral and Facial Function*. New York: Plenum.

DUNCAN, G.W., SHAHANI, B.T. and YOUNG, R.R. (1976) An evaluation of blofen treatment for certain symptoms in patients with spinal cord lesions. A double cross-over study. *Neurology,* 26, 441–6.

ENDERBY, P.M. (1980) Frenchay dysarthria assessment. *British Journal of Disorders of Communication,* 15, 165–73.

ENDERBY, P.M. (1983a) The standardized assessment of dysarthria is possible. In W.R. Berry (Ed.), *Clinical Dysarthria.* San Diego: College Hill.

ENDERBY, P.M. (1983b) *Frenchay Dysarthria Assessment.* San Diego: College Hill.

EVARTS, E.V. (1981) Role of motor cortex in voluntary movements in primates. In V.B. Brooks (Ed.), *Handbook of Physiology, Section 1, Vol II: Motor Control, Part 2.* Maryland: American Physiological Society.

GRACCO, V.L. and ABBS, J.H. (1984) Sensorimotor dysfunction in Parkinson's Disease: Observations from a Multiarticulate Speech Task. *Society for Neuroscience Abstract.*

GUBBAY, S.S., KAHANA, E., ZILBER, J., COOPER, G., PINTOV, S. and LEIBOWITZ, Y. (1985) Amyotrophic lateral sclerosis: A study of its presentation and prognosis. *Journal of Neurology,* 232, 295–300.

HARDY, J.C. (1967) Suggestions for physiological research in dysarthria. *Cortex,* 3, 128–56.

HIRANO, A. (1982) Aspects of the ultrastructure of ALS. In L.P. Rowland (Ed.), *Human Neuron Diseases.* New York: Raven Press.

HIXON, T.J. (1975) *Respiratory-Laryngeal Evaluation.* Paper presented at the Veterans Administration Workshop in Motor Speech Disorders, Madison, Wisconsin.

HOFFMAN, D.S. and LUSCHEI, E.S. (1980) Responses of monkey precentral cortical cells during a controlled jaw bite task. *Journal of Neurophysiology,* 44, 333—48.

HUGHES, J.T. (1982) Pathology of ALS. In L.P. Rowland (Ed.), *Human Motor Neuron Diseases.* New York: Raven Press.

HUNKER, C.J., ABBS, J.H. and BARLOW, S.M. (1982) The relationship between Parkinsonian rigidity and hypokinesia in the orofacial system: A quantitative analysis. *Neurology,* 32, 7, 740–54.

HUNKER, C.J. and ABBS, J.H. (1984) Physiological analyses of Parkinsonian tremors in the orofacial system. In M.R. McNeil, J.C. Rosenbek and A. Aronson (Eds), *The Dysarthrias: Physiology-Acoustics-Perception-Management.* California: College Hill.

KIMURA, J. (1973) The blink reflex as a test for brain-stem and higher central nervous system function. In J.E. Desmedt (Ed.), *New Developments in Electromyography and Clinical Neurophysiology, Vol. 3.* Basel: Karger.

KUSHNER, M.J., PARRISH, M., BURKE, A., BEHRENS, M., HAYS, A.P., FRAME, B. and ROWLAND, L.P. (1984) Nystagmus in motor neuron disease. Clinicopathological study of two cases. *Annals of Neurology,* 16, 71–7.

LABUSZEWSKI, T. and LIDSKY, T.I. (1979) Basal ganglia influences on brain stem trigeminal neurons. *Experimental Neurology,* 65, 471–7.

LANCE, J.W. (1980) Pathophysiology of spasticity and clinical experience with baclofen. In R.G. Feldman, R.R. Young, and W.P. Koella (Eds), *Spasticity: Disordered Motor Control.* Chicago: Year Book Medical Publishers.

LANDAU, W.M. (1974) Spasticity: The fable of a neurological demon and the emperor's new therapy. *Archives of Neurology,* 31, 217–9.

LANDAU, W.M. (1980) Spasticity: What is it? What is it not? In R.G. Feldman, R.R. Young, and W.P. Koella (Eds), *Spasticity: Disordered Motor Control.* Chicago: Year Book Medical Publishers.

LAWYER, T. and NETSKY, M.G. (1953) Amyotrophic lateral sclerosis: A clinicoanatomic study of fifty-three cases. *Archives of Neurology and Psychiatry*, 69, 171–92.

LIDSKY, T.L., ROBINSON, J.A., DENARO, F.J. and WEINHOLD, P.M. (1978) Trigeminal influences on entopeduncular units. *Brain Research*, 141, 227–34.

LOGEMANN, J.A., BLONSKY, E.R. and BOSHES, B. (1975) Dysphagia in Parkinsonism. *Journal of the American Medical Association*, 231, 1, 69–70.

LOGEMANN, J.A., FISHER, H.B., BOSES, B. and BLONSKY, E. (1978) Frequency and co-occurrence of vocal tract dysfunctions in the speech of a large sample of Parkinson patients. *Journal of Speech and Hearing Disorders*, 43, 47–57.

LOVE, R.J., HAGERMAN, E.L. and TAIMI, E.G. (1980) Speech performance, dysphagia and oral reflexes in cerebral palsy. *Journal of Speech and Hearing Disorders*, 45, 59–75.

LYBOLT, J., NETSELL, R. and FARRAGE, F. (1982) *A Bite-Block Prosthesis in the Treatment of Dysarthria*. Paper presented at the annual convention of the American-Speech-Language-Hearing Association, Ontario, Canada.

McNAMARA, R.D. (1983) A conceptual holistic approach to dysarthria treatment. In W.R. Berry (Ed.), *Clinical Dysarthria*. California: College Hill.

MARSDEN, C.D. (1982) The mysterious motor function of the basal ganglia. *Neurology*, 32, 515–39.

MORTIMER, J.A. and WEBSTER, D.D. (1978) Relationships between quantitative measures of rigidity and tremor and the electromyographic responses to load perturbations in unselected normal subjects and Parkinson patients. In J.E. Desmedt (Ed.), *Cerebral Control in Man: Long Loop Mechanisms, Vol. 4*. Basel: Karger.

MORTIMER, J.A., PIROZZOLO, F.J., HANSCH, E.C. and WEBSTER, D.D. (1982) Relationship of motor symptoms to intellectual deficits in Parkinson disease. *Neurology*, 32, 133–7.

NIELSON, P.D., ANDREWS, G., GUITAR, B.E. and QUINN, P.T. (1979) Tonic stretch reflexes in lip, tongue and jaw muscles. *Brain Research*, 178, 311–27.

NETSELL, R. and DANIEL, B. (1979) Dysarthria in adults: Physiological approach to rehabilitation. *Archives of Physical and Medical Rehabilitation*, 60, 502–8.

PALMER, E.D. (1974) Dysphagia in Parkinsonism. *Journal of American Medical Association*, 220, 1, 1349.

PHILLIPS, C.G. and PORTER, R. (1977) *Corticospinal Neurons. Their Role in Movement*. London: Academic Press.

ROBBINS, J., LOGEMANN, J.A. and KIRSHNER, H.S. (1986) Swallowing and speech production in Parkinson's disease. *Annals of Neurology*, 19, 283–7.

ROSENBEK, J. and LaPOINTE, L.L. (1978) The dysarthrias: Description, diagnosis and treatment. In D.F. Johns (Ed.), *Clinical Management of Neurogenic Communicative Disorders*. Boston: Little, Brown.

RUBOW, R.T. and NETSELL, R. (1979) *EMG Biofeedback Rehabilitation in Facial Paralysis: Ten Year Follow-Up of a Case Study*. Proceedings of the Tenth Annual Meeting of the Biofeedback Society of America, San Diego, California.

RUBOW, R.T. (1981) *Biofeedback in the Treatment of Speech Disorders*. Biofeedback Society of America Task Force Reports.

SAHRMAN, S.A. and NORTH, B.J. (1977) The relationship of voluntary movement to spasticity in the upper motor neuron syndrome. *Annals of Neurology*, 2, 460–5.

SCHLIESSER, H.F. (1982) Alternate motion rates of the speech articulators in adults with cerebral palsy. *Folia Phoniatrica*, 34, 258–64.

SHAWKER, T.H. and SONIES, B.C. (1984) Tongue movement during speech: A real time ultrasound evaluation, *Journal of Clinical Ultrasound,* 12, 125–33.

SHIRAKI, H. and YASE, Y. (1975) Amyotrophic lateral sclerosis in Japan. In G.W. Bruyn, P.J. Vincken and J.M. DeJong (Eds), *Handbook of Clinical Neurology.* Vol 2, New York: Elsevier Publishing Co.

TATTON, W.G. and LEE, R.G. (1975) Evidence for abnormal long-loop reflexes in rigid Parkinsonian patients. *Brain Research,* 100, 671–6.

VINCKEN, W.G., GAUTHIER, S.G., DOLLFUSS, R.E., HANSON, R.E., DARAUAY, C.M. and COSIO, M.G. (1984) Involvement of upper-airway muscles in extrapyramidal disorders; a cause of airflow limitation. *New England Journal of Medicine,* 311, 438–42.

WELZL, H., SCHWARTING, R. and HUSTON, J.P. (1984) Substantia nigra efferents and afferents in the control of the perioral biting reflex. In R. Bandler (Ed.), *Modulation of Sensorimotor Activity During Alterations in Behavioral States.* New York: Alan R. Liss.

WYKE, B. (Ed.), (1974) *Ventilatory and Phonatory Control Systems.* London: Oxford University Press.

14   Apraxia of Speech

Niklas Miller

Apraxia of speech is found discussed under numerous other labels, including speech dyspraxia, verbal dyspraxia, aphemia, efferent motor dysphasia, etc. Darley, Aronson and Brown (1975) and Messerli (1983) provide a more extensive discussion of the labelling problem. Apraxia of speech is only one of a range of disorders associated with disturbances of action. Others include the limb dyspraxias, constructional dyspraxia, ocular motor dyspraxia and many more (see Miller, 1986 for detailed discussion of these).

The classical definition of apraxia is a disorder of motor planning and/or execution in the presence of an otherwise normally functioning motor system. Thus there is no loss of power or change in tone; reflexes are normal as are the range and speed of movements. Sensory functions are also normal; there is no change in auditory, visual and tactile perception. It can be demonstrated that the person's failure to carry out a motor task correctly is not due to non-cooperation, low motivation, non-comprehension, or any generalised intellectual deficit. Of course, apraxia may co-occur with any one or more of the above problems. For example, the speech apraxic often has a (right) facial weakness; the limb apraxic may have a hemiparesis or loss of sensation. In such cases the clinician's task is all the more difficult since the problem then is to unravel which disability is contributing in what way and to what degree to the person's disability. The presence of a marked dysphasia may render differential diagnosis and the treatment approach difficult.

Following this line, a bare definition of apraxia of speech would be an (acquired) disorder of articulation due to dysfunction in the planning and/or execution of speech motor control in the presence of an otherwise normal motor system. Whilst it commonly occurs with dysphasia and/or evidence of muscle weakness and sensory changes, it is not *caused* by them though it *interacts* with them.

For anyone grappling to come to an understanding of apraxia of speech, it is sad to relate that even such a general definition contains many controversial implications.

What Does Apraxia of Speech Sound Like?

In mild cases there is full or nearly full intelligibility. Speech might sound slow, deliberate, halting, with minor apparent dysfluencies and dysprosody. Speakers sound as if they are talking with a foreign accent (Kent and Rosenbek, 1982; Square and Mlcoch, 1983; Graff-Radford, Cooper, Colsher and Damasio, 1986; Tonkonogy, 1986). The acoustic and articulatory correlates of this are mentioned below.

The dysfluency and dysprosody increase as severity increases. Unexpected pauses appear between, and even within words. These silences may be filled with visible oral-facial struggle. The impression of foreign accent gives way to definite distortions. Atypical allophones are heard: e.g., unaspirated [t] in two. Distortion might be so marked as to suggest another sound has been substituted. At other times unwanted sounds seem to be added, or expected ones omitted. This pattern of distortion, apparent substitution, addition and omission is characteristically inconsistent, so that in the same phonetic context on repeated occasions, a quite different production ensues. 'A tea please' could be realised as [ə'ti pliz], ['əe 'tipfliz], [ə 'dalə bɬIs], and so on.

In more severe cases unintelligible utterances take over. In the severest speech apraxia there may not even be any utterances. Patients may be mute, aphonic. Attempts at spontaneous conversation or even imitating single syllables end after effortful struggle in frustrated silence.

Language picture in apraxia of speech

Lecours and Lhermitte (1976) and Square, Darley and Sommers (1982) report cases with no language disorder or a negligible disorder which usually remits spontaneously over a period of days or weeks (Mohr, 1980). More typically the profile is of relatively good comprehension accompanied by poor or absent expression. Writing may be (relatively) spared, but in severer cases provides no scope as an immediate communication channel. Apraxia of speech, being found with all the classical dysphasic types may be associated with agrammatism, dysgrammatism, word finding difficulty and so on.

Arguments in the past have raged over whether apraxia of speech is a language or a speech disorder. Martin, 1974; Martin and Rigrodsky, 1974a, 1974b; Aten, Darley, Deal and Johns, 1975; Darley *et al.,* 1975; Klich, Ireland and Weidner, 1979; Kent and Rosenbek, 1983; Keller, 1984; Wolk, 1986; and Square, 1987 provide the relevant reading. The focus of attention has passed now to a consideration of the way language and (motor) speech are united rather than divided to produce spoken utterances. This theme is resumed below, but it is noted here that language factors do influence speech patterns (Wertz, LaPointe and Rosenbek, 1984; Elman and

McClelland, 1984; but see Mlcoch, Darley and Noll, 1982).

Speech apraxics are more likely to be derailed the more complex the syllable structure; on polysyllabic words; on more unfamiliar words, especially content words; and errors might rise with increased grammatical complexity.

The above offers a thumbnail sketch of what the speech apraxic sounds like. But there is more to it than meets the ear, so to speak. Instrumental examination has offered deeper insights.

Instrumental descriptions of apraxia of speech

Workers have approached the subject using a variety of techniques. Washino, Kasai and Uchida (1981) and Hardcastle, Morgan-Barry and Clark (1985) used electropalatography for a moment by moment view of tongue and palate relationship. Shankweiler, Harris and Taylor (1968) and Fromm, Abbs, McNeil and Rosenbek (1981) monitored muscle activity by electromyography. The latter also utilised simultaneous sensors to trace lip and jaw movements. Itoh and fellow workers (Itoh, Sasanuma and Ushijima, 1979; Itoh, Sasanuma, Hirose, Yoshioka and Ushijima, 1980; Itoh and Sasanuma, 1984) used fibre-optic techniques to study velar function and X-ray microbeam apparatus to follow tongue activity. Keller (1987) has outlined the potential of ultra-sound recording.

Sound spectrographic and laryngographic studies have also been used to look at voice onset time (VOT) and termination, vowel duration, formant transitions and co-articulation in speech apraxics (Itoh, Sasanuma, Tatsumi, Murakami, Fukusako and Suzuki, 1982; Kent and Rosenbek, 1983; Ziegler and von Cramon, 1985; 1986a 1986b).

A detailed review of all the above studies is not possible here. The trend in conclusions though points towards a disorder in the timing patterns needed to produce sounds and move from one sound to the next. For instance the dissolution of relative timing of voice onset with plosive release correlates with the impression of voiced-voiceless confusions.

Dysfunction in the timing as opposed to the speed and range of movement of velar activity relates to what are heard as inconsistencies in nasal-oral distinctions. What are heard as stopping and affricatisation difficulties tie in with problems of controlling contact force and time/duration. In milder cases these distortions and vowel duration and formation alterations give the impression of foreign accent and lie behind the atypical coarticulation (heard as additions, distortions and omissions) common to apraxia of speech.

McNeil, Caligiuri, Weismer and Rosenbek (1986) investigated acceleration and velocity times for apraxics. They too emphasised that in apraxia it is relative and not absolute values that are disturbed. They found, despite delayed initiation and considerable inter- and intra-individual variation, that apraxics and normals behaved similarly regarding speed and range of movements. Dysarthrics were characterised by failure to reach peak velocities and to attain the desired range of movement (Ziegler *et al.,* 1986c).

Two significant findings not apparent to the naked ear, are that even during 'silent' pauses considerable abortive articulatory activity may be taking place, and that many sounds that appear correct to the listener are actually produced with abnormal articulatory postures (Fromm *et al.,* 1982; Hardcastle *et al.,* 1985).

Theoretical Basis of Intervention

Despite hiding behind countless labels the clinical characteristics of apraxia of speech have always been agreed upon. Real controversy, still unresolved, arises when investigators go beyond description, to explanation of the disorder. The dispute over language versus motor dysfunction was mentioned previously. Currently the question is phrased more around how language and praxis are linked to produce speech.

Earlier scholarship sharply divided a pre-motor language (phonological) planning stage from the phonetic, motor, executive stage. The latter was linked to apraxia of speech whereas the former was designated a dysphasia. While adhering to recognition of an 'earlier' and 'later' stage in speech sound realisations, recent argument, both theoretical, linguistic and clinical has challenged such rigid compartmentalisation to stress the much closer interaction and interdependence of these phases.

Buckingham (1983) has spoken of apraxia of speech for the executive and apraxia of language for the planning stages. He discusses the same clinical–theoretical issues in relation to perseveration in aphasics and to a theoretical model of production (Buckingham 1985; 1986). Miller (1986) draws parallels with other areas of dyspraxia (gestural, constructional) where the notion of an unfolding action passing from an abstract ideational frame to concrete action is well established. Just as one views underlying visual-spatial disruption as crucial to planning in constructional praxis, so language can be considered in the same light for pronunciation. Gestural dyspraxias include ideational and ideomotor types, arguably parallel to planning and executive dyspraxias. A third type, midway between dyspraxia and paresis, is limb-kinetic dyspraxia. Interestingly, instrumental and clinical descriptions of speech point to an equivalent to this (Keller, 1984; Hardcastle *et al.,* 1985, and the debate between Schiff, Alexander, Naeser and Galaburda, 1983 and Crary, Hardy and Williams, 1985). Kimura (1982) and Roy and Square (1985) amongst others have drawn attention to commonalities in breakdowns across the different dyspraxic syndromes (gestural, speech, etc.).

Within a linguistic context, Hewlett (1985), Grunwell (1985) and Milroy (1985) have argued convincingly against a strict phonological-phonetic demarcation, especially in speaker oriented study. Hewlett advocates a tripartite view of interdependent phonological, phonetic and articulatory disorders which closely reflect the clinical suggestions made above. In assessment this results in looking for clusters of deficits along a continuum rather than strictly demarcated disorders; also in therapy, features that interact can be manipulated along a continuum instead of being treated in isolation.

Making these claims is a step towards understanding apraxia of speech but it is no solution. More questions are raised. For example, if there is a planning stage, where does the plan originate? What is planned? What processes are passed through from intention to speak to actual production of speech sounds? Labels such as plan, stage, process, programme, scheme, levels and so on are all highly contentious terms. How is the programming and execution (again a debatable dichotomy or continuum) organised? Is it a unidirectional, hierarchical, linear flow command system, where orders are dictated from the top down, or is it a heterarchically organised system where there is cross talk backwards, forwards and across in the chains of command (Kelso and Tuller, 1981; Kelso, Tuller, Harris, 1983; Fowler, 1985)? From all the possible movements the human body could make, how does the action control system restrict occurrences to only those that need to be produced, yet at the same time maintain the option of creating actions and sequences of actions never before performed? A similar question arises with language — how, with finite units (phonological, syntactic, etc.) is the facility retained of an infinite number of novel utterances? Other questions raised include whether oral verbal and non-verbal movements are under the same control system and patterns; how the speech production system arrives at a constant set of relative output values, heard as the same sound, word and sentence on repeated occasions, despite varying roads of arriving at the time-space relationships needed to produce the utterances? Consider for instance the movement variations introduced by different speeds and loud-nesses, talking with food in the mouth, lying down as opposed to standing, or all the sound-movement contexts that any given sound can occur in. These are not idle theoretical questions. They all ultimately have bearing on clinical practice.

If there is a programming and an execution difference, then assessment must be geared to highlight this, both for sounds in isolation and combination (Mateer and Kimura, 1977; Guyard, Sabouraud and Gagnepain, 1981). Not only must it distinguish cases at either end of this claimed continuum, but it must be able to sort out the varying degrees along the continuum of any one case. Therapy must, in turn, recognise elements of the different underlying tendencies. Rehabilitating selection and ordering of segments in an overall semantic-syntactic matrix versus realisation of these as actual sound producing concatenations of movements and the control of relative time and space variables is necessary. In effect, the transition between segments will require separate therapeutic approaches.

If all or parts of the action control system operate hierarchically, then ways of restoring or compensating for shortcomings will be different if one is dealing with a heterarchy. The notion of intra- and inter-systemic reorganisation (Luria, 1970; Wertz *et al.*, 1984) matches well with the concept of the heterarchy, where interactions and locus of control within the system can be manipulated to bypass or boost a deficit. Thus one could envisage exploiting the idea of motor equivalence, arriving at the same target via numerous means, as one way of compensation. Visual or tactile control may bypass deficient motor control, or verbal planning might support action organisation. Increased auditory monitoring may compensate for reduced tactile-kinaesthetic awareness, or vice versa. These aspects are taken up again below in the discussion of treatment approaches.

Causative Factors

The immediate causative factors are clear — anything which causes damage to the structures and functions of the brain — be it stroke, head injury or various disease processes. There is consensus on where damage associated with apraxia of speech is located. The language dominant hemisphere is involved, and within it the areas most often implicated are the parietal or temporal-parietal lobe, the frontal lobe (especially frontal operculum and insula) (Mohr, 1980; Marquardt and Sussman, 1984; Abbs and Welt, 1985), and various subcortical structures (Kertesz, 1984; Basso, Della Sala and Farabola, 1987; Poncet, Habib and Robillard, 1987 for conduction dysphasia). There any semblance of agreement ends.

Are different areas linked with different types/manifestations of dyspraxia? Strong argument (Deutsch, 1984; Tonkonogy, 1986) exists for seeing fluent apraxia of language breakdown as essentially a (temporal) parietal disorder and the more non-fluent phonetic apraxia of speech as essentially a frontal one. So-called limb-kinetic dyspraxia is seen in lesions believed to compromise pyramidal fibres from Brodmann's Area 4, giving a (right) hemiparesis, but also catching (left-right) intercortical fibres, or their origins in Brodmann's Area 6. Possible subcortical lesion sites have included the (dominant hemisphere) thalamus and basal ganglia.

Why are these areas involved in apraxia? The answer to this is intimately bound up with what apraxia is. Until the intricacies of motor control are disentangled answers to this question can only be tentative and speculative. Luria (1973), Abbs and Welt (1985), and Tonkonogy (1986) approach the question. It will not be pursued any further here. Students are merely reminded of Hughlings Jackson's caveat that localisation of symptoms is not synonymous with localisation of function.

Assessment Considerations

In assessment the questions are: has the person got apraxia of speech, or something else? If they have apraxia what features do they show, and how severely? What other problems might be influencing the apraxic picture? Can anything be done about it?

Differential diagnosis

Not only will clinicians require to sort out which symptoms are due to dyspraxia and which due to dysarthria and/or dysphasia, but they will need to remember that there are subtypes of each of these categories. Teasing out speech dyspraxia from ataxic dysarthria (Kent *et al.*, 1981; Gillmer and van der Merwe, 1983; Wertz, 1985) will pose a different problem to differentiating it from Parkinsonian (Kent *et al.*, 1982; Weismer, 1984) or spastic dysarthric features (Hardcastle *et al.*, 1985; Ziegler *et al.*, 1986c). Which hesitations and dysprosody come from speech dyspraxia and which from word finding or syntax problems, will be a central question when planning treatment in cases with co-existing dysphasia.

Other works deal in detail with the diagnostic process (Darley *et al.*, 1975; Dabul, 1979; Wertz *et al.*, 1984; Miller, 1986). There is just space here to mention a few clinical rules of thumb.

Table 14.1: Some Clinical Rules of Thumb for Looking for Dysarthric Versus Speech Dyspraxic Symptoms

Dysarthrics' 'errors' tend to have:	*Dyspraxics tend to have:*
1. Consistency for a given sound across time, contexts and stimulus conditions.	1. Inconsistent realisation including islands of fluency for a given sound or word.
2. Comparable severity in verbal and non-verbal modes.	2. Better in less volitional (automatic, imitation) than highly volitional. Better on sense than non-sense tasks.
3. Links to overall medical physical condition.	3. Dissociation ± verbal. Possible oral non-verbal dyspraxia not necessarily correlating with speech symptom severity.
4. Visible struggle consistent with muscle tone, power, co-ordination disorder.	4. Severity inconsistent with observable physical disability. Inconsistent struggle related to psychomotor complexity.
5. Visible struggle to reach necessary range and velocity of movement.	5. Visible struggle to achieve overall articulatory postures.

Table 14.2: Some Rules of Thumb for Gauging the Degree of Co-existing Dysphasia

1. Greater the degree of comprehension loss.
2. Greater the degree of errors on responses (word, letter arranging; ABC board; writing) not demanding a verbal response
3. Lesser the awareness of articulatory errors.
4. Lesser the attempts to communicate by any means (gesture, mime).

Other conditions affecting assessment and treatment planning include:

1 Co-existing limb and/or constructional apraxia
2 Perceptual (auditory, visual, tactile) deficit
3 Intellectual deterioration

These guidelines only create a subjective impression. For more objective measurement performance on a series of tasks that tap areas in which patients with apraxia of speech experience difficulty is necessary. The dimensions typically chosen are:

1 Sounds in isolation through to sounds in words (nonsense and real) and sentences, with words increasing both in number and complexity of syllables
2 Repetitive production of a single syllable versus alternating production of two or three different syllables (pa-pa-pa v. pa-ta-pa-ta-pa-ta)
3 Execution of these spontaneously and to repetition/imitation
4 Comparison of these in varying contexts — free speaking, reading and writing; semi-automatic tasks such as familiar phrase or word pair completion; supposedly automatic tasks (counting, passages known by heart).

Instrumental assessments are not generally available, but if used can supply objective data on voice onset time (VOT), vowel length, formant transitions, co-articulatory behaviour and electromyographic correlates of these. Such clinical and instrumental data are supplemented and placed in perspective by a language and oral physical examination and any other tests which the person's situation warrants (perceptual; psychometric evaluation). It is vital to complement formal assessments with an informal functional assessment: i.e., what can the person do with the communicative means at their disposal? Two people with identical formal profiles may have markedly different success as communicators (Miller, 1989).

Basically, the search is for evidence that the person's problems with articulation stem from disability in selecting a correct sound or difficulty realising a target sound despite indications that they have the range and power of movement to product it, and 'know' the word that they wish to put it in. The clinician looks for tell-tale signs of these difficulties being exacerbated by increase in length and complexity of utterance, on less familiar words, and the other dimensions mentioned above.

The more the disability lies in struggling transition from one segment to the next, with variable, inconsistent distortions of sound and co-articulation, even when occurring in same or similar contexts, the more one suspecs a dysfluent ideomotor apraxia of speech or limb-kinetic dyspraxia-dysarthria. The more the tendency is to contamination of sounds across syllable and word boundaries in the form of effortless frank substitutions, anticipations or perseverations, the more likely one is dealing with elements of fluent apraxia of language (Buckingham's 1983 term; Mateer and Kimura, 1977; Guyard, Sabouraud and Gagnepain, 1981; Nespoulous, Lecours and Joanette, 1983).

Treatment

Some issues in neurological rehabilitation

Design and implementation of treatment begs several theoretical and practical questions. What is the relationship between therapy and recovery? Does improvement come through spontaneous recovery or not at all? Can therapy directly restore lost or impaired function? Is reorganisation and substitution by retained skills the only means of effecting change after brain injury? Can therapy influence outcome of spontaneous recovery, or is the therapist's role restricted to short-circuiting emerging self-defeating or limiting practices? Is relearning only task specific or is generalisation possible? Are there optimum times for introducing different types of therapy in different ways? There are no straightforward answers to these problems yet, but the issues are pertinent to speech therapy and must be borne in mind.

Clinicians, ever ones to hedge their bets, tend to cover all possibilities until studies indicate better ways. Currently most therapists initiate intervention during spontaneous recovery, even if only to counsel patient and family on forestalling maladaptive trends. In the chronic phase direct retraining is paired with compensatory reorganisation to cover deficiencies.

Aims of therapy

Some of the essential principles involve knowing where you are going and how to get there, sharing this knowledge with patient and family, setting realistic goals in terms of likely speech–language outcome, and functional usefulness of attainments.

This will demand prognostic evaluation not only in the context of speech and language assessment, but also of the person's general neuropsychological and social circumstances.

Mapping out a path to the end-goal in manageable and worthwile stages is important and therapy must target crucial areas that are (a) amenable to change, and (b) if changed will produce a significant difference in the person's performance. Each substep must be an end in itself or provide access to more significant performance. That is why each programme must be tailored to individuals' needs, even when the therapy (e.g., Melodic Intonation Therapy — Sparks and Holland, 1976; Tonkovich and Marquardt, 1977) comes as an off-the-shelf package. When focus is on the minutiae of voice onset time or whatever, the whole person and total communication perspective must not be lost. Efficient therapy knows when and how to stop.

Mainstream Treatment Practices

Fashions in therapy are continually evolving. To-day's clinical spring collection is tomorrow's old hat. Therapy content is shaped by clinicians' views on what they believe to be the cause and course of the disorder, what has seemed to work in the past, by their training background, and the organisation of their rehabilitation services.

The following outlines some methods which have been associated with success against apraxia of speech by North American and British Isles speech clinicians. Whether the actual content and methods were what truly brought about improvement still awaits experimental confirmation, as does whether there might be more optimal therapy. Clinicians should not close their eyes to methods not mentioned here, nor novel combinations of those mentioned. If careful monitoring is built into therapy it should soon become clear whether a particular path is the treatment of choice.

Before planning in detail remember that communication involves listeners as well as speakers. Speakers need to remain included, to have a sympathetic listener (Enderby and Crow, 1987) but importantly, too, to have an active, constructively facilitative listener (Miller, 1989). In aiming for maximum support, visual tactile and non-speech communication always remain important channels. Experience has shown that successful apraxics are those able to take over their own therapy, and therapy that is ever dependent on the clinician is of limited or no value. Therapy must teach the person not only what to do, but how to *use* it. If a technique, content or goal has no use it is redundant.

Some therapeutic practices

Intervention varies with severity of the disorder. In very severe cases the person will be mute. Efforts will be directed towards eliciting any sound and establishing some (alternative) communication channel. Methods available for the former include stimulation: via so-called automatic actions (singing, humming, over-learned material and series, etc.); via paralinguistic and non-verbal gestures (tut-tut; yawning; blowing a kiss, etc.); by physical placement of the articulators by the therapist; through imitation (+/− verbal); and by following static or moving pictograms/articulograms (Hill, 1978).

Emphasis will be on looking, feeling, listening as much as speaking (Simmons, 1980). The why and how of following pictograms, copying clinicians and using mirrors all need to be trained. They are not magic wands. As soon as a sound is possible it should be given a use. Elicitation techniques must also be taught to the family. Mystique about apraxia and its therapy should not become an added symptom to combat.

Less severe cases may manage approximations to sounds. The above techniques can be used to stabilise and extend the repertoire. Once a sound is stable it can be used to derive other positions/sounds, and to stand in contrast with another element. Except in extreme instances when problems arise even in producing isolated sounds, apraxia of speech manifests itself more when concatenation of sounds and syllables commences. Sounds/syllables in isolation tend to be relatively preserved.

Which sound do you start with? Group data suggest a gradient of difficulty rising through vowels, plosives, nasals, laterals and fricatives to affricates. Individual people do not necessarily conform. Hence the need to establish each individual's patterns. Order of teaching will then depend on this and factors such as: visibility, feelability, direct manipulability, usability, and frequency of occurrence in familiar words and phrases (family names, pets, over-learned and social words). Debate exists concerning whether it is better to proceed through nonsense or meaningful syllables. Programmes employing nonsense syllables (Rosenbek, Lemme, Ahern, Harris and Wertz, 1973; Dabul and Bollier, 1976; Holtzapple and Marshall, 1977; Deal and Florance, 1978) aim to tackle the actual motor speech dysfunction more directly. Because meaningful syllables are tied to linguistic and situational variables there may be less generalisability. There are no hard data to support either way. Functionally, for the apraxic, it is hard to wait months before meaningful stimuli are introduced, and many would say if a technique works (meaningful syllables), then why ignore it? Either way therapy progresses through increasing syllabic complexity, moving from familiar single syllable words to uncommon (for the person) polysyllabic words in simple then complex grammatical utterances, in situations of increasing propositionality and decreasing external (visual, tactile, contextual, etc.) support.

With the attainment of stable syllables progressing to multisyllables, several more important ways of extending communicative competence are available. Tonal variation offers scope for saying the same utterance with an imperative, questioning, doubting, etc., tone. Different nuances can be expressed by contrasting stress on different syllables. Contrastive stress drills take a phrase and practise it with alternative stress and intonational patterns — e.g., /gI mI maI ti/, give me my tea, as '*give* me my tea', 'give *me* my tea', give me my *tea*'. In some cases intelligibility might be improved considerably simply by concentration on suprasegmental features.

Relearned or intact 'chunks' can serve as carrier phrases. Gonna, wanna, /Isa/ (it's a. .) /w z / (where's the . . .) especially if combined with other (approximations to) familiar utterances (ta/thanks; næŋks/no thanks, etc.) can boost communicative morale.

The gap can be bridged between single and polysyllabic words by first introducing longer words composed of well rehearsed single syllable elements; toe-ma-toe for tomato; pan-D-mow-knee-M for pandemonium; car-ten for carton and curtain.

Another method of deriving connected speech is by approximation of propositional language from less volitional. An often cited example is fried egg from Friday. Others would be 'want to' from 1, 2; deaf from D.E.F.

As an especial difficulty of apraxia of speech is smooth transition from syllable to syllable, techniques which ease this by teaching with co articulations incorporated, modifying transitional complexity, or permitting a degree of distortion, are useful. The production of curtain as car-ten (above) is a brief example of the latter. The area is dealt with more extensively by Miller (in press). In using such methods, apraxic and therapist are seeking the best trade-off between articulatory precision and functional intelligibility.

Mention has been made of direct therapy, various ways of reorganising intact functions to replace lost skills and gaining access to utterances through alternative channels. For some patients speech will always remain elusive or inadequate and substitution or augmentation through other media will be necessary.

Replacement therapies

Some apraxics are fortunate enough to have (relatively) intact writing. Others will be able to utilise alphabet charts or mechanical equivalents to these. Concurrent language problems, alas, often mean that use of such equipment will be as limited as spoken communication. Machines that employ pictographic, prerecorded messages associated with a single button, or synthesised speech as alternative or augmentative expression (Bennett, 1987; Easton, 1987) may be more suitable here.

Gestural sign systems from ad hoc personal choices to complete systems provide another avenue of expression (Dowden, Marshall and Tomkins, 1981; Bennett, 1987). The presence of limb dyspraxia may inhibit learning in some subjects (Roy, 1981; Rothi and Heilman, 1985). Also, as Coelho and Duffy (1985) point out, there are people who acquire manual gestures but who just do not or cannot use them. Code and Gaunt (1986) report a case without encouraging success. Underlying language disability may impair sign language too (Thomson, 1982).

This has been a very fleeting skim over some central principles in apraxia of speech therapy. One is aware that as much has been left out as included, especially regarding treatment of fluent apraxia of language and the potential of instrumental techniques (EPG, laryngograph). The concerned clinician must consult the more detailed references for closer guidance.

Effectiveness of Treatment

There are no large scale studies on the efficacy of apraxia of speech therapy equivalent to reviews attempted on dysphasia intervention. LaPointe (1984) conducted a single case multiple baseline study and Wertz (1984) reported on the performance of dyspraxic-dysphasic people in a larger survey of dysphasics. Additionally, there exist numerous investigations into the usefulness or not of various components of overall apraxia treatment. These include the viability of melodic intonation therapy (Tonkovich and Marquardt, 1977); fading of integral stimulation (Holtzapple and Marshall, 1977); a hierarchical continuum of integrated stimulation (Rosenbek, *et al.,* 1973; Deal *et al.,* 1978); the strategy of rehearsal (Warren, 1977; Bugbee and Nichols, 1980); the pairing of vibrotactile stimulation with speech production (Rubow, Rosenbek, Collins, Longstreth, 1982); and numerous others summarised in major works (e.g., Wertz *et al.,* 1984) on apraxia of speech.

The patient of LaPointe demonstrated improvement and the patients in the study reported by Wertz improved if they received motor speech training, but not from general language therapy. Given the controlled conditions stipulated in the studies concerning the different approaches (as opposed to diluted, haphazard application, which is always a danger in clinic), it has been shown that apraxics of speech can and do respond to therapy.

All approaches have involved an intensive pattern of therapy. Even if not being seen daily by a therapist, patients have carried out daily practice. Experimental and clinical experience (Hill, 1978; Wertz *et al.,* 1984; Rosenbek, 1985) suggest that patients with apraxia of speech who cannot take over responsibility for daily drills, whether this be due to concurrent neuropsychological disabilities, or for social or clinical organisational reasons, have a poor prognosis for improvement and reaching beyond what spontaneous central nervous system repair and reorgani-sation bring.

However, with each person the clinicians need to become researchers — establishing baselines and controls, systematically manipulating variables (input, response demands, etc.) and monitoring which mode and combination of therapies are proving most effective for the individual. Only in this way will unproductive practice be eliminated and the apraxic reap maximum benefit from intervention.

Conclusion

The centre ground of a definition and description of apraxia of speech is relatively uncontroversial. It is a disorder in the unfolding of an action at a higher cortical level, bringing about mistiming and misplacement of articulators despite normal tone, power and sensation. Speakers sound dysprosodic, and appear to distort, omit, misorder and struggle to produce sounds, even though at other times they pronounce the same sound in the same context with ease. In severe cases spoken expression may be completely banished. Despite instrumental techniques having added greatly to our descriptive knowledge, many issues of explanation remain undecided. Evidence was cited supporting the notion that the central disruption in what is traditionally considered to be apraxia of speech lies in a breakdown in the temporal and spatial cohesion of speech action. But how do these actions originate, how are they organised and carried out within the central nervous system and what exactly is disrupted? What should be the units of analysis? Are there different types of apraxia of speech according to which aspects in the assembly and unfolding of actions are disordered?

Suggestions for solutions point towards an interplay between an ideational, conceptual, cognitive-linguistic planning disorder (traditionally termed phonological dysfunction), an ideomotor executive production breakdown (traditional apraxia of speech) and a so-called limb-kinetic dyspraxic-dysarthria. These arise from different disruptions to a heterarchically organised speech motor system.

Within this scheme the strict division between mental and physical (action, motor) constructs is clinically and neuroanatomically unreliable, even erroneous. Apraxia of speech may be a motor disorder, but it exists within a linguistic framework, which exists within social interaction. Elements of planning and execution may be higher cortical, but this activity interacts and is in turn dependent on subcortical organisation. Hence apraxia may be influenced by, and simultaneously itself influence, co-existing language and dysarthric disorders. Therapy may be via direct attention to (assumed) underlying apraxic breakdown, but manipulation of other aspects of planning and communication can also be used to influence speech output. A philosophy of intervention was introduced that was aware of and exploited all these interdependencies.

Accordingly therapy, at different times, or through different approaches, might concentrate on (1) direct, so-called intrasystemic, attempts to restore malfunctioning areas; (2) indirect, so-called intersystemic reorganisation of intact functions to compensate for or circumvent deficits; and (3) creation of an optimal communication environment. This chapter has suggested first steps in these directions.

Acknowledgments

The author is grateful to Rachel Simmons and Margaret Stoves, who provided helpful comments on earlier versions of this chapter. Shortcomings remain the author's responsibility.

References

ABBS, J. and ROSENBEK, J. (1985) Some motor control perspectives on apraxia of speech and dysarthria. In J. Costello (Ed.), *Speech Disorders in Adults*. San Diego: College Hill.

ABBS, J and WELT, C. (1985) Structure and function of the lateral precentral cortex: Significance for speech motor control. In R. Daniloff (Ed.), *Speech Science*. London: Taylor and Francis.

ATEN, J., DARLEY, F., DEAL, J. and JOHNS, D. (1975) Comments on Martin's 'Some Objections to the Term Apraxia of Speech'. *Journal of Speech and Hearing Disorders*, 40, 416–20.

BASSO, A., DELLA SALA, S. and FARABOLA, M. (1987) Aphasia arising from purely deep lesions. *Cortex*, 23, 29–44.

BENNETT, J. (1987) Talk about low technology. In P. Enderby (Ed.), *Communication Aids*. Edinburgh, Churchill.

BROOKS., V. (1986) *Neural Basis of Motor Control*. Oxford: Oxford University Press.

BUCKINGHAM, H. (1983) Apraxia of language vs. apraxia of speech. In R. Magill (Ed.), *Memory and Control of Actions*. Amsterdam: Elsevier.

BUCKINGHAM, H. (1985) Perseveration in aphasia. In S. Newman *et al.* (Eds), *Current Perspectives in Dysphasia*. Edinburgh: Churchill.

BUCKINGHAM, H. (1986) Scan copier mechanism and the positional level of language production. *Cognitive Science*, 10, 195–217.

BUGBEE, J. and NICHOLS, A. (1980) Rehearsal as a self-correction strategy for patients with apraxia of speech. In R. Brookshire (Ed.), *Clinical Aphasiology Conference Proceedings*. Minneapolis: BRK.

CODE, C. and GAUNT, C. (1986) Treating severe speech and limb apraxia in a case of aphasia. *British Journal of Disorders Communication*, 21, 11–29.

COELHO, C. and DUFFY, R. (1985) Communicative use of signs in aphasia: Is acquisition enough? In R. Brookshire (Ed.), *Clinical Aphasiology*. Minneapolis: BRK.

CRARY, M., HARDY, T. and WILLIAMS, W. (1985) Aphemia with dysarthria or apraxia of speech. In R. Brookshire (Ed.), *Clinical Aphasiology*. Minneapolis: BRK.

DABUL, B. (1979) *Apraxia Battery for Adults.* Tigard, Oregon: C.C. Publications.

DABUL, B. and BOLLIER, B. (1976) Therapeutic approaches to apraxia. *Journal of Speech and Hearing Disorders,* 41, 268–76.

DARLEY, F., ARONSON, A. and BROWN, J. (1975) *Motor Speech Disorders.* Philadelphia: Saunders.

DEAL, J. and FLORANCE, C. (1978) Modification of the eightstep continuum for treatment of apraxia of speech in adults. *Journal of Speech and Hearing Disorders,* 43, 89–95.

DEUTSCH, S. (1984) Prediction of site of lesion from speech apraxic error patterns. In J.C. Rosenbek, M. McNeil, and A.E. Aronson (Eds), *Apraxia of Speech.* San Diego: College Hill.

DOWDEN, P., MARSHALL, R. and TOMKINS, C. (1981) Amer-Ind sign as a communicative facilitator for aphasic and apraxic patients. In R. Brookshire (Ed.), *Clinical Aphasiology Conference Proceedings.* Minneapolis: BRK.

EASTON, J. (1987) Aid user or effective communicator: Developing effective communication in aid users. In P. Enderby (Ed.), *Communication Aids.* Edinburgh, Churchill.

ELMAN, J. and McCLELLAND, J. (1984) Speech perception as a cognitive process: The interactive activation model. *Speech and Language,* 10, 337–74.

ENDERBY, P. and CROW, E. (1987) Raising awareness of speech disability. *Speech Therapy in Practice,* 2, 26–7.

FREEMAN, F., SANDS, E. and HARRIS, K. (1978) Temporal co-ordination of phonation and articulation in a case of verbal apraxia: A voice onset time study. *Brain Language,* 6, 106–11

FROMM, D., ABBS, J., McNEIL, M. and ROSENBEK, J. (1982) Simultaneous perceptual-physiological method for studying apraxia of speech. In R. Brookshire (Ed.), *Clinical Aphasiology Conference Proceedings.* Minneapolis: BRK.

FOWLER, C. (1985) Current perspectives on language and speech production — a critical review. In R. Daniloff (Ed.), *Speech Science.* London: Taylor and Francis.

GILLMER, E. and VAN DER MERWE, A. (1983) Die Stemaanvangstyd van Apraktiese en Disartriese Sprekers. *South African Journal of Communication Disorders,* 30, 34–9.

GRAFF-RADFORD, N., COOPER, W., COLSHER, P. and DAMASIO, A. (1986) Unlearned 'foreign accent' in a patient with aphasia. *Brain and Language,* 28, 86–94.

GRUNWELL, P. (1985) Comment on the terms phonetics and phonology as applied in the investigation of speech disorders. *British Journal of Disorders of Communication,* 20, 165–70.

GUYARD, H., SABOURAUD, O. and GAGNEPAIN, J. (1981) A procedure to differentiate phonological disturbances in Broca's aphasia and Wernicke's aphasia. *Brain and Language,* 13, 19–30.

HARDCASTLE, W., MORGAN-BARRY, R. and CLARK, C. (1985) Articulatory and voicing characteristics of adult dysarthric and verbal dyspraxic speakers: An instrumental study. *British Journal of Disorders of Communication,* 20, 249–70.

HEWLETT, N. (1985) Phonological vs. phonetic disorders: Some suggested modifications to the current use of the distinction. *British Journal of Disorders of Communication,* 20, 155–64.

HILL, B. (1978) *Verbal Dyspraxia in Clinical Practice.* Melbourne, Australia: Pitman.

HOLTZAPPLE, P. and MARSHALL, N. (1977) Application of multiphonemic articulation therapy with apraxia patients. In R. Buckingham (Ed.), *Clinical*

Aphasiology Conference Proceedings. Minneapolis, BRK.

ITOH, M. and SASANUMA, S. (1984) Articulatory movements in apraxia of speech. In J.C. Rosenbek *et al., Apraxia of Speech.* San Diego: College Hill.

ITOH, M., SASANUMA, S., HIROSE, H., YOSHIOKA, H. and USHIJIMA, T. (1980) Abnormal articulatory dynamics in a patient with apraxia of speech: X-ray microbeam observation. *Brain and Language,* 11, 66–75.

ITOH, M., SASANUMA, S., TATSUMI, I., MURAKAMI, S., FUKUSAKO, Y. and SUZUKI, T. (1982) Voice onset time characteristics in apraxia of speech. *Brain and Language,* 17, 193–210.

ITOH, M., SASANUMA, S and USHIJIMA, T. (1979) Velar movements during speech in a patient with apraxia of speech. *Brain and Language,* 7, 227–39.

KELLER, E. (1984) Simplification and gesture reduction in phonological disorders of apraxia and aphasia. In J.C. Rosenbek *et al.* (Eds), *Apraxia of Speech.* San Diego: College Hill.

KELLER, E. (1987) Factors underlying tongue articulation in speech. *Journal of Speech Hearing Research,* 30, 223–9.

KELSO, J. and TULLER, B. (1981) Toward a theory of apractic syndromes. *Brain and Language,* 12, 224–45.

KELSO, J., TULLER, B. and HARRIS, K. (1983) A 'dynamic pattern' perspective on the control and co-ordination of movement. In P. MacNeilage (Ed.), *Production of Speech.* Heidelberg: Springer.

KENT, R. (1983) Segmental organisation of speech. In P. MacNeilage (Ed.), *Production of Speech.* Heidelberg: Springer.

KENT, R. and ROSENBEK, J.C. (1982) Prosodic disturbance and neurologic lesion. *Brain and Language,* 15, 259–91.

KENT, R. and ROSENBEK, J.C. (1983) Acoustic patterns of apraxia of speech. *Journal of Speech Hearing Research,* 26, 231–49.

KERTESZ, A. (1984) Subcortical lesions and verbal apraxia. In J.C. Rosenbek, *et al.* (Eds), *Apraxia of Speech.* San Diego: College Hill.

KIMURA, D. (1982) Left hemisphere control of oral and brachial movements and their relation to communication. *Phil. Transacts. Royal Society, London* B298, pp. 135–49.

KLICH, R., IRELAND, J. and WEIDNER, W. (1979) Articulatory and phonological aspects of consonant substitutions in apraxia of speech. *Cortex,* 15, 451–70.

LA POINTE, L. (1984) Sequential treatment of split lists: A case report. In J.C. Rosenbek *et al.* (Eds), *Apraxia of Speech.* San Diego: College Hill.

LECOURS, A. and LHERMITTE, F. (1976) The 'pure form' of the phonetic disintegration syndrome (pure anarthria): Anatomico-clinical report of a historical case. *Brain and Language,* 3, 88–113.

LURIA, A. (1970) *Traumatic Aphasia.* Hague: Mouton.

LURIA, A. (1973) *The Working Brain.* Harmondsworth: Penguin.

MARQUARDT, T. and SUSSMAN, H. (1984) The elusive lesion — apraxia of speech link in Broca's aphasia. In J.C. Rosenbek *et al.* (Eds), *Apraxia of Speech.* San Diego: College Hill.

MARTIN, A. (1974) Some objections to the term apraxia of speech. *Journal of Speech Hearing Disorders,* 39, 53–64.

MARTIN, A. and RIGRODSKY, S. (1974a) An investigation of phonological impairment in aphasia, I. *Cortex,* 10, 317–28.

MARTIN, A. and RIGRODSKY, S. (1974b) An investigation of phonological impairment in aphasia, II: Distinctive feature analysis of phoneme commutation errors in aphasia. *Cortex,* 10, 329–46.

MATEER, C. and KIMURA, D. (1977) Impairment of non-verbal oral movements in aphasia. *Brain and Language,* 4, 262–76.

NCNEIL, M., CALIGIURI, M., WEISMER, G. and ROSENBEK, J. (1986) *Labio-mandibular kinematic durations velocities and dysmetrias in apraxic adults.* Paper presented at Annual Convention American Speech-Language and Hearing Association, Detroit.

MESSERLI, P. (1983) De l'Aphemie a l'Apraxia of Speech, ou les Tribulations d'une Notion. In P. Messerli, P. Lavorel and J.L. Nespoulous (Eds), *Neuro-psychologie de l'Expression Orale.* Paris: Edition du Centre National de la Recherche Scientifique.

MILLER, N. (1986) *Dyspraxia and its Management.* Beckenham: Croom Helm.

MILLER, N. (1989) Strategies of language use in assessment and therapy for acquired dysphasia. In P. Grunwell *et al.* (Eds), *Functional Evaluation of Language Disorders.* Beckenham: Croom Helm.

MILLER, N. (in press) Acquired speech disorders — applying linguistics to treatment. In K. Grundy (Ed.), *Linguistics in Clinical Practice.* London: Taylor and Francis.

MILROY, L. (1985) Phonological analysis and speech disorders: A comment. *British Journal of Disorders of Communication,* 20, 171–9.

MLCOCH, A., DARLEY, F. and NOLL, J. (1982) Articulatory consistency and variability in apraxia of speech. In R. Brookshire (Ed.), *Clinical Aphasiology Conference Proceedings* Minneapolis: BRK.

MLCOCH, A. and NOLL, J. (1980) Speech production models as related to the concept of apraxia of speech. *Speech and Language,* 4, 201–38.

MLCOCH, A. and SQUARE, P. (1984) Apraxia of speech: Articulatory and perceptual factors. *Speech and Language,* 10, 1–57.

MOHR, J. (1980) Revision of Broca aphasia and the syndrome of Broca's area infarction and its implications in aphasia theory. In R. Brookshire (Ed.), *Clinical Aphasiology Conference Proceedings.* Minneapolis: BRK.

NESPOULOUS, J.L., LECOURS, A. and JOANETTE, Y. (1983) La Dichotomie 'Phonetique-Phonemique', a-t-elle une Valeur Nosologique. In P. Messerli *et al.* (Eds). *Neuropsychologie de l'Expression Orale.* Paris: CNRS.

PONCET, M., HABIB, M. and ROBILLARD, A. (1987) Deep left parietal lobe syndrome: Conduction dysphasia due to a small subcortical lesion. *Journal of Neurology, Neurosurgery and Psychiatry,* 50, 709–13.

ROSENBEK, J.C. (1985) Treating apraxia of speech. In D. Johns (Ed.), *Clinical Management of Neurogenic Communicative Disorders.* (2nd ed.). Boston: Little, Brown.

ROSENBEK, J.C., KENT, R. and LAPOINTE, L. (1984a) Apraxia of speech: An overview and some perspectives. In J.C. Rosenbek *et al.* (Eds), *Apraxia of Speech.* San Diego: College Hill.

ROSENBEK, J.C., LEMME, M., AHERN, M., HARRIS, E. and WERTZ, R. (1973) A treatment for apraxia of speech in adults. *Journal of Speech Hearing Disorders,* 38, 462–72.

ROSENBEK, J.C., MCNEIL, M. and ARONSON, A. (Eds) (1984) *Apraxia of Speech.* San Diego: College Hill.

ROTHI, L.G. and HEILMAN, K. (1985) Ideomotor apraxia: Gestural discrimination, comprehension and memory. In E. Roy, (Ed.), *Neuropsychological Studies of Apraxia and Related Disorders*. Amsterdam: Elsevier.

ROY, E. (1981) Action sequencing and lateralised cerebral damage evidence for asymetries in control. In J. Long (Ed.), *Attention and Performance*. Hillsdale: Lawrence Erlbaum.

ROY, E. and SQUARE, P. (1985) Common considerations in the study of limb, verbal and oral apraxia. In E. Roy (Ed.), *Neuropsychological Studies of Apraxia and Related Disorders*. Amsterdam: Elsevier.

RUBOW, R., ROSENBEK, J.C., COLLINS, M. and LONGSTRETH, D. (1982) Vibrotactile stimulation for intersystemic reorganization in the treatment of apraxia of speech. *Archives of Physical Medicine and Rehabilitation*, 63, 150–3.

SANDS, E., FREEMAN, F. and HARRIS, K. (1978) Progressive changes in articulatory patterns in verbal apraxia: A longitudinal case study. *Brain and Language*, 6, 97–105.

SCHIFF, H., ALEXANDER, M., NAESER, N. and GALABURDA, A. (1983) Aphemia: clinical–anatomic correlations. *Archives of Neurology*, 40, 720–7.

SHAIMAN, S., ABBS, J. and GRACCO, V. (1986) *Evidence for Comparable Neural Control of Speech and Non-Speech Movement*. Paper presented ASHA Convention, Detroit, Michigan.

SHANKWEILER, D., HARRIS, K. and TAYLOR, M. (1968) Electromyographic studies of articulation in aphasia. *Archives Physical Medicine Rehabilitation*, 49, 1–8.

SIMMONS, N. (1980) Choice of stimulus modes in treating apraxia of speech: A case study. In R. Brookshire (Ed.), *Clinical Aphasiology Conference Proceedings*. Minneapolis: BRK.

SPARKS, R. and HOLLAND, A. (1976) Melodic intonation therapy for aphasia. *Journal of Speech Hearing Disorders*, 41, 287–97.

SQUARE, P. (1987) Acquired apraxia of speech. In H. Winitz (Ed.), *Human Communication: A Review, Vol. I*. New York: Ablex.

SQUARE, P., DARLEY, F. and SOMMERS, R. (1982) Analysis of the productive errors made by pure apractic speakers with differing loci of lesions. In R. Brookshire (Ed.), *Clinical Aphasiology Conference Proceedings*. Minneapolis: BRK.

SQUARE, P. and MLCOCH, A. (1983) Syndrome of subcortical apraxia of speech: An acoustic analysis (Abstract). In R. Brookshire (Ed.), *Clinical Aphasiology Conference Proceedings*. Minneapolis: BRK.

THOMSON, F. (1982) The use of sign language and the Makaton Vocabulary with adults with acquired speech and language disorders — a review of current literature and clinical practice. *Bulletin College of Speech Therapists*, 361, 1–3.

TONKONOGY, J. (1986) *Vascular Aphasia*, Cambridge, Mass: MIT Press.

TONKOVICH, J. and MARQUARDT, T. (1977) Effects of stress and melodic intonation on apraxia of speech. In R. Brookshire (Ed.), *Clinical Aphasiology Conference Proceedings*. Minneapolis: BRK.

WARREN, R. (1977) Rehearsal for naming in apraxia of speech. In R. Brookshire (Ed.), *Clinical Aphasiology Conference Proceedings*. Minneapolis: BRK.

WASHINO, K., KASAI, Y. and UCHIDA, Y. (1981) Tongue movement during speech in a patient with apraxia of speech: A case study. *Language Sciences*, Suppl, 125–59.

WEISMER, G. (1984) Articulatory characteristics of Parkinsonian dysarthria: Segmental and phrase-level timing, spirantisation, and glottal-supraglottal coordination. In M. McNeil *et al.* (Eds), *The Dysarthrias.* San Diego: College Hill.

WERTZ, R. (1984) Response to treatment in patients with apraxia of speech. In Rosenbek, J.C. *et al.* (Eds), *Apraxia of Speech.* San Diego: College Hill.

WERTZ, R. (1985) Neuropathologies of speech and language: An introduction to patient management. In D. Johns (Ed.), *Clinical Management of Neurogenic Communicative Disorders* (2nd ed.). Boston: Little, Brown.

WERTZ, R., LAPPOINTE, L. and ROSENBEK, J.C. (1984) *Apraxia of Speech in Adults: The Disorder and its Management.* New York: Grune Stratton.

WOLK, L. (1986) Markedness analysis of consonant error productions in apraxia of speech. *Journal of Communication Disorders,* 19, 133–60.

ZIEGLER, W. and VON CRAMON, D. (1985) Anticipatory co-articulation in a patient with apraxia of speech. *Brain and Language,* 26, 117–30.

ZIEGLER, W. and VON CRAMON, D. (1986a) Disturbed coarticulation in apraxia of speech: Acoustic evidence. *Brain and Language,* 29, 34–47.

ZIEGLER, W. and VON CRAMON, D. (1986b) Timing deficits in apraxia of speech, *European Archives Psychiatry Neurological Sciences,* 236, 444–9.

ZIEGLER, W. and VON CRAMON, D. (1986c) Spastic dysarthria after acquired brain injury: An acoustic study. *British Journal of Disorders of Communication,* 21, 173–87.

ZIEGLER, W. (in press) On the phonetic realisation of phological contrast in aphasic patients. In J. Ryalls (Ed.), *Phonetic Approaches to Speech Production in Aphasia and Related Disorders.* San Diego: College Hill.

15   Voice Disorders in Adults

Joseph Stemple

In technical terms, voice is the major element of speech production that provides the speaker with the vibration signal upon which speech is carried. In practical terms, it is much more than this. For voice provides the melody of speech and, beyond the spoken meaning of words, it provides additional expression, intent and mood to our spoken thoughts (Stemple and Holcomb, 1988). We all share an intimate relationship with our own voices. The way we feel, both physically and emotionally, will often be reflected in the quality of our voices. Therefore vocal disorders will often cause significant personal, social and vocational difficulties which may affect the quality of our lives.

The normal voice will fall within a very wide range of acceptability, and thus it is easier to define the abnormal voice. A voice disorder is said to exist when the quality, pitch and loudness of the voice differ from those of other persons of similar age, sex, cultural background and geographic location (Stemple, 1984; Aronson, 1980; Boone, 1977; Greene, 1972; Moore, 1971). In other words, if the voice is deviant enough to draw attention to the speaker, a voice disorder is said to be present. Indeed, no-one is more sensitive to normal voice production than the owner of the voice.

Successful management of the voice disorder will depend upon recognition of the problem by the owner of the voice and acceptance of the need for improvement. The effects of a voice disorder on the lives and the livelihoods of individuals will vary considerably. Those with a great need for normal, effective production may be unusually concerned with very minor vocal difficulties. People with low vocal needs may not be greatly concerned with even more severe vocal problems.

Our study will focus upon the speech and language clinician's role in the evaluation and management of voice disorders commonly seen in the adult population. The role of the clinician includes the identification and modification or elimination of the causes that have led to the development of the voice disorder (if the causes continue as precipitating factors), as well as the evaluation and modification of specific deviant voicing components (i.e., pitch, loudness, breathiness, and so on).

Common Causative Factors in Voice Disorders

Discovering the causes of voice disorders is a major first step in the remediation of the disorder. Categories of vocal misuse, medically-related causes, primary disorders and personality-related causes will be discussed here.

Vocal misuse

Vocal misuse refers to functional voicing behaviours that contribute to the development of voice disorders. Indeed, functional misuse of voice is the most common cause for the development of voice disorders. We will divide this category into two major parts, behaviours of vocal abuse and the use of inappropriate voice components.

Vocal abuse

Often, when we think of voice abuse, we focus our attention on children who shout, scream and make unusual vocal noises. Adults also have many opportunities to abuse the voice and demonstrate many vocally abusive behaviours. Vocal abuse occurs whenever the vocal folds are forced to adduct too vigorously causing hyperfunctioning of the laryngeal musculature. This vocal hyperfunction may take the form of excessive shouting or loud talking such as a mother with her child, cheering at a sporting event, or shouting over noise in a factory. Vocal abuse is also present in screaming, as during an argument, and in excessive harsh crying or laughing.

One of the most prevalent forms of voice abuse in adults which must be extinguished is incessant, habitual, non-productive throat clearing. This behaviour may be a primary cause of a voice disorder or throat clearing may be secondary to the presence of a voice disorder. Coughing is also a vocally abusive behaviour. Because coughing is a symptom of many physical ailments, a persistent cough must always be examined medically and is most often treated by a physician.

Inappropriate voice components

The production of voice is dependent upon the balanced relationship of many different components. The major voice components include respiration, phonation, resonation, pitch and loudness. Any component that is used in a functionally inappropriate manner may be the direct cause of a voice disorder. Let us examine each component.

Respiration

Breathing for speech is dependent upon the appropriate passage of air through the approximated vocal folds. You will find that the vast majority of patients use anatomically and physiologically adequate respiration for the support of speech. They may expand the thoracic cavity for the exchange of air through thoracic or chest breathing or through downward diaphragm contraction (diaphragmatic breathing). Either air exchange method is adequate for providing the necessary respiratory support for voice. Some patients, however, may use a shallow, thoracic, non-supporting breathing pattern with poor vocal fold adduction. The resultant voice quality will be breathy with a low intensity. Long term use of poorly supported phonation may lead to laryngeal strain and laryngeal pathology. Another functional breathing pattern which may lead to vocal strain is the habit of speaking on residual air. This occurs when a person continues to speak when the normal tidal expiration has been completed.

Phonation

Inappropriate phonation, as a functional cause of voice disorders, may be present in patients who utilise hard glottal attacks, breathy phonation and glottal fry phonation. A hard glottal attack is accomplished by approximating the vocal folds, building subglottic air pressure, and exploding the folds while phonating initial vowel sounds. When done excessively this phonatory habit will have a negative impact on the vocal mechanism. On the other hand, breathy phonation is accomplished by an incomplete approximation of the vocal folds causing the voice to sound weak and breathy due to the excessive escape of air. This problem of phonation may often be associated with poor respiratory support as well.

Glottal fry refers to an aperiodic phonation of the vocal folds in a lower frequency range than the normal pitch of the individual. This splutter-like phonatory pattern causes a grinding of the vocal processes of the arytenoid cartilages and is often produced by persons attempting to demonstrate a deep, authoritative sounding voice.

Resonation

There is a wide variation of acceptable resonance patterns in voice with acceptability often being determined by geographic location. Certain resonation disturbances occur on a functional or an organic basis due to the improper coupling of the pharyngeal, oral or nasal cavities or the improper positioning of the tongue or larynx.

Hypernasality is present when excessive nasal emission occurs during phonation. This behaviour results when the velopharyngeal port remains open during the production of sounds other than the nasal consonants /m/, /n/, and /ng/. Another form of hypernasality is assimilative nasality. Assimilative nasality occurs when the phonemes adjacent to the three nasal consonants are nasalised along with these sounds. A mild form of hypernasality is called *cul de sac* nasality. With this resonance disturbance, the velopharyngeal port remains open permitting all sound to be resonated through the nose. Much less nasal emission is present with this form of hypernasality. Denasality, or hyponasality, occurs when normal nasal resonance is not present on the phonemes /m/, /n/, and /ɳ/. The acoustic result sounds as if the speaker has a head cold.

Pitch

Inappropriate use of the voice component of pitch may lead to a voice disorder. Pitch is the perceptual correlate of the fundamental frequency of voice. Misuse refers to pitch levels that are either too high or too low or monotonous during conversation speech. Habitual use of an inappropriate pitch places great strain on the laryngeal musculature to produce the tone.

Habitual pitch is a term that refers to the range that an individual uses the majority of the time for conversational speech. Optimal pitch refers to the most appropriate pitch range for use by an individual. Only when the use of an inappropriate pitch level has been isolated as the primary cause of a voice disorder should therapeutic attempts be made to modify pitch. It is very common for pitch change to be a symptom of a voice disorder and not necessarily the cause. Time spent in direct pitch modification may not be the most appropriate approach in this circumstance.

Loudness

Loudness is the perceptual term that relates to vocal intensity. The inappropriate use of loudness is demonstrated in voices that are habitually too soft, too loud or monotonous in their loudness variability. Vocal intensity is determined by the volume of airflow through the vocal folds and the amplitude of the vibration. Less than adequate breath support or a limited lateral excursion of the vocal folds on a habitual basis will increase the laryngeal muscle effort which may lead to the development of a voice disorder.

Combination of causative factors

Rarely will a speech and language clinician be presented with a voice disorder in which a single voice component is isolated as the primary cause. If inappropriate components are found to be the cause of the disorder, then a combination of components will usually be identified with misuse of one being the predominant causative factor. Inappropriate voice components may also be the result of laryngeal pathologies that were caused by other etiological factors. When inappropriate voice components are a result of the voice disorder they are recognised as the acoustic symptoms such as low pitch, glottal fry phonation, breathiness and so on.

Vocal misuse represents the most common etiological factor identified in patients with voice disorders. Cooper (1973) found that of 1,406 patients, 36.6 per cent had disorders associated with vocal misuse; Brodnitz (1971) reported a figure of 25.8 per cent. Voice therapy is particularly effective in the remediation of voice disorders caused by vocal misuse.

Medically-related causes

Many medical/surgical conditions and situations exist which may lead to the development of a voice disorder. These conditions may be the result of direct or indirect surgeries which affect the larynx such as laryngectomy or thyroid surgery respectively. The causes may also be the result of chronic illnesses or disorders such as allergies, sinusitis, smoking, alcohol or other substance abuses. In addition, a number of other primary medical problems produce vocal difficulties as a secondary symptom along with the major disorder. For example, people who are deaf may not be able to monitor their voices well; people with neurological disorders such as a stroke, Parkinson's disease or Huntingdon's chorea may have many problems with voice as well as speech.

Personality-related causes

The way we feel, both physically and emotionally, is often directly reflected in the quality of our voices. The tensions and stresses of everyday life may contribute directly to the ineffective functioning of the sensitive laryngeal mechanism. One term used to describe the many occurrences in human life that can cause emotional and psychological stresses is environmental stress. Personal, work, school, social or family situations may well create difficulties that increase whole body and laryngeal muscle tension to a level that causes a hyperfunctioning of the voice. This hyperfunction may lead to the development of a voice disorder.

At times, environmental stress may become so severe that avoidance behaviours develop to counteract stressful situations. These avoidance behaviours, called *psychological conversion reactions,* permit people to draw attention away from the emotional stress or conflict. Conversion behaviours associated with voice disorders include aphonia (whispering), muteness (inability to speak or produce voice), or unusual dysphonias.

The final personality-related cause of a voice disorder is that of identity conflict. Persons who experience difficulty in establishing their own identities and personalities may develop specific voice disorders in the presence of normal laryngeal mechanisms. These disorders may include the high pitched voice of the post-adolescent male or the weak, thin, juvenile-sounding voice of an adult female. The many causes of voice disorders lead to the development of very specific laryngeal pathologies.

Laryngeal Pathologies Common to Adults

Traditionally, laryngeal pathologies have been classified as either organic or functional depending upon their specific causes. Organic pathologies may be laryngeal diseases or congenital anomalies that develop with little or no contributory laryngeal behaviours on the part of the speaker. Functional pathologies, however, are caused by factors directly attributed to the laryngeal behaviours and habits of the patient. Historically, pathologies such as laryngeal carcinoma, leucoplakia and hyperkeratosis have been classified as organic pathologies. However, we now know that the habits and behaviours of many individuals lead directly to the development of these laryngeal pathologies.

Organic laryngeal pathologies

Acute laryngitis: The term *laryngitis* is used to describe an inflammation of the vocal fold mucosa. Symptoms of acute laryngitis (Fig. 15.1) include mild to severe dysphonia, a nonproductive cough, and a local pain or soreness that is aggravated by phonation. The causes of acute laryngitis may be bacterial infections, inhalation of hot gases or flames, aspiration of caustic solutions, and less commonly, acute vocal abuse. Typical treatments include steam inhalation, anaesthetic lozenges, medications and voice rest. Voice therapy is not indicated for acute cases of laryngitis.

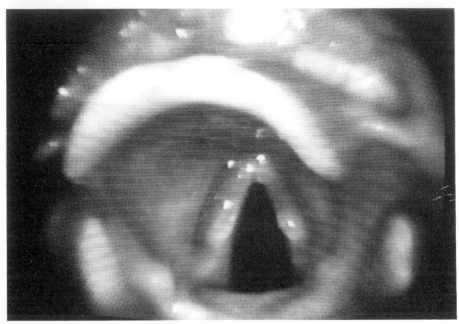

Figure 15.1: Acute Laryngitis
(Rick Berkey, Medical Photographer, St Elizabeth Medical Center, Dayton, Ohio)

Hyperkeratosis and leukoplakia: Two pathologies typically classified as organic are *leukoplakia* (Fig. 15.2) and *hyperkeratosis* (Fig. 15.3). They are considered premalignant growths, but the causes of these disorders may be more functional in nature. They include the chronic irritations of the chemicals in tobacco smoke, the irritation of alcohol abuse, incessant coughing and throat clearing, and general voice abuse.

Leucoplakia appears as a patchy white membrane and is usually located on the anterior one-third of the true vocal folds. Hyperkeratosis is a layered buildup of keratinised cell tissue. Treatment for both pathologies includes elimination of the irritants and surgical excision of the abnormal tissue. Voice therapy prior to surgery is helpful in reducing behaviours of vocal abuse and for vocal hygiene counselling. Therapy after surgery will aid in re-establishing normal strength and tone of the laryngeal musculature.

Laryngeal carcinoma: *Cancer* of the larynx (Fig. 15.4) is potentially the most devastating of all laryngeal pathologies due to the implications of the disease itself and the initial devastating effect on communication. The most common symptom of this pathology is persistent hoarseness. There is little if any pain or soreness,

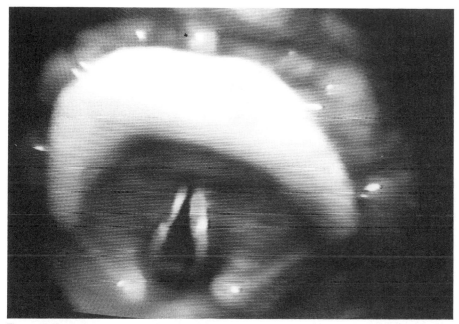

Figure 15.2: Leukoplakia

(Rick Berkey, Medical Photographer, St Elizabeth Medical Center, Dayton, Ohio)

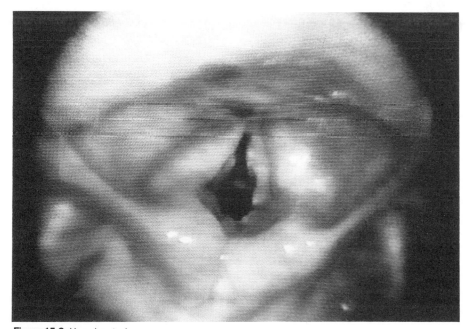

Figure 15.3: Hyperkeratosis

(Rick Berkey, Medical Photographer, St Elizabeth Medical Center, Dayton, Ohio)

although either may occur at later stages in the development of the disease and be referred to the ears. In advanced disease, the patient may experience both swallowing and respiratory problems.

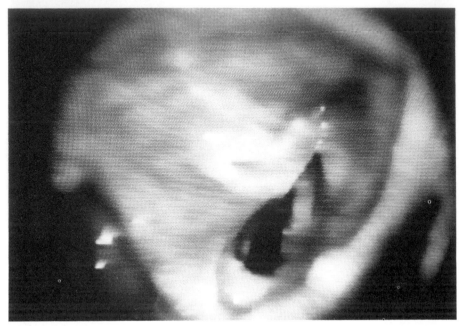

Figure 15.4: Cancer of the Larynx
(Rick Berkey, Medical Photographer, St Elizabeth Medical Center, Dayton, Ohio)

Laryngeal carcinoma is thought to be caused by chronic irritation to the laryngeal mucosa by such agents as tobacco smoke and alcohol. Treatment modalities include radiation therapy or surgical excision, or both. Vocal symptoms are characterised by a mild to severe dysphonia depending on the location and the extent of the lesion. The speech and language clinician plays an extremely important role in preparing the patient and the family for the consequences of the various forms of surgery and in the subsequent speech rehabilitation.

Vocal fold paralysis

The symptoms of vocal fold paralysis may vary from no dysphonia (when, for example, only one vocal fold is paralysed at the midline) to severe dysphonia (for example, when both vocal folds are paralysed in a paramedian position). Vocal fold paralysis may be bilateral or unilateral and is typically caused by peripheral involvement of the recurrent laryngeal and, less commonly, the superior laryngeal nerves.

There are many possible etiologies of vocal fold paralysis, including surgical trauma, such as thyroidectomy, endarterectomy, and heart, lung and breast surgeries that may involve the laryngeal nerves. Other causes include cardiovascular diseases, neurological diseases, accidental trauma, endotracheal intubation, and bronchoscopy. It is also important to note that the cause of approximately 30 to 50 per cent of all vocal fold paralysis is idiopathic.

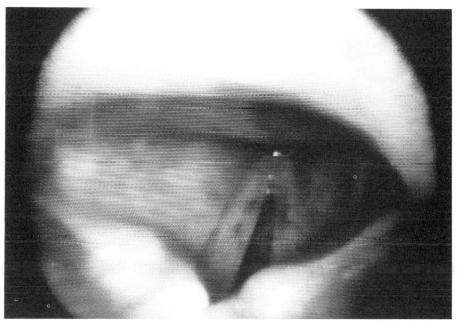

Figure 15.5: Bilateral Adductor Paralysis
(Rick Berkey, Medical Photographer, St Elizabeth Medical Center, Dayton, Ohio)

Bilateral abductor paralysis (Fig. 15.5) is the most serious form of vocal fold paralysis in its relation to the respiratory function. With this pathology, both vocal folds are positioned near the midline and are unable to abduct, requiring that an adequate airway be established. This may involve a tracheostomy or a surgical procedure in which one arytenoid cartilage is either removed or tied off laterally in an effort to open the airway. The role of voice therapy, following medical treatment, is in the establishment of the patient's most efficient voice.

Bilateral adductor paralysis results in both vocal folds resting in a paramedian position, not able to adduct to close the glottis. Individuals with this paralysis will obviously be aphonic, but the primary concern is aspiration. After 6 to 9 months the folds may migrate to the midline position, creating a bilateral abductor paralysis. Voice therapy is not effective for bilateral adductor paralysis.

Unilateral adductor paralysis (Fig. 15.6) is the most common type of vocal fold paralysis with the paralysed fold resting in the paramedian position while the other fold approximates the midline normally. As might be expected, phonation is characterised by the breathiness due to air wastage between the nonapproximating folds. The ability to build subglottic air pressure is also impaired resulting in a decrease in vocal intensity. Patients with this pathology often complain of physical fatigue resulting from the increased effort to approximate the folds for phonation.

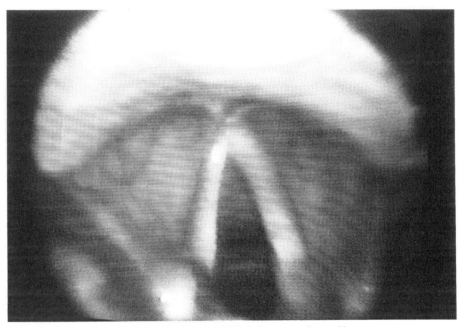

Figure 15.6: Left Unilateral Adductor Paralysis. Left fold is in the paramedian position
(Rick Berkey, Medical Photographer, St Elizabeth Medical Center, Dayton, Ohio)

The most common medical treatment for unilateral adductor paralysis is to wait 6 to 9 months for possible spontaneous recovery of nerve function. If this does not occur, then the paralysed fold is injected with surgical Teflon, or more recently, with a synthetic collagen substance, which increases its bulk thus decreasing the size of the glottal opening and improving phonation. Voice therapy attempts various methods to encourage the non-paralysed fold to over-adduct decreasing the size of the glottal airway.

Bilateral and unilateral superior nerve paralyses

These two types of vocal fold paralysis occur with involvement of the superior laryngeal nerve which is much less frequent than involvement of the recurrent laryngeal nerves due to a much shorter course. Bilateral superior nerve paralysis causes paralysis of the cricothyroid muscles bilaterally. The voice, therefore, decreases in pitch and lacks the ability to add inflection to the speaking voice or to sing. There is no medical treatment for this pathology. Voice therapy focuses on educating the patient regarding the causes and implications of the pathology.

Unilateral superior nerve paralysis causes an unequal rocking of the cricoid and thyroid cartilages leaving the vocal folds in an overlapped, oblique position. The resultant voice quality is flat and monotonous in pitch, with breathiness and a loss in vocal intensity due to the oblique positioning of the folds. Most patients with this pathology complain of vocal fatigue, which results from their efforts to phonate and inability to sing. There is no medical treatment. The author has utilised voice therapy to explain the causes and implications of the pathology and to teach vocal conservation to patients who were required to use their voices daily in their work.

Spastic dysphonia

One of the more curious and serious voice disorders is that of spastic dysphonia. Although researched and debated for many years, the cause of this disorder is yet to be understood, though evidence is strong regarding a possible neurogenic cause (Dordain and Dordain, 1972; Dedo, Townsend and Izdebski, 1978; Harrman, 1980) Spastic dysphonia occurs equally in men and women and normally has an onset at middle age (Brodnitz, 1976; Aronson, Brown, Litin and Pearson, 1968). The syptoms of this disorder differ depending on the type. Adductor, abductor, and mixed spastic dysphonia have been described.

Adductor spastic dysphonia is the most common type. The laryngeal behaviour is characterised by an intermittent, tight adduction of the vocal folds creating a strained, staccato vocal pattern. When examined through indirect laryngoscopy, the vocal folds appear normal in structure and function. Intermittent, brief periods of normal phonation may occur especially during laughter and anger and while attempting to sing. The severity of the disorder may vary depending on the frequency and strength of the laryngospasm. Many patients with this disorder complain of physical fatigue, tightness of the chest, back, and shoulder muscles and shortness of breath due to their efforts to phonate through the closed glottis. In the more severe cases, patients may compensate by whispering or phonating on inspired air. Secondary behaviours similar to those observed in stutterers, such as head jerking and eye blinking, may also develop.

The only treatment to date that has effected some measure of success in relieving the symptoms of adductor spastic dysphonia has been a surgical method suggested by Dedo (1976). This method involves sacrificing a recurrent laryngeal nerve to create a unilateral fold paralysis. With one fold paralysed in a paramedian position, the non-paralysed fold would not be able to attain adequate closure to ceate the laryngospasm.

Abductor spastic dysphonia is a mirror image of the adductor type. Phonation is characterised by sudden, involuntary periods of aphonia accompanied by a release of air. The vocal folds appear to be in spasm primarily during the production of unvoiced consonants, although Hartman (1980) reported breathy moments during all positions of words, on whole words, and on several words in succession. Merson and Ginsberg (1979) reported some success in modifying voice quality utilising relaxation training and teaching patients to raise their pitch and use hard glottal attacks. Patients have also been observed who exhibit vocal qualities of both abductor and adductor spastic dysphonia (Aronson, 1980; Hartman, 1980). This 'mixed' spasticity has not been researched in any detail.

Functional Laryngeal Pathologies

Chronic laryngitis

By far the most common form of laryngeal pathology is chronic laryngitis (Fig. 15.7). Laryngitis is the laryngeal condition which occurs when the vocal folds are

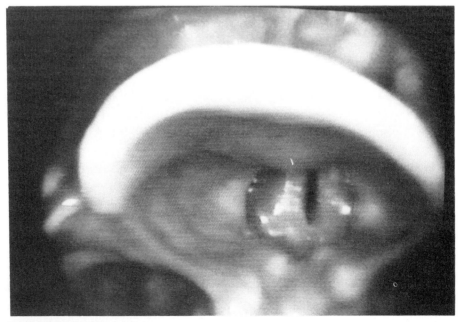

Figure 15.7: Chronic Laryngitis
(Rick Berkey, Medical Photographer, St Elizabeth Medical Center, Dayton, Ohio)

swollen (edemic) and red (erythema). Chronic laryngitis results from chronic misuse of voice and the vocal folds remain edematous and red. Seldom is pain present though the person with the condition will experience hoarseness. People who smoke and drink, shout, talk over noise and generally misuse their voices, will likely develop this condition. Treatment involves elimination of the misuse of voice.

Vocal nodules

Vocal nodules (Figs. 15.8a and b) are also a fairly common benign laryngeal growth. Sometimes described as vocal fold callouses, singer's nodes or screamer's nodules, these hard fibrous nodules develop as a result of vocal abuse. Vocally abusive behaviours cause friction which breaks down the normal vocal fold tissue and creates the build-up of layered hard tissue between the anterior one-third and posterior two-thirds of both vocal folds. These hard, fibrous nodules, similar to callouses that might build-up on your hands, interfere with the normal vibrations of the vocal folds causing the voice to sound hoarse. Treatment would include elimination or modification of the vocal misuse, training a more appropriate voice production and possible surgical excision of the nodules should therapy not prove successful in their resolution.

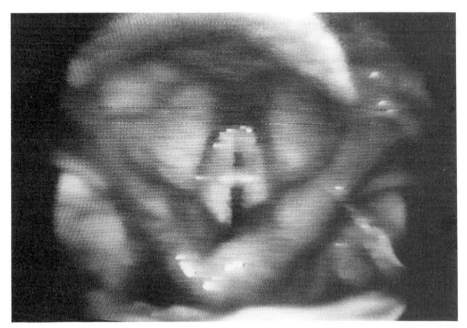

Figure 15.8a: Vocal Nodules (Adducted Folds)
(Rick Berkey, Medical Photographer, St Elizabeth Medical Center, Dayton, Ohio)

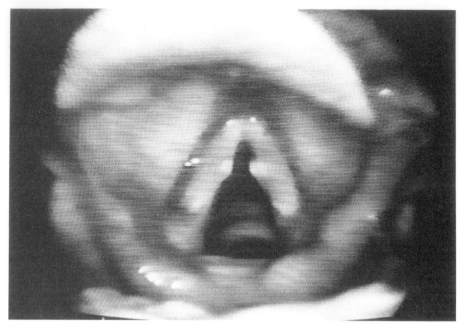

Figure 15.8b: Vocal Nodules (Abducted Folds)
(Rick Berkey, Medical Photographer, St Elizabeth Medical Center, Dayton, Ohio)

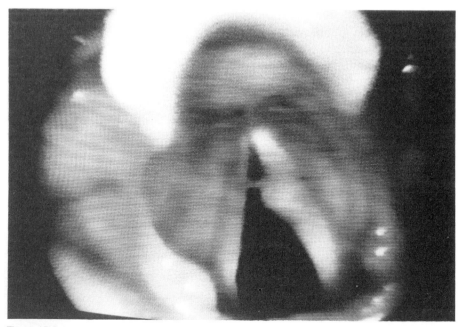

Figure 15.9: Laryngeal Polyp
(Rick Berkey, Medical Photographer, St Elizabeth Medical Center, Dayton, Ohio)

Polyps

Another laryngeal pathology, similar in origin to vocal nodules are laryngeal polyps (Fig. 15.9). Polyps develop as a result of voice misuse and abuse. They have been described as being similar to blisters in that they are fluid-filled sacs. These sacs may develop as a breakdown of normal vocal fold tissue and occur anywhere along the medial edge of one or both of the vocal folds. Their presence interferes with vibration causing the voice to be dysphonic. Polyps may resolve with the tissue and fluid being reabsorbed by the normal tissue if the vocal misuse is discontinued. If they do not resolve then they must be surgically excised. Again smoking and alcohol abuse, as well as general voice abuse, are implicated in the development of polyps.

Reinke's edema/polypoid degeneration

Reinke's edema (Fig. 15.10) is a diffuse, watery swelling that may run the entire length of the vocal fold. Because of voice abuse or other forms of laryngeal irritation, fluid will fill Reinke's space giving the fold a floppy, water-balloon appearance. Mild Reinke's edema may resolve with the elimination of the causative behaviours. More severe edema often requires surgical aspiration of the affected fold or folds.

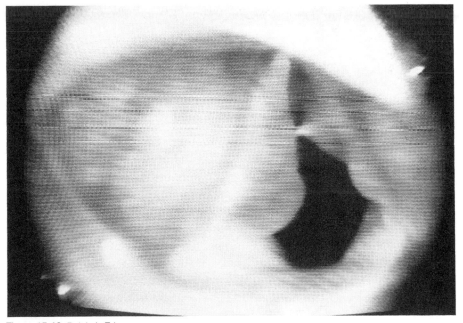

Figure 15.10: Reinke's Edema
(Rick Berkey, Medical Photographer, St Elizabeth Medical Center, Dayton, Ohio)

Contact ulcers/granuloma

Contact ulcers are a less common laryngeal pathology than nodules or polyps. Again, caused by voice misuse, their development results from a breakdown of the normal vocal fold tissue that course the area around the arytenoid cartilages. Voice quality will be hoarse. A common vocal behaviour which may lead to the development of contract ulcers is talking while using a pitch level that is too low. Constant use of a low pitch will cause the arytenoid cartilages to grind together, thus breaking down the tissue lining and developing the ulcers. Sometimes the ulcerated tissue will proliferate forming granulation tissue. Contact ulcers are one functional pathology in which pain may be present. Treatment again will be the identification and modification of vocal misuse and the possible surgical excision of the ulcerated tissue.

Ventricular phonation

Occasionally a large enough amount of muscle tension is created in the laryngeal area to cause the ventricular folds (False vocal folds) to approximate for phonation. Normally the ventricular folds will simply rest quietly while the true vocal folds vibrate. False vocal fold vibration, as a functional behaviour may be caused by physical or emotional tension. This form of voicing has also been used as a compensatory voice when other serious pathologies make it too difficult for the true vocal folds to vibrate. Treatment for functional ventricular phonation involves counselling and vocal re-education through direct voice therapy.

Conversion aphonia and dysphonia

As discussed earlier, some voice disorders may result from environmental stress or out of psychological needs. The conversion voice problems are evident when a person whispers or produces an inappropriate voice in the presence of normal vocal folds and entirely normal laryngeal mechanism and vocal tract. The conversion voice problems have numerous possible vocal symptoms and the onset is often quite sudden. More women present with conversion problems than men. The conversion pathology is normally the person's unconscious method of avoiding a strong interpersonal conflict that may cause stress, anxiety or depression. Treatment for conversion voice pathologies will involve counselling and direct voice manipulation. It must be noted that people who present with these disorders truly do not believe that they are capable of producing normal voice. They are not joking or malingering and need to be handled delicately.

Assessment Considerations

Prior to being evaluated by the speech and language clinician, the patient should have been seen by an otolaryngologist who is an ear, nose and throat specialist. The otolaryngologist would have examined the patient through indirect laryngoscopy, fiberoptic laryngoscopy, a rigid scope, direct microlaryngoscopy or videostroboscopy. This process is necessary to rule out the possibility of life threatening pathological conditions or conditions which cannot be remediated therapeutically.

The primary objectives of the voice evaluation performed by the speech and language clinician are to: (1) identify the causes, (2) describe the present vocal components, and (3) develop an individualised management plan. Secondary objectives include: (1) patient education, (2) patient motivation, and (3) to establish the credibility of the examiner.

The voice evaluation should be viewed not only as a diagnostic tool, but also as a major part of the therapeutic process. It is the first stage of therapy. It helps to establish the rapport and understanding between the therapist and the patient. It serves to develop the patient's awareness and understanding of the disorder and develops the motivation for change.

The typical voice evaluation will be accomplished through a systematic interview including information regarding the history of the development of the problem, associated medical history, information related to personal, work and social lives of the patients and a formal assessment of the present voice components. When completed, the clinician should have identified all the causes associated with the development of the problem and behaviours which serve to continue the problem. Inappropriate vocal components will be identified, and the management plan will be developed. During the interview, your knowledge of anatomy and physiology, causative factors and pathological conditions becomes extremely important. At the beginning of each evaluation you want to establish that the patient understands the reason for the referral and make sure you know why the patient was referred to you. Therefore, you will develop the patient's knowledge of his/her pathological condition through an explanation of the pathology and common reasons for its development. This will lead the patient to think about his/her own causative factors and help to develop your own credibility.

The history of the disorder as well as the medical and social history of the patient have to be systematically evaluated in the interview to learn about the causative and maintaining factors relating to the disorder. Such an interview is followed by the physical oral-peripheral examination and the subjective voice analysis to determine the present state of the various vocal components.

Oral-peripheral examination

The oral-peripheral examination will determine the physical condition of the oral mechanism and the peripheral speech system. At this point the examiner checks for laryngeal area or whole body tension and difficulties with swallowing. Swallowing difficulties may be present in some patients because of the close relationship between the physical structures associated with voice and swallowing. Laryngeal sensations such as dryness, tickling, aching, burning, soreness or a 'lump in the throat feeling' are also questioned. Some or all of these sensations are often present with laryngeal hyperfunction.

Voice Analysis

The subjective voice analysis will then examine each vocal component in detail to determine its appropriateness. At times, a particular voice component, such as pitch, may be used habitually in an inappropriate manner (such as too low) and will be identified as the primary cause of the voice disorder. This cause must then be directly modified. At other times, an inappropriate low pitch may simply be the vocal symptom of the voice disorder and not the actual cause. Often, if the actual cause is eliminated or modified, the voice component will indirectly improve.

To begin the voice analysis simply jot down the significant voice qualities you heard during the interview. Using a five-point scale, state 'the quality was a (1) mild, (2) mild to moderate, (3) moderate, (4) moderate to severe, (5) severe dysphonia characterised by . . .' At this point, list the purely subjective terms that will be meaningful to you at a later time for comparison. These terms may include hoarse, harsh, strident, tinny, breathy, raspy and so on. Then test or comment on the seven major components of respiration, phonation, resonation, pitch, loudness, and rate and rhythm.

Respiration

1   Describe the breathing pattern as abdominal or thoracic and as supporting or non-supportive of voice.
2   Sustain and time the /s/ sound and /z/ sound for as long as possible. The times for both sounds should be fairly equal. Healthy vocal folds do not require more air to sustain voice on /z/ than to produce the voiceless /s/.
3   Sustain and time the /a/ sound for as long as possible. This establishes your respiratory baseline.

Phonation

Report on the presence of (1) hard glottal attacks, (2) breathiness, (3) glottal fry, (4) diplophonia, (5) phonation breaks. If you are not sure from the interview process whether these behaviours are present, simply have the patient recite the alphabet at a moderate loudness level.

Resonation

Report on the presence of (1) hypernasality, (2) hyponasality, (3) assimilative nasality, (4) cul de sac nasality. You may wish to compare contrasting pairs such as: beat/meat, bit/mit, bait/mate, bet/met, bat/mat.

Pitch

1 Test the present pitch range by singing, in whole notes from the lowest to highest note. Match each note to a pitch pipe or piano and record the note for future reference.
2 Describe adequacy of conversational inflection — monotone, adequate, too great.
3 Subjectively judge where the habitual pitch falls in the present range — bottom, middle, top. We would suggest that an optimum pitch cannot be identified yet in the pathological voice.

Loudness

1 Determine whether the voice is too loud, too soft or has appropriate loudness for the speaking situation.
2 Check the patient's ability to shout. This will yield good information regarding the ability of the vocal folds to adequately adduct and build appropriate sub-glottic air pressure to produce voice.

Rhythm and rate

1 Describe whether the rate of speech was too fast, too slow or adequate.
2 Decribe any vocal characteristics which may have interrupted the normal rhythm of the voice production. These may be frequent voice breaks, hesitations or spasms.

In examining the history of the problem, the medical and social histories, conducting the oral-peripheral examination and subjectively evaluating the vocal components, you have gathered together many pieces of the diagnostic puzzle. Now, examine the pieces and assemble them in the order which identifies the causes of the disorder, and describes the present vocal components. Report your results under a section of the evaluation titled 'Impressions'. Based on these results, develop an individualised management plan under 'Recommendations' which is designed to remediate the problem. In so doing, you will have completed the three major goals of the voice evaluation.

Objective Voice Analysis

The reader should be aware that it is now possible to objectify the voice analysis procedure with special instrumentation. This instrumentation, which depends on computer technology, quickly and objectively analyses both acoustic and aerodynamic parameters of voice. As the instrumentation becomes more affordable and available, its routine use will become the standard of the voice analysis component of the evaluation. Instrumentation, however, will never be able to replace the systematic, detailed patient interview which offers the most important information regarding the psychosocial aspects of the patient's voice disorder.

Voice Therapy Techniques

The diagnostic voice evaluation not only served to discover the causes of the voice disorder, but also prepared the patient for the therapeutic process. Since the patients now understand how voice is produced, aspects of the pathology and causes of their specific disorders, they are better able to comprehend the reasoning behind the specific therapy techniques to be employed.

One chapter cannot adequately describe all of the available therapeutic techniques for remediation of voice disorders. Therefore, our discussion is meant to be a sample introduction to a few remediation approaches for voice disorders which are caused by voice abuse, inappropriate voice components, medically-related causes and personality-related causes.

Management of voice abuse

Hyperadduction of the vocal folds is vocally abusive, especially when the abuse occurs frequently. The most effective way of dealing with vocal abuse is through vocal hygiene counselling. Once the abuses have been identified, the first step of this approach is patient education. This involves making the patient aware of the effects that abuse has on the laryngeal mechanism by utilising graphic pictures and descriptions of the anatomy and physiology. The more that patients understand about the problem, the more likely it is that they will resolve the problem. After the general abuses have been identified and explained, it is important to determine exactly why the patient demonstrates those abuses. For example, if the abuse is shouting, the speech and language clinician will want to know when and why it occurs and whether it is required. Once these factors are determined the management plan will involve (1) eliminating those abusive behaviours that may be eliminated; (2) modifying those abusive behaviours that cannot be eliminated to reduce the impact on the vocal mechanism; and (3) environmental manipulation to secure more favourable voicing conditions.

We may synthesise the vocal hygiene approach to a four-step outline:

1   Identify the abuse (e.g., shouting, throat clearing)
2   Describe the effects (e.g., accomplished with illustration and discussion of physiology)
3   Define the specific occurrences (e.g., shouting to discipline children, shouting at sporting events, chronic throat clearing), and
4   Modify the behaviour (e.g., attempt to discipline through discussion and deprivation; substitute mechanical noise maker for vocal enthusiasm at sporting events; eliminate throat clearing).

Vocal hygiene counselling is vital to teach modification of vocal abuse habits. Direct therapy may be utilised to eliminate throat clearing through substitution of a forceful swallow. Any abusive behaviours may be modified or eliminated by using the four step hygiene plan.

Management of inappropriate voice components

Previously we described the components of voice that include respiration, phonation, resonation, pitch, and loudness. The inappropriate use of any one voice component or combination of components may lead directly to the development of a voice disorder or may result from laryngeal pathologies. For example, the voice of the vocal nodule patient may be breathy and low in pitch. Although these vocal components are inappropriate, they are not the primary cause of the pathology. Modification of the primary etiology is the first line of treatment, with symptom modification following when necessary. The following outline introduces the major problems which might exist in utilising the primary voice components and suggests methods for modification.

Respiration modification

An efficient exchange of air is necessary for the production of normal voice. Problems in the respiratory support of voice may exist when the patient uses shallow breathing by not using enough of their lung capacity, or if the patient talks using residual air. With regard to the first problem, expand and improve respiratory lung capacity through abdominal breathing. Give the following instructions:

1   Stand upright. Place one hand on your chest and the other hand on your abdomen. Sharply inhale. The hand on your chest should remain relatively still while the hand on the abdomen should move out with the expansion of the abdominal muscles. Relax the abdominal muscles; lightly and slowly exhale. Repeat the inhalation and exhalation until you are able to easily maintain the proper movement of the abdomen — out during inhalation, in during exhalation.

2   Lie flat on your back on the floor. Place a hard-backed textbook on your upper abdomen. Inhale by expanding the abdominal muscles and contracting the diaphragm. Exhale through relaxation of the muscles. Watch the text rise during inhalation and fall during exhalation.

3   Add speech to the first two exercises. Begin by counting, saying one number per inhalation/exhalation. Then say two numbers, and then three, and so on. Say only as many numbers as you can comfortably say while the air is flowing easily. Do not push or strain.

4   Continue using speech with abdominal breathing by reading short phrases and sentences. Inhale before each sentence and build your ability to produce each sentence through nine- and ten-syllable phrases on one controlled inhalation and exhalation. Continue this through paragraph reading.

To eliminate the use of residual air for speech the clinician may:

1   Refer to a series of sentences graduated by length. Begin with two syllable phrases. Ask the patient to inhale and exhale lightly while reading each phrase. Continue building through longer phrases. When the patient loses the relaxed inhalation/exhalation — stop. This will represent the number of syllables that the patient can comfortably produce without utilising residual air.

2   Utilising paragraph reading, ask the patient to read aloud. Determine where you think appropriate phrase markers should be and place them in the text. Have the patient practice reading this paragraph while breathing only at the markers. Make sure no strain is placed on the respiratory system.

3 Continue the previous exercise, with the patient marking his own appropriate phrases in paragraphs. Expand to conversational speech.

Phonation modification

Phonation is the term that described the actual vibration of the vocal folds. Characteristics of phonation that may cause this component of voice to be inappropriate may be (1) hard glottal attacks caused by too great a buildup of air pressure beneath the vocal folds or too much laryngeal area muscle tension; (2) breathy phonation caused by inefficient vocal fold closure or a lack of proper breath support; (3) glottal fry phonation normally associated with two other ineffective voice components, respiration and pitch.

To eliminate hard glottal attacks the clinician may:

1 Teach the patient to produce vowel sounds using an easy onset or a soft glottal attack. Ask the patient to say each vowel preceded by the sound /h/. Gradually drop the /h/ until the vowel may be said lightly and easily without the hard attack. Expand this ability by reading phrases, sentences, paragraphs, and eventually conversational speech.

2 Utilise negative practice. Ask the patient to produce each vowel with a soft glottal attack followed by a hard attack, and then soft again. This practice will develop control over their laryngeal behaviour.

3 Because increased laryngeal area tension may be a cause of hard glottal attack productions, excercises designed to reduce laryngeal tension may be necessary. For example, progressive relaxation, the chewing method or the yawn/sigh method.

To eliminate breathiness, the following procedures may be used:

1 Mild breathiness may be improved simply by using more precise articulation, especially on the plosive sounds /p/, /t/, and /k/. Ask the patient to practice reading phrases and paragraphs while using an exaggerated articulation pattern. The increased intraoral air pressure required for more precise articulation will decrease the mild laryngeal breathiness.

2 A moderate amount of breathiness may be modified by increasing vocal intensity. Louder voice production requires that the vocal folds approximate more firmly, thus decreasing the amount of wasted air.

3 A greater amount of breathiness may require a more aggressive exercise programme consisting of glottal attack exercises. Hard glottal attacks were previously described as an inappropriate phonatory behaviour. However, a

person with poor glottal closure may use this vocal behaviour as an exercise to develop improved glottal closure. To purposely produce a hard glottal attack ask the patient to breathe in deeply; close the vocal folds and squeeze them together as if lifting a heavy object and then release the buildup of subglottic air pressure while saying the vowels /a/, /e/, /i/, /o/, and /u/, one vowel at a time. These vowels should be said aloud, using the hard glottal attack, three times each, three times per day.

4   The most aggressive exercise to use with moderate to severe breathiness is the isometric push. The pushing exercise is accomplished by pushing the palms of your hands together while producing the vowel sounds using Exercise 3. The combination of these two exercises will cause normal vocal folds to adduct vigorously and decrease breathiness.

To eliminate glottal fry phonation:

1   Review respiratory problem 1. Practice all associated exercises needed.
2   Refer to pitch problem 1. Practice associated exercises to raise pitch; this will help to eliminate the glottal fry.

Resonation modification

Once the voice leaves the larynx it begins the journey through the vocal tract. The vocal tract is made of cavities that either dampen or enhance the voice vibration, giving each of us our own distinctive sounds. The resonance cavities include the pharynx, the oral cavity, and the nasal cavity. Effective resonance is dependent upon the proper coupling of these cavities. The following characteristics of resonance may be ineffective:

1   Permitting too much air to pass through the nasal cavity. An extreme amount of air passage through the nasal cavity is called hypernasality. Too much nasal resonance but with less air passage through the nose is called cul de sac or dead-end nasality. When vowel sounds are inappropriately resonated through the nasal cavity following the normal nasal consonants (/m/, /n/, /ŋ/), assimilative nasality is said to occur.
2   Not permitting normal nasal resonance on the nasal consonants /m/, /n/, and /ŋ/. When this occurs, the person is said to produce voice with too little resonance or hyponasality (denasality). This voice quality may be evident when someone has a head cold.
3   Attempting to speak with a retracted tongue and jaw and an elevated larynx, which essentially pinches or traps the voice in the pharynx. The resultant quality is weak and lacks a full resonant sound.

To decrease hypernasality, cul de sac and assimilative nasality caused by a lack of palatal-pharyngeal closure (the assumption is made here that lack of closure is a functional disturbance and not organic in nature):

1 Maximise the precision and correctness of articulation. Work on articulatory drills with exaggerated oral movements. Precise articulation will decrease the perception of hypernasality.

2 Utilise all the loudness exercises for increasing loudness level. Inappropriate nasal resonance may be decreased with a slightly increased loudness level.

3 Do the obvious, ask the patient to produce voice as 'if you have a cold'. In other words, practice a hyponasal resonance — the opposite extreme of the problem. A slight modification of the 'cold' voice will then yield a normal nasal resonation.

4 Practice contrasting pairs while attempting to produce a definite and distinct difference for each word. Use words such as beat/meet; boot/moot, etc.

5 Use negative practice by repeating all the /b/ words in Exercise 4 with too much nasal resonance. Then produce each word with the normal amount of resonance.

6 Expand the patient's ability to produce a decreased hypernasality by practising phrases, sentences, and paragraphs.

To decrease hyponasality caused by completely or partially blocked nasal passage. Assuming this blockage is not caused by a cold, allergies, or a growth such as nasal polyps, the problem is generally the result of fixing the soft palate too high against the pharyngeal wall.

1 Chill a small mirror in the refrigerator. Place the mirror under the patient's nose. With lips pressed tightly together, ask the patient to hum the sound mmm. When lips are together, the airflow must go through the nose and the mirror will steam. Slowly modify the hummed mmm by (a) opening the mouth while humming and saying /ma/, (b) expanding to other vowel sounds (/ma/, /me/, /may/, /mo/, /moo/), and (c) eliminating the hum and then expanding into words, phrases, sentences and paragraphs.

2 Utilise a hypernasal resonance. Ask the patient to practice the words in resonance problem 4, using an exaggerated hypernasal resonation. Slowly decrease the degree of nasality until a normal coupling of the cavities is reached.

By reducing tension of the jaw, tongue, and laryngeal strap muscles, one increases the size of the resonating cavities and frees the laryngeal vibration.

1   Ask the patient to consciously loosen the jaw at the hinges next to the ears. With the loose jaw, open and close the mouth with wide jaw excursions. Continue to exaggerate this movement while repeating the vowel sounds /a/, /e/, /i/, /o/, and /u/. Now add an /m/ before each sound while continuing to use wide jaw movements. Then practice reading short phrases while exaggerating the jaw movement on every word. Expand this into sentences and short paragraphs. Gradually decrease the exaggerated jaw movements into a more normal open jaw position. To guarantee that the jaw does not become fixed during practice, ask the patient to place a finger between the front teeth during practice. Do not let the teeth come any closer than the finger width for practice purpose.

2   The retracted tongue should be helped by loosening the fixed jaw position. An additional exercise for gaining more natural tongue placement is to exaggerate the movements necessary for producing the vowel /e/. Say the /e/ several times by protruding the tongue far forward through and between the teeth. Add the five vowel sounds to each /e/: /e/-/a/, /e/-/e/, /e/-/i/, /e/-/o/, and /e/-/u/. Then gradually decrease the extension of the tongue until it is no longer protruding between the teeth but remains orally in a forward position.

3   Improved forward placement of the tongue and increased jaw mobility should help to place the larynx in a less elevated position in the neck. Another way to lower the larynx in the neck is through gentle massage. Identify the edges of the thyroid cartilage of the patient's larynx. Grasp the cartilage with your thumb on one edge and your finger on the other and gently massage downward in a circular manner. When you feel the larynx loosening, begin saying the vowel sound slightly and easily while not permitting the larynx to stiffen and elevate. Also, make sure the jaw is loose and the tongue is forward. Expand this by saying the short phrases, sentences and paragraphs (Aronson, 1980).

Pitch modification

An inappropriate use of the pitch component may exist when (1) a patient uses a pitch range that is either too high or too low for his or her laryngeal anatomy to successfully produce (we often see this problem in individuals who while attempting to sound more authoritative, will artificially lower the voice), or (2) a person uses a rather flat, or monotonous, pitch pattern, decreasing the effectiveness of the vocal variety.

To determine appropriate optimum pitch range, ask the patient to sing the sound /o/ on a comfortable level. Now, in whole-note steps, sing down the scale until you reach the lowest note that the patient can produce comfortably. If a piano or pitch pipe is available, match this tone and document the note. Now from the lower note, ask the patient to sing up the scale as high as possible in whole notes. Count the number of notes. If possible, match the highest note to a piano. This is the patient's pitch range. A range of 14–16 notes would be considered adequate for conversational voice production. The optimum pitch range would be located approximately one-fourth of the way up the entire range given a normal vocal fold condition. (Remember, if a laryngeal pathology exists, the patient will probably not be able to demonstrate the full pitch range which would make the concept of optimum range invalid.).

To some people, the concept of notes and singing to find the optimum pitch range is very difficult. If you find this to be the case, ask the patient, in a natural conversational voice to say um-hum, as if answering 'yes' to a question (Cooper, 1973). The hum part of this production is usually produced in a very relaxed tone near the optimum pitch level. Once you have determined the appropriate pitch range for the patient, practice phrases, sentences and paragraphs within that range. One way of confirming the use of the optimum pitch range is through negative practice. Practice saying exercise sentences using pitch levels that are too high and too low. The patient will soon see that it is more comfortable and takes less effort to utilise the optimum pitch range.

To improve pitch inflection, you may demonstrate the use of inflection by asking the patient to say one phrase in different ways to express different meanings (e.g., 'I love you', using a robot voice or asking a question, making a simple statement, a declaration, etc.). It is easy to see how meaning can change simply by changing pitch patterns used with the exact same words.

Loudness modification

Another determinant of normal voice production is the use of an appropriate loudness level in various situations as well as the ability to use loudness changes for inflectional purposes. Problems associated with the voice component of loudness may include: speaking too softly as dictated by the situation; speaking with an habitual loud level in most situations; or permitting the loudness level to be monotonous, thus decreasing vocal variety and expression.

It may be necessary to raise the patient's level of awareness of volume by tape recording a conversation with you. Compare the loudness levels. Explain that people who talk too softly are constantly asked to repeat themselves, they may be ignored or they may project a bashful or backward image.

Similar approaches may be used to decrease habitual speaking loudness level. It is necessary to raise the patient's level of awareness of volume. This may be done similarly to the above using a tape recorder. Compare the loudness level of the patient to yourself. Ask the patient to pay attention to the reactions of those with whom he/she talks. Do people back away or look away? Understand that people who talk too loudly often project an image of being overbearing. Monitor as above using the loudness metre. (Sometimes, when people have difficulty monitoring loudness levels, the problem may be associated with hearing loss. All voice patients should be screened for normal hearing.)

Improving loudness variation may be accomplished by (1) practicing loudness variation by counting from 1 to 10, beginning very softly and ending very loudly (then perform the same task from loud to soft); (2) sustaining the vowel /o/ beginning very softly and ending loudly (try to maintain one pitch level, then perform the task from loud to soft); (3) practicing reading phrases, sentences and paragraphs, changing stress markers to modify intent, mood and meaning.

Management of Medically-related Disorders

Several voice disorders caused by medical conditions or surgical intervention are amenable to modification through voice therapy. These include unilateral adductor vocal fold paralysis, superior laryngeal nerve paralysis, adductor spastic dysphonia, various neurologic voice disorders, and those caused by head and neck surgeries.

Unilateral adductor vocal fold paralysis

Varied vocal symptoms characterise patients with unilateral adductor vocal fold paralysis. These may be mild to severe dysphonias characterised by breathiness, low intensity, low pitch, and diplophonia, or a two-toned voice. These vocal properties occur when the normal functioning vocal fold approximates the midline upon closure, while the paralysed fold remains lateral to the midline in a fixed retracted position. Severity of the vocal symptoms is dependent upon the exact position of the paralysed fold. The closer it rests to the glottal midline, the less severe the dysphonia and the more effective voice therapy may be.

The goal of voice therapy with unilateral vocal fold paralysis is to strengthen the normal vocal fold and to encourage it to overadduct across the midline to better approximate the paralysed fold. The most popular, and to date, the most successful method of increasing laryngeal strength and movement, is the pushing exercise, which was first suggested by Froeschels, Kastein and Weiss (1955). This method essentially combines the production of vowel sounds with isometric pushing involving the arms. By pushing the palms of the hands together, lifting up on the arms of a chair or interlocking the fingers and pulling, the patient increases the muscular activity of laryngeal effort closure. This forces the normal vocal fold to adduct vigorously. When done routinely as a systematic exercise, pushing helps to strengthen the muscles of adduction. Progression of the exercises continues utilising vowels, syllables, words, and phrases.

Other vocal exercises that have proved helpful are the use of hard glottal attack exercises for strengthening laryngeal muscles; turning the head to one side or the other to increase tension on the paralysed vocal fold; and digital manipulation of the thyroid cartilage for the same purpose. Many of these approaches, along with EMG biofeedback, have proven to be highly successful in improving the vocal qualities of patients with this disorder.

The effects of vocal fold paralysis may have a strong emotional impact on many patients. Besides the positive effects of direct mechanical intervention, voice therapy may also be effective as a time to monitor and discuss the emotional, social, and job-related difficulties the patient may be experiencing as a result of the pathology. Occasional referral to mental health professionals may be required.

Superior laryngeal nerve paralysis

Patients with a diagnosis of superior laryngeal nerve paralysis may occasionally be referred to speech and language clinicians. While it is somewhat unusual for this type of paralysis to occur, the vocal symptoms may be extremely frustrating. The superior laryngeal nerve innervates the cricothyroid muscle. Unilateral paralysis causes an uneven rocking motion of the thyroid cartilage in relation to the cricoid cartilage. This could cause the vocal folds to overlap each other slightly in an oblique relationship upon adduction. The vocal symptoms are a flat, monotonous conversational pitch with the pitch range grossly limited. Patients also report that laryngeal fatigue also occurs quickly, especially in those who depend on their voices in the job setting.

Unfortunately, direct voice therapy is not effective in improving the function of the laryngeal mechanism or in improving voice quality. The speech and language clinician does, however, have a role in the management of these patients. This role involves (1) explaining the nature of the disorder by utilising illustrations and diagrams; (2) exploring how the pathology is affecting everyday communication abilities and the subsequent emotional state of the patient; (3) establishing strategies for dealing with the negative communication effects such as environmental manipulation and vocal rest periods; and (4) making the appropriate referrals to deal with depression that may be a result of this disorder.

Adductor spastic dysphonia

The actual cause or causes of adductor spastic dysphonia have yet to be determined. One of the more debilitating, yet non-life-threatening laryngeal pathologies, it has proved extremely resistive to many modification approaches including voice therapy, drug therapy, psychotherapy, hypnosis, acupuncture, relaxation therapy, and biofeedback training. It was not until 1975 that patients with adductor spastic dysphonia were offered any kind of relief from this disorder. This relief came in a most unusual form, that being the resection of one recurrent laryngeal nerve, creating a unilateral vocal fold paralysis (Dedo, 1976). This radical therapy approach has proved successful in reducing laryngospasm in many patients.

The rationale of this approach is based on the fact that when a laryngospasm occurs, the vocal folds meet at the midline with great force. When one vocal fold is paralysed in a paramedian position, the force of the spasm will enable the normal fold to cross the glottal midline and approximate the paralysed fold. This essentially eliminates the laryngospasm, releasing the patient from the strained, strangled quality. Return of spasticity may occur following surgery. This return appears to occur for one of two reasons: either the paralysed vocal fold migrates too close to the midline, thus re-establishing the laryngospasm, or the nonparalysed fold overcompensates, crossing too far beyond the glottal midline and again creating the laryngospasm.

In discussing the possibility of using this procedure with a patient, it is the responsibility of the laryngologist and speech and language clinician to detail all factors, positive and negative. The most positive factor is that after surgery the voice is normally produced with much less effort and strain. The patient should be aware, however, that it will not be the same voice that was present prior to the onset of spasticity. Because of the paralysis, it is likely to be mildly dysphonic, characterised by low intensity and breathiness. Another negative factor is the necessity for surgical intervention. No matter how simple the surgical procedure, general anaesthesia always presents risks. Finally, at least 39 per cent of those who choose this form of therapy may have a return of spasticity within one and one-half years after surgery (Aronson and DeSanto, 1981).

If, after examining these issues, the patient chooses to explore this procedure further, the laryngologist will temporarily paralyse the recurrent laryngeal nerve with an injection of a paralysing agent such as xylocaine. This temporary paralysis will cause a simulation of the approximate vocal quality following surgery. It has been our experience that most patients are more impressed with the lack of laryngeal strain than with the improved vocal quality. The quality of voice during the presurgical test will be very close to that of the postsurgical voice. Tape recordings of a standard voice sample should be taken both before and during temporary paralysis.

When the temporary paralysis has resolved, the patient, laryngologist, and speech and language clinician should take time to evaluate critically the tape recordings and the patient's reaction to the 'new' voice. Family members may be included in the process if the patient desires. Following this evaluation, the patient is given as much time as needed to decide whether to proceed with surgery. Even with the negative issues involved with this approach, the majority of patients choose to undergo surgery. Surgery is relatively simple taking only 35 to 45 minutes. After recovering from the anaesthesia, the patient will notice a mild to moderate breathy dysphonia. The strain and tension of phonation will not be present. The speech and language clinician will tape-record the postsurgical voice for future reference.

The return of normal voicing with this approach has effected many gratifying experiences as well as several heartbreaking experiences. Its positive impact for many patients cannot be denied. However, from personal and legal aspects, it is essential that all patients being considered for this procedure go through the rigorous evaluation described.

Neurological voice disorders

Some excellent publications describe and classify various neurologic voice, speech and language disorders (Darley, Aronson and Brown, 1975; Aronson, 1980). Many vocal symptoms are evident in the majority of these disorders. These symptoms are, however, only a part of the larger disorder and often are of minor consideration in the overall treatment of the disorder. For example, almost all dysarthrias involve impairment of articulation, resonation, respiration, and phonation, most of which are voice components. The primary thrust of therapy, however, is to improve the muscular incoordination of the articulation component. Voice therapy has seldom proved of significant benefit with the neurologic disorders. Currently, it is most important for the speech and language clinician to understand these disorders in order to distinguish them for non-neurologically based pathologies.

Head and neck surgeries create a range of voice disorders; these are discussed in Chapter 17.

Management for Personality-related Causes

Patients who develop pathologies as a result of personality disorders are among the more interesting in voice therapy. The major types of laryngeal pathologies caused by personality conflicts in the adult population are conversion aphonia and dysphonia. The management plans for these pathologies include four major stages. The first stage is the medical evaluation. As with all voice disorders, it is essential that the presence of organic pathology be ruled out prior to the initiation of therapy. The report of normal laryngeal structures will also confirm the diagnosis of a personality-related disorder, in the presence of inappropriate and often unusual vocal symptoms.

The second management stage is the diagnostic evaluation. During the evaluation, the speech and language clinician will develop the history of the pathology and will learn how the patient functions socially and physically within the environment. An impression of the patient's personality will evolve. The diagnostic time is also used to prepare the patient for vocal change. This is accomplished by explaining to the patient how the vocal mechanism works and by describing what is happening physiologically within the larynx to create the present voice. Although no attempt is yet made to explain why this is occurring, the physiological description provides the patient with a rationale for the vocal problems.

The third stage of vocal management is the direct manipulation of the voice. The type of manipulation will vary, depending on the non-speech phonation abilities demonstrated by the patient. Vocal manipulation most often begins during the diagnostic evaluation. The expected result is a dramatic change in the voice toward normal phonation. Greene (1972) and Boone (1977) both report that these patients often attain normal voicing during the first treatment session. This has also been my experience.

The final stage of management involves counselling to determine why the disorder was present. Conversion voice disorders present themselves in patients who have undergone some physical or emotional trauma. It is the patient's subconscious effort to escape the unpleasant situation or the memory of the situation that promotes the reaction. Aronson (1980) suggests that the most appropriate professional to deal with this type of disorder is the speech and language clinician, whose complete understanding of the vocal processes and counselling background provide the basic skills and abilities to remediate these pathologies. Once normal voicing has been achieved, it is a natural transition to begin examining why the problem existed. By this time the clinician has gained an excellent trust and rapport with the patient. With interview questions that are structured in a non-threatening manner, the clinician can usually determine the cause. Patients frequently volunteer the necessary information, which often opens a floodgate of emotion.

Once the cause or causes have been identified and discussed, the clinician needs to determine if further professional counselling is advisable. If so, the appropriate referral should be discussed with the patient and should be made with the patient's consent. Let us now examine therapy strategies for conversion voice disorders.

Traditional management approaches examine the patient's ability to phonate during nonspeech phonatory behaviours such as coughing, throat clearing, laughing, crying, or sighing. When clear phonation is identified on one of these behaviours, it is then shaped into vowel sound, nonsense syllables, words, and short phrases. The speech and language clinician must demonstrate much patience at this time. Most patients have not phonated for several weeks. The possibility of proceeding too quickly and frightening the patient away from phonation is present. Once good consistent phonation is established under practice conditions, the clinician begins to insist gently that it be used during the therapy conversations. When voice is regained in this manner, it is seldom lost again, and patients do not substitute other conversion symptoms.

Another management technique utilises the falsetto voice. The patient is instructed in the basic physiology of the laryngeal mechanism and how it relates to the vocal difficulties. It is explained that we are going to manipulate the vocal mechanism in a manner that will force the muscles to pull the vocal folds together. The clinician then produces a falsetto tone on the sound /ai/. The patient is told in a matter-of-fact manner that everyone can produce this tone, even those who are having vocal difficulties. The falsetto is again demonstrated by the clinician, and the patient is then told to produce the same sound. Of more than fifty patients treated by the author, only two, both of whom resisted all forms of voice therapy, would not or could not produce the falsetto tone. The falsetto is then stabilised briefly on vowels.

It is explained to the patient that we are going to use the muscle tension created by producing the falsetto tone to force the vocal folds to pull together normally. The patient is then given a list of 150 two-syllable phrases and asked to read them in the falsetto voice. During this exercise the patient is constantly encouraged to read swiftly and loudly. After the voice stabilises in a relatively strong falsetto, the patient is halted and asked to match the clinician singing down the scale about three to four notes from the original falsetto tone. The patient is then asked to continue reading the phrases at this new pitch level. The same procedure is repeated two or three more times until the patient is fairly closely approximating a normal pitch level. The patient is continually encouraged to produce these phrases louder and faster until eventually the voice 'breaks' into normal phonation.

It is extremely important that the clinician be patient when utilising this technique. The normal time frame from aphonia to normal voice is approximately 30 to 45 minutes. The clinician must not only be patient but also must present a very matter-of-fact, confident manner.

Why do these techniques work? Possibly because the patient is ready to change; the clinician has given a reasonable explanation for what the vocal folds are doing and has demonstrated confidence in the therapeutic technique.

Following return of voice, it is necessary to explore the actual cause for the conversion. It is desirable to do this in a direct manner. By this time the patient has developed strong confidence in the clinician and quite often opens up a floodgate of information about deaths, family problems, work problems, and the like. In discussing these problems, the clinician attempts to accomplish two major objectives: (1) to give the patient total and final control over the laryngeal mechanism; and (2) to determine the patient's general emotional state to decide the need for further professional counselling. If the clinician feels the problem is not resolved and further counselling is in order, the suggestion should be discussed with the patient and appropriate referrals should be made.

Conclusion

You have now been introduced to the five major areas of knowledge necessary for undertaking the treatment of patients with voice disorders. The term 'introduction' is important in this discussion because your understanding of voice disorders is dependent upon in-depth study of anatomy/physiology, causes of voice disorders, laryngeal pathologies, diagnostic procedures and therapy techniques. Because of space consideration, it is not possible to include more than introductory comments regarding each of these areas of knowledge. Indeed, entire texts are devoted to these topics with many of the texts referenced throughout this chapter. Students are encouraged to read further and to develop the theoretical knowledge necessary for the practical treatment of voice disorders.

Acknowledgments

The author sincerely thanks Charles E. Merrill Publishing Co., for the permission of liberal use of materials from the texts *Clinical Voice Pathology: Theory and Management* and *Effective Voice and Articulation,* with both texts referenced within this chapter. The patience of Margaret Leahy during the preparation of this chapter is also greatly appreciated.

References

ARONSON, A.E. (1980) *Clinical Voice Disorders: An Interdisciplinary Approach.* New York: Brian C. Decker.

ARONSON, A.E., BROWN, J.R., LITIN, E.M. and PEARSON, J.J. (1968) Spastic dysphonia. 1. Voice, neurologic and psychiatric aspects. *Journal of Speech and Hearing Disorders,* 33, 203–18.

ARONSON, A. and DESANTO, L. (1981) Adductor spastic dysphonia: 1½ years after recurrent laryngeal nerve section. *Annals of Otology, Rhinology and Laryngology,* 90, 11–6.

BAKEN, R.J. (1987) *Clinical Measurement of Speech and Voice.* Boston: Little, Brown.

BOONE, D. (1977) *The Voice and Voice Therapy* (2nd ed.). Englewood-Cliffs, NJ: Prentice Hall.

BRODNITZ, F. (1971) *Vocal Rehabilitation.* Rochester, MA: American Academy of Ophthalmology and Otolaryngology.

BRODNITZ, F.F. (1976) Spastic dysphonia. *Annals of Otology, Rhinology and Laryngology*, 85, 210–4.

COOPER, M. (1973) *Modern Techniques of Vocal Rehabilitation.* Springfield, IL: Charles C. Thomas.

DARLEY, F.L., ARONSON, A.E. and BROWN, J.R. (1975) *Motor Speech Disorders.* Philadelphia: W.B. Saunders.

DEDO, H. (1976) Recurrent laryngeal nerve section for spastic dysphonia. *Annals of Otology, Rhinology and Laryngology*, 85, 451–9.

DEDO, H., TOWNSEND, J.J. and IZDEBSKI, K. (1978) Current evidence for the organic etiology of spastic dysphonia. *Transactions of Otolaryngology*, 86, 875–80.

DORDAIN, M. and DORDAIN, G. (1972) L'epreuve du (a) tenu au course des tremblements de la voix (tremblement ideopathique et dyskinesie volitionnelle, leurs rapports avec la dysphonic spasmodique). *Revised Laryngology*, 93, 167–82.

FROESCHELS, E., KASTEIN, S and WEISS, D. (1955) A method of therapy for paralytic conditions of the mechanisms of phonation, respiration and glutination. *Journal of Speech and Hearing Disorders*, 20, 365–70.

GREENE, M.(1972) *The Voice and its Disorders* (3rd ed.). Philadelphia: J.B. Lippincott.

HARTMAN, D.E. (1980) *Clinical Investigations of Abductor Spastic Dysphonia (Intermittent Breathy Dysphonia).* Paper presented at the American Speech-Language-Hearing Association Convention, Detroit.

MERSON, R.M. and GINSBERG, A.P. (1979) Spasmodic dysphonia: Abductor type. A clinical report of acoustic, aerodynamic and perceptual characteristics. *Laryngoscope*, 89, 129–39.

MOORE, G.P. (1971) *Organic Voice Disorders.* Englewood Cliffs, NJ: Prentice Hall.

STEMPLE, J. and HOLCOMB, B. (1988) *Effective Voice and Articulation.* Columbus: Charles E. Merrill.

STEMPLE, J. (1984) *Clinical Voice Pathology: Theory and Management.* Columbus, OH: Charles E. Merrill.

16 Adult Stuttering

Margaret M. Leahy

The vast majority of adults who stutter will have been stuttering since childhood. The disruptions, which are the central core of the disorder, remain, and are often compounded or truncated, and around this central core layers of learned responses to stuttering will have grown. The symptoms which the adult stutterer presents differ markedly from those of the children.

Horsley (Chapter 9) stresses the involuntary disruption in the flow of speech as a characteristic of stuttering, but problems remain in providing an adequate definition (Bloodstein, 1981; Perkins, 1983; Van Riper, 1982). There is general agreement about the abnormally high frequency of intra-phonemic breaks that disrupt transitions between sounds (Stromsta, 1986) and in the adult, these disruptions are often accompanied by excessive tension and struggle. Dalton and Hardcastle (1977) point out that dysfluency affects not only the segmental aspects of speech but prosodic, syntactic, lexical and semantic levels of communication. The interaction process may also be disrupted (Krause, 1982) and adult stutterers may be socially maladjusted (Cox, 1986; Prins, 1972). An important aspect of stuttering is its cyclic or variable nature (i.e., people who stutter will tend to stutter less for long periods or in some situations) (Gregory, 1987; Andrews, Craig, Feyer, Hoddinott, Howie and Neilson, 1983). Avoidance is considered a feature of confirmed or advanced stuttering (Starkweather, 1987).

Causative Factors

Adults who have stuttered since childhood share the causative factors of childhood stuttering which have already been discussed in Chapter 9. However, the theories of the origins of stuttering may not bear much relevance to the adult form of stuttering as the disorder will have grown and changed significantly during its development. It is estimated that as many as 78 per cent of children who have ever stuttered will recover by age sixteen (Andrews *et al.,* 1983), but those who will persist in stuttering will typically follow patterns of development described by Van Riper (1982) and by Starkweather (1987). These patterns are generally episodic and they provide insight into a major causative factor of developing stuttering: learning.

While there is increasing evidence to support theories that consider stutterers to be constitutionally different to nonstutterers (Kidd, 1985; Moore, 1985; Moore and Boberg, 1987), learning theories may be readily applied to the development of the disorder. Among the most notable of these theories are Brutten and Shoemaker's (1967) two-factor learning theory and Sheehan's (1968) approach-avoidance theory. Brutten and Shoemaker propose that the intraphonemic disruptions are influenced and precipitated by classically conditioned negative emotion. In learning to cope with the threat and experience of stuttering, the stutterer reacts by using 'helping' or avoiding behaviours which are instrumentally conditioned by reinforcing consequences. Thus the secondary behaviours such as severe blocking and limb movements accompanying stuttering are learned because they seem to relieve, albeit temporarily, the core stuttering behaviour. These coping behaviours become part of the stutterer's symptomatology.

Sheehan's approach-avoidance theory centres on the conflict experienced by the stutterer when he wants to speak but fears speaking (because of stuttering) and also, he wants to remain silent but fears silence (because of its undesirable consequences, i.e., failure to communicate). The resolution of the conflict lies in one urge becoming stronger than the other and as the unpleasantness associated with the conflict is reduced, the behaviour ensuing — either stuttering or avoidance — is reinforced.

According to Sheehan (1968), the conflict is not only related to speech and speech situations, but to the social presentation of the self. So the stutterer is more likely to stutter when he feels low in self-esteem or when he is in awe of his listener or where he perceives the threat of penalty for stuttering. In this theory, stuttering is self-reinforcing as anxiety levels drop when the stuttering occurs.

The 'histories of intermittent reinforcement which we may never know' (Van Riper, 1984, p. 220) account for the range of abnormal behaviours that the adult stutterer presents. Resistance to therapy is also a common feature because of past failure, as many will have attended fluency therapy, achieved some level of fluency and regressed to stuttering again.

Acquired stuttering in adults

Stuttering, or dysfluency reminiscent of stuttering, appearing subsequent to central nervous system damage is reported in the literature. It is not considered a unitary disorder, 'anymore than aphasia is a unitary disorder' (Helm-Estabrooks, 1986, p.

193). Canter (1971) identified three types which he designated as dysarthric, dyspraxic and dysnomic, providing subtypes of dysarthric stuttering. The problem of defining neurogenic stuttering is discussed by Rosenbek (1985), who differentiates it from the dysfluencies that occur with any speech-language disorder, stressing the 'involuntary repetition primarily of the correct sounds and syllables any place in a word' (p. 46). Lebrun, Retif and Kaiser (1983), also describe a case of stuttering as a forerunner of motor-neuron disease and Deal (1982) describes sudden onset of stuttering, apparently idiopathic stuttering, in an adult.

Assessment Considerations

Assessment is a dynamic process that is often inextricably linked to therapy. It involves the collection of as much relevant information as is necessary to describe and delimit the presenting problem and arrive at a decision regarding therapy. The adult stutterer will be directly involved in the identification and analysis of his stuttering, although objective measures of stuttering should also be used (Edwards and Harcastle, 1987). Ingham and Costello (1984) suggest that there should be at least four once-weekly within- and beyond-clinic assessments of stuttering over the base rate period, with the rationale of providing a basis for evaluating treatment outcome and terminating therapy. While this may seem time consuming, there is reason to doubt the representativeness of severity ratings estimated from the initial sessions, as stutterers tend to seek therapy when they are particularly dysfluent (Van Riper, 1982). In our experience, some may even deliberately stutter more severely because of their anxiety to be accepted on a course of therapy, having been previously told that their dysfluency was 'mild' or 'within normal limits'.

Measures of stuttering severity

Minimal requirements for estimating severity of stuttering include sampling speech under different conditions, estimating the frequency of stuttering and rate of speaking, and describing the tension and struggle associated with speaking. Observing extraneous movements during speaking may be included in estimates of struggle. Because of the variability of stuttering, many authors suggest that speech should be sampled in different modes and under different conditions (Ingham and Costello, 1984; Riley, 1982; Ryan and Van Kirk, 1974). The Stuttering Severity Instrument (SSI) (Riley, 1982) uses reading and monologue as the base measures together with a system for estimating tension and degree of struggle. The procedure presented by Ingham and Costello includes measures of stuttering frequency, rate of speech and quality of speech, including ratings of naturalness, prosody and fluency.

As mentioned above, beyond-clinic measures are considered very important in their approach.

Motivation

Low motivation and resistance to therapy is not uncommon in the stutterer, as a result of a history of failure both with self-therapy and with other therapies. Motivation fluctuates, not only the client's but the clinician's also, and low motivation on the part of the clinician is likely to have a negative effect on the client (Ragsdale and Ashby, 1982; St. Louis and Lass, 1981; Woods and Williams, 1976). Continuous monitoring of motivation is called for. Direct and indirect methods may be utilised (e.g., the clinician can estimate degrees of motivation by noting attendance records, punctuality and cooperation in completing assignments). As well as this, asking the client how improved fluency will affect current status in work, social life, etc. may also provide insight into motivation. Secondary gains from stuttering also have to be taken into consideration — if stuttering is rewarding in any way, motivation to change will not be constant. Furthermore, low motivation to cooperate in fluency therapy may indicate that the stuttering is not the primary problem but perhaps secondary to anxiety in social situations or relationships.

Areas directly and indirectly associated with stuttering

Social skills and nonverbal behaviour are integral to successful communication and there has long been an emphasis on specific aspects of these skills in the stuttering literature, most notably of eye contact and avoidance behaviours. More recently, following developments in research in the area of social skills (see for example, Argyle, 1984; Argyle, Furnham and Graham, 1981) the nonverbal behaviours of stutterers have been receiving attention, both in assessment (Seymour, Ruggiro and McEneaney, 1983) and in therapy (Levy, 1983). There are indications that some stutterers differ from nonstutterers in expression of affect and in the use of nonverbal behaviours when speaking and when listening (Krause, 1980, 1982). A checklist of social skills, including nonverbal behaviours, may be useful for indicating those stutterers who have deficiencies in this area.

Avoidance behaviours may be assessed using questionnaires such as the Johnson, Darley and Spriestersbach (1963) but we have also found it useful to assess assertive behaviour as it may be directly influenced by avoidance. A schedule for assessing assertive behaviour such as the Rathus (1973) or that provided by Trower, Bryant and Argyle (1978) may be used.

Attitudes

Controversy about focusing on attitudes in stuttering therapy reflects the unsatisfactory state of attitude assessment (Guitar and Bass, 1978; Hayhow, 1983; Ulliana and Ingham, 1984) as well as the basic controversy about attitude change and its role in stuttering therapy (Gregory, 1979; Howie and Andrews, 1985). The attitude scale most widely used in speech clinics and in research with stutterers is the S24 (Andrews and Cutler, 1974). This procedure has been criticised by Preus (1981) because of inconsistency in item pairs and resultant inconsistency in responses. Ulliana and Ingham (1984) also criticised the S24 on the basis that scores reflected the type and quality of speech in situations actually mentioned rather than attitudes to communication as such. Using an amended version of the scale, the AS24, they found that stutterers regarded their responses to the scale items as largely influenced by their judgements about their stuttering and speech behaviour, and that stuttering frequency was consistently higher in situations associated with item responses implying negative attitudes.

Change in attitude seems to be important for long-term maintenance of fluency (Sheehan, 1979; Van Riper, 1982) so some assessment of attitudes is indicated, either by using the S24, the AS24 or more informally, i.e., by asking pertinent questions, or perhaps with the use of repertory grids.

Repertory grids as assessment procedures

The repertory grid was devised as a means of analysing relationships and inter-relationships among constructs and elements in applying Kelly's (1955) personal construct theory. Grids have been used successfully in facilitating a delineation of the issues likely to be concentrated on in therapy, and as a means of evaluating changes that occur during therapy (Evesham and Fransella, 1985; Leahy and O'Sullivan, 1987). Although grids are by no means necessary to personal construct therapy, they are useful for introducing the notion of reconstruction and the possible implications of change for an individual client. The issues highlighted by using grids may be less easily articulated by other means, and points of similarity between members of a group provide an immediate focus for discussion. The role relationship grid and the situations grid (see Fransella and Bannister, 1977) allow for development of insight into the attitudes to and construing of important roles people play in situations that are frequently encountered.

Theoretical Basis of Intervention

Just as learning plays a major role in the development of stuttering, learning and unlearning play major roles in therapy for the adult stutterer, regardless of the school of thought one follows regarding either the origins of the disorder, or the principal approach to therapy. Initially, the identification process involves learning. Fluency techniques using delayed auditory feedback, masking, prolonged speech or smooth speech all involve learning. Transfer and generalisation involve learning. In many instances, however, although learning is considered to be of great importance for changes to be maintained, it is not the basic premise of therapy. Therapies that derive from an understanding of stuttering as an operant behaviour provide the theoretical basis for systematic conditioning in stuttering therapy.

Fluency shaping therapies: underlying principles

The objective of the fluency shaping therapies is the reduction in frequency, and finally the elimination of stuttering without direct focus on negative attitudes, feelings or perceptions. Fluency change is brought about mainly by manipulating the consequences of various behaviours of stutterers. Fluency behaviours are reinforced and stuttering behaviours punished and in some instances, a combination of both reinforcement and punishment have been used (Ingham and Andrews, 1973; Ingham and Packman, 1977; Ryan and Van Kirk, 1974; Howie, Tanner and Andrews, 1981; Webster, 1979). Although it is acknowledged that some change in attitude is desirable for change in fluency to be maintained, there is evidence to suggest that attitudes will change as a result of increased fluency (Ryan, 1979; Webster, 1979). The underlying principles of operant conditioning are deftly illustrated by Costello and Ingham (1985, p. 188), showing possible response contingent arrangements of stimuli that identify operant behaviours and how the frequency of behaviours may be increased or decreased. (More detailed descriptions are provided by Costello, 1982; Shames and Florance, 1986.)

Stuttering modification therapies: underlying principles

The objective of the stuttering modification therapies is change in the *form* of stuttering with accompanying change in feelings, attitudes and perceptions. This entails direct focus on stuttering with the aim of producing 'fluent stuttering' (Van Riper, 1982) as opposed to fluent speech. But the focus on the person who stutters is no less important than the speech process itself, as adjustment to stuttering, albeit in a more controlled and fluent form, is seen as a major goal in therapy. This adjustment to stuttering has been criticised for producing 'happy stutterers' as some levels of stuttering behaviour are considered acceptable (Stromsta, 1986). However, the stated principle of those who support this approach is that by accepting stuttering, one is in a better position to deal constructively with it, as tension and anxiety related to stuttering are reduced. Furthermore, the possibility of constitutional differences amongst stutterers is recognised in this approach.

Mainstream Treatment Practices

Phases in intervention

Typically, intervention procedures for stuttering are described in a series of phases of therapy and this holds true whether the fundamental approach follows fluency shaping, stuttering modification therapies, or perhaps, a combination of both (see Gregory, 1979). With the possible exception of some programmes based on operant principles, phases are not necessarily rigidly adhered to but they have a function in the organisation and orientation of therapy. The phases in intervention outlined here serve such functions. (More detailed descriptions may be found in Cooper, 1984; Shames and Florance, 1986; Stromsta, 1986; and Van Riper, 1982.)

Initial contact: interview and information exchange

The initial contact between clinician and client sets the scene for all that follows and is important for instilling in the client a sense of confidence and trust in the clinician and in therapy. Although many authors focus on generating an atmosphere that will help the client provide 'the information he (the clinician) wants' (Nation and Aram, 1977, p. 276), it is incumbent on the clinician to be able and willing to provide information to the client as well as collect it. In this way the initial sessions can become a genuine exchange of data and ideas that immediately invite the active participation of the client. As well as collecting case history data, including a history of the development of the stuttering and a description of its current status, the clinician can present information regarding his experience with stuttering (or lack thereof); the client's and clinician's understanding of the problem of stuttering can be discussed, and the cyclic nature of the disorder within and without therapy examined. Stromsta (1986) rcommends that the complexity of speech and language acquisition be a topic during these early stages. He presents a model of speech production and focuses on the concept of fluent speech as continual movement and co-articulation using examples from sound spectography. Such a focus represents for Stromsta the essential aspects of fluency that lead to the development of 'a practical definition of stuttering' (p. 120).

Assessment: identification, analysis and understanding

Assessment considerations have already been discussed above. It is important to reiterate the client's involvement in identifying and analysing his stuttering which will be facilitated by knowledge of the speech process and the nature of fluency. Discriminating between core features of stuttering and associated reactive features is necessary, as it leads to a better understanding of the disorder, both for the clinician and the client. With the developing understanding both of the nature of fluency and stuttering and the nature of therapy, a contract may be drawn up that specifies among other things, commitment to therapy (including follow-up) and an undertaking to share responsibility in therapy and to dedicate time and attention to change outside the clinic. Fluctuating fluency may also be specified to allow for strategies to be implemented when stuttering increases. Gregory (1987) refers to the initial reluctance of stutterers to become involved in the analysis of stuttering, but its importance is recognised afterwards as the desire to deny the existence of the problem is reduced.

Technique selection: trials and practice

Because of the individuality of each person who stutters as well as the uniqueness of the stuttering presentation, selecting a technique is largely an individual matter. Costello and Ingham (1985) recommend the use of probes to help in selecting a technique, and Ryan (1986) proposes that his Delayed Auditory Feedback (DAF) programme be used with more severe and older stutterers and the Gradual Increase in Length and Complexity of Utterance (GILCU) programme with less severe and younger stutterers. Composite techniques such as prolonged speech and slowed speech help regulate breathing, pausing, articulatory contact and continuity or co-articulation and allow for the client to develop aspects of the technique that he finds most helpful. Others, such as airflow or easy onset techniques, focus largely on one aspect of behaviour and the development and regulation of that behaviour to reduce dysfluency. The Van Riperian concepts of *preparatory set, pullout* and *cancellation* with the emphasis on the stuttering moment and what happens before and after it, can be implemented into a programme of therapy to supplement the primary technique being used. Although the clinician acts as model, teacher and initially chief monitor of the client's performance, it is the responsibility of the client not only to become proficient in the use of a particular technique, but also to learn to evaluate it. Regardless of the school of thought one adopts in therapy, reward as reinforcement of desired behaviour and withdrawal of reward and time-out as punishment schedules may be used extensively during this phase and regulated for the following phases.

Transfer: the initial stage

Transfer of the use of a technique within the clinic begins as soon as the client has begun to learn the technique. Within-clinic practice may be seen as technique transfer where:

1   the amount of speech, and
2   the speaking mode changes (reading, monologue, conversation, asking questions, etc.) and it is furthered by
3   changing the composition and size of the audience (speaking with receptionist, within a group, on the telephone, etc.).

Transfer schedules for outside the clinic are drawn up either from avoidance reports or speaking logs, but in the early stages only 'safe' situations are considered, i.e., with selected friends or family. As therapy progresses, roleplay of more difficult situations outside the clinic can be done in groups and video recorded. This facilitates transfer and is also useful for analysis of other communication skills. Transfer programmes generally exploit behavioural principles to some degree in establishing fluency outside the clinic. (See Ingham and Andrews, 1973; Mowrer, 1975; and Boberg, 1976.)

Transfer in action

As fluency develops it is appropriate to consider other aspects of relationship and situational anxiety that may inhibit the transfer process. In this regard issues that are highlighted through the use of repertory grids or with discussion and/or questionnaires may be discussed in detail and roleplay begun in individual and/or group sessions. The broad spectrum of communication and more effective use of nonverbal skills, including listening skills can be introduced in such sessions. Wilkinson and Canter (1982), and Ellis and Whittington (1981, 1983), present useful data for assessment and management of social skills. Self-regulation of fluency with occasional monitoring by the clinician becomes the order of the day during this phase.

Maintenance and preventing relapse

The final phase of therapy is arguably the most important phase as it represents the ultimate goal of fluency therapy: maintenance and development of newly acquired skills and attitudes. Despite this, it is one of the least well researched areas in the literature. Boberg, Howie and Woods (1986, p. 496) provide a brief overview of four categories of procedures used during this phase. These are:

1 regular clinical contact following treatment
2 emphasis on client self-responsibility
3 emphasis on the need for changes in attitudes to speech, self-concept, etc. and
4 intensive 'refresher programmes' or recycling through the initial programme.

Whatever the procedure chosen, a major point of attention is the client's ability to recognise and deal with fluctuations in fluency. Strengthening the fluency and fluency-enhancing behaviours is an important commitment for the client. As Sheehan (1984, p. 93) states: 'When two habits are of approximately equal strength but are unequal in age, at any given time in the future the older will be stronger, provided that neither is practised in the meantime. All the stutterer has to do to relapse is to rest on his oars'. Boberg, Howie and Woods (1979) examine possible reasons for poor practice and concludes that practice is punishing for the stutterer whose fluency has improved dramatically with therapy. Spontaneity is lost because of the careful monitoring that is necessary and feelings of self-acceptance may be reduced. The inherent abnormality of a technique requiring practice may be rejected and the rewards of practice are delayed and not always obvious to the client who is fluent most of the time anyway. Genetic influences may also increase the risk of relapse.

Facing up to failure and admitting defeat is not easy for either client or clinician and relapse represents failure for both parties. This fact alone may account for the small number of studies on relapse. Kuhr and Rustin (1985) reported an in-patient programme for clients who had failed in 'multiple treatments' and indicated that along with 'booster sessions' with the therapist, help from the social environment of the client (i.e., spouse and friends), was important. The depressing effect of fluency on some participants was also noted as a factor that may influence relapse. (Gregory (1979; 1987) refers to 'personality characteristics' that may influence a person's response to therapy and Leahy and O'Sullivan (1987) to the ' "safety" of stuttering', factors that have to be considered when therapy is undertaken and when fluency has been established. Commitment to the practice of skills learned in therapy is a point that needs to be stressed throughout therapy.

Effectiveness of Therapy

There is no doubt that therapy for stuttering can produce long-term, positive effects with time spent in therapy the single best predictor of outcome (Andrews, Guitar and Howie, 1980; Bloodstein, 1981). However, as we have seen, neither is there any doubt that degrees of relapse occur for many clients. In reviewing therapy effects, Andrews *et al.,* (1983) conclude that only the prolonged speech (Perkins 1973; Perkins, Rudas, Johnson, Michael, Curlee, 1974) and precision fluency shaping (Webster, 1979) strategies have reported sufficient follow-up data on clients to allow claims of success to be made and evaluated. Attitude therapy alone was considered unlikely to be of benefit (Van Riper, 1982; Andrews *et al.,* 1983) and airflow therapy alone, taught over a short term, is also unlikely to have any long-term positive effect (Andrews and Tanner, 1982). Nevertheless substantial gains can be made in therapy: the average treated stutterer is more normal speaking than 90 per cent of untreated stutterers (Andrews *et al.,* 1980). While such a report is optimistic, Boberg (1986, p. 510) adds a caveat 'to postpone our victory celebrations' while some methodological issues are addressed and new strategies tested. St. Louis and Westbrook (1987) and Purser (1987) echo this call for increasing attention to evaluating effectiveness and they highlight the fact that effectiveness is not a simple unitary phenomenon.

Although stuttering is probably one of the most researched areas in speech pathology, and recent research has greatly improved our understanding of the disorder, there are many unresolved issues and areas of uncertainty which invite and even demand further research. Foremost among these is therapeutic success with adults. While it is evident that there are many divergent opinions about the nature of the disorder and consequently the nature of therapy, every clinician shares the goal of reducing stuttering, increasing fluency and maintaining the improvement. Despite this, the amount of research on therapy, most particularly on maintenance and follow-up, is relatively small but increasing. The research that has been presented in the past does not present analyses of the essential components of treatment processes and why they work (Andrews *et al.,* 1980) and often findings cannot be generalised because of the small number of subjects involved or failure to replicate findings (Starkweather, 1987). Another area concerns the different subgroups of stutterers that are encountered (see Preus, 1981; St. Louis, 1986).

Conclusion

Working with people who stutter demands a great deal of expertise, time, energy and most of all longterm commitment from clinicians and clients. Despite its demands, reward in the form of successful fluency is not guaranteed. Nevertheless we have reason to be optimistic. Research into the nature (or natures) of the disorder is flourishing. Evaluations of studies of effectiveness of therapy clearly indicate vast improvement in maintenance of fluency over long periods. The future looks bright for understanding the processes of stuttering behaviours and most importantly for working with people who stutter so that they too can understand and acquire the fluency they seek.

References

ANDREWS, G., and CUTLER, J. (1974) Stuttering therapy: the relation between changes in symptom level and attitudes. *Journal of Speech and Hearing Disorders,* 39, 312–9.

ANDREWS, G., GUITAR, B. and HOWIE, P. (1980) Meta-analysis of the effects of stuttering treatment. *Journal of Speech and Hearing Disorders,* 45, 287–307.

ANDREWS, G., CRAIG, A., FEYER, A.M., HODDINOTT, S., HOWIE, P. and NEILSON, M. (1983) Stuttering: A review of research findings and theories c. 1982. *Journal of Speech and Hearing Disorders,* 48, 226–46.

ANDREWS, G. and TANNER, S. (1982) Stuttering treatment: Replication of the regulated breathing method. *Journal of Speech and Hearing Disorders,* 47, 138–40.

ARGYLE, M. (1984) *The Psychology of Interpersonal Behaviour* (4th ed.). Harmondsworth: Penguin.

ARGYLE, M., FURNHAM, J. and GRAHAM, A. (1981) *Social Situations.* Cambridge: Cambridge University Press.

BLOODSTEIN, O. (1981) *A Handbook of Stuttering* (3rd ed.). Chicago: National Easter Seal Society.

BOBERG, E. (1976) Intensive Group Therapy Program for Stutterers. *Human Communication,* 1, 29–42.

BOBERG, E. (1986) Postscript: relapse and outcome. In G.H. Shames and H. Rubin (Eds), *Stuttering Then and Now.* Columbus: OH: Merrill.

BOBERG, E., HOWIE, P. and WOODS, L. (1979) Maintenance of fluency: A review. *Journal of Fluency Disorders,* 4, 93–116.

BOBERG, E., HOWIE, P. and WOODS, L. (1986) Maintenance of fluency: A review. In G.H. Shames and H. Rubin (Eds), *Stuttering Then and Now.* Columbus, OH: Merrill.

BRUTTEN, E.J. and SHOEMAKER, D.J. (1967) *The Modification of Stuttering,* Englewood-Cliffs, NJ: Prentice Hall.

CANTER, G.J. (1971) Observations on neurogenic stuttering: A contribution to differential diagnosis. *British Journal of Disorders of Communication,* 6, 139–43.

COOPER, E.B. (1984) Personalised Fluency Control Therapy: A status report. In M. Peins (Ed.), *Contemporary Approaches in Stuttering Therapy.* Boston: Little, Brown.

COSTELLO, J.M. (1982) Techniques of therapy based on operant theory. In W.H. Perkins (Ed.), *Current Therapy of Communicative Disorders.* New York: Decker.

COSTELLO, J.M. and INGHAM, R.J. (1985) Stuttering as an operant disorder. In R.F. Curlee and W.H. Perkins. *Nature and Treatment of Stuttering.* New Directions, San Diego: College Hill.

COX, M.D. (1986) The psychologically maladjusted stutterer. In K.O. St. Louis (Ed.), *The Atypical Stutterer.* Orlando, FL: Academic Press.

DALTON, P. and HARDCASTLE, W. (1977) *Disorders of Fluency and Their Effects on Communication.* London: Arnold.

DEAL, J.L. (1982) Sudden onset of stuttering: A case report. *Journal of Speech and Hearing Research,* 47, 301–4.

EDWARDS, S. and HARDCASTLE, W. (1987) Linguistic profiling of stuttering behaviour. In L. Rustin, H. Purser and D. Rowley (Eds), *Progress in the Treatment of Fluency Disorders.* London: Taylor and Francis.

ELLIS, R. and WHITTINGTON, D. (1981) *A Guide to Social Skills Training*. Beckingham: Croom Helm.

ELLIS, R. and WHITTINGTON, D. (1983) *New Directions in Social Skills Training*. Beckingham: Croom Helm.

EVESHAM, M. and FRANSELLA, F. (1985) Stuttering relapse: The effect of a combined speech and psychological reconstruction programme. *British Journal of Disorders of Communication*, 20, 237–48.

FRANSELLA, F. and BANNISTER, D. (1977) *A Manual for Repertory Grid Technique*. New York: Academic Press.

GREGORY, H. (1979) Controversial issues: Statement and review of the literature. In H. Gregory, (Ed.), *Controversies about Stuttering Therapy*. Baltimore: University Park Press.

GREGORY, H. (1987) *Handling Relapse*. Paper presented at Clinical Management of Chronic Stuttering Conference. Washington DC.

GUITAR, B. and BASS, C. (1978) Stuttering therapy: The relation between attitude change and long-term outcome. *Journal of Speech and Hearing Disorders*, 43, 392–400.

HAYHOW, R. (1983) The assessment of stuttering and the evaluation of treatment. In P. Dalton (Ed.), *Approaches to the Treatment of Stuttering*. Beckingham: Croom Helm.

HELM-ESTABROOKS, N. (1986) Diagnosis and management of neurogenic stuttering in adults. In K.O. St. Louis (Ed.), *The Atypical Stutterer*. Orlando, FL: Academic Press.

HOWIE, P. and ANDREWS, G. (1985) Treatment of adults: managing fluency. In R.F. Curlee and W.H. Perkins (Eds), *Nature and Treatment of Stuttering: New Directions*. San Diego: College-Hill.

HOWIE, P., TANNER, S. and ANDREWS, G. (1981) Short- and long-term outcome in an intensive treatment program for adult stutterers. *Journal of Speech and Hearing Disorders*, 46, 104–9.

INGHAM, R. and ANDREWS, G. (1973) An analysis of a token economy in stuttering therapy. *Journal of Applied Behavior Analysis*, 6, 219–29.

INGHAM, R. and COSTELLO, J. (1984) Stuttering treatment outcome evaluation. In J. Costello (Ed.), *Speech Disorders in Adults*. San Diego: College Hill.

INGHAM, R. and PACKMAN, S. (1977) A further analysis of stutterers during chorus- and nonchorus- reading conditions. *Journal of Speech and Hearing Research*, 22, 784–93.

JOHNSON, W., DARLEY, F. and SPRIESTERSBACH, D.C. (1963) *Diagnostic Methods in Speech Pathology*. New York: Harper and Row.

KAMHI, A.G. (1982) The problem of relapse in stuttering: some thoughts on what might cause it and how to deal with it. *Journal of Fluency Disorders*, 7, 459–68.

KELLY, G. (1955) *The Psychology of Personal Constructs, Vols. 1 and 2*. New York: Norton.

KIDD, K. (1985) Stuttering as a genetic disorder. In R.F. Curlee and W.H. Perkins (Eds), *The Nature and Treatment of Stuttering: New Directions*. San Diego: College Hill.

KRAUSE, R. (1980) Stuttering and nonverbal communications: Investigations about affect inhibition and stuttering. In H. Giles, W.P. Robinson and P.M. Smith (Eds), *Language: Social Psychological Perspectives*. Oxford: Pergamon.

KRAUSE, R. (1982) A social psychological approach to the study of stuttering. In C. Fraser and K.R. Sherer (Eds), *Advances in the Social Psychology of Language.* Cambridge: Cambridge University Press.

KUHR, A. and RUSTIN., L. (1985) The maintenance of fluency after intensive in-patient therapy: Long-term follow up. *Journal of Fluency Disorders,* 19, 229–36

LEAHY, M. and O'SULLIVAN, B. (1987) Psychological change and fluency therapy: A pilot project. *British Journal of Communication Disorders,* 22, 245–51.

LEBRUN, Y., RETIF, J. and KAISER, G. (1983) Acquired stuttering as a forerunner of motor-neuron disease. *Journal of Fluency Disorders,* 8, 161–7.

LEVY, C. (1983) Group therapy with adults. In P. Dalton (Ed.), *Approaches to the Treatment of Stuttering.* Beckingham: Croom Helm.

MOORE, W.H. and BOBERG, E. (1987) Hemispheric processing and stuttering. In L. Rustin, H. Purser and D. Rowley (Eds), *Progress in the Treatment of Fluency Disorders.* London: Taylor and Francis.

MOORE, W.H. (1985) Central nervous system characteristics of stutterers. In R.F. Curlee and W.H. Perkins (Eds), *Nature and Treatment of Stuttering: New Directions.* San Diego: College Hill.

MOWRER, D.E. (1975) An instrumental program to increase fluent speech of stutterers. *Journal of Fluency Disorders,* 1, 25–35.

NATION, J.E. and ARAM, D.M. (1977) *Diagnosis of Speech and Language Disorders.* St. Louis: C.V. Mosby.

PERKINS, W.H. (1973) Replacement of stuttering with normal speech: 1 rationale and 2 clinicial procedures. *Journal of Speech and Hearing Disorders,* 37, 295–303.

PERKINS, W.H., RUDAS, J., JOHNSON, L., MICHAEL, W.B. and CURLEE, R.F. (1974) Replacement of stuttering with normal speech. III: Clinical Effectiveness. *Journal of Speech and Hearing Disorders,* 39, 416–29.

PERKINS, W.H. (1983) The problem of definition: commentary on 'stuttering'. *Journal of Speech and Hearing Disorders,* 48, 246–9.

PREUS, A. (1981) *Identifying Subgroups of Stutterers.* Oslo: Universitetsforlaget.

PRINS, D. (1972) Personality, stuttering severity and age. *Journal of Speech and Hearing Research,* 15, 148–54.

PURSER, H. (1987) The psychology of treatment evaluation studies. In L. Rustin, H. Purser and D. Rowley (Eds), *Progress in the Treatment of Fluency Disorders.* London: Taylor and Francis.

RAGSDALE, J.D. and ASHBY, J.K. (1982) Speech-Language pathologists connotations of stutterers. *Journal of Speech and Hearing Disorders,* 25, 75–80.

RATHUS, S.A. (1973) A 30-item schedule for assessing assertive behaviour. *Behaviour Therapy,* 4, 398–406.

RILEY, G. (1982) *The Stuttering Severity Instrument.* Tigard, Oregon: C.C. Publications.

ROSENBEK, J.C. (1985) Stuttering secondary to nervous system damage. In R.F. Curlee and W.H. Perkins (Eds), *Nature and Treatment of Stuttering: New Directions.* San Diego: College Hill Press.

RYAN, B. (1974) *Programmed Therapy for Stuttering in Children and Adults.* Springfield, IL: Chas. C. Thomas.

RYAN, B. (1979) Stuttering Therapy in a framework of operant conditioning and programmed learning. In H. Gregory (Ed.), *Controversies about Stuttering Therapy.* Baltimore: University Park Press.

RYAN, B. (1986) Operant therapy for children. In G.H. Shames and H. Rubin (Eds), *Stuttering Then and Now*. Columbus, OH: Merrill.

RYAN, B. and VAN KIRK, B. (1974) The establishment, transfer and maintenance of fluent speech in 50 stutterers using delayed auditory feedback and operant conditioning procedures. *Journal of Speech and Hearing Disorders*, 39, 3–10.

SEYMOUR, C., RUGGIERO, A. and MCENEANEY, J. (1983) The identification of stuttering — can you look and tell? *Journal of Fluency Disorders*, 8, 215–20.

SHAMES, G.H. and FLORANCE, C.L. (1986) Stutter-free speech: A goal for therapy. In G.H. Shames and H. Rubin (Eds), *Stuttering Then and Now*. Columbus, OH: Chas C. Merrill.

SHEEHAN, J.D. (1958) Conflict theory of stuttering. In J. Eisenson (Ed.), *Stuttering: A Symposium*. New York: Harper and Row.

SHEEHAN, J.D. (1968) In H. Gregory (Ed.), *Learning Theory and Stuttering*. Evanston, IL: Northwestern University Press.

SHEEHAN, J.D. (1979) Current issues on stuttering and recovery. In H. Gregory (Ed.), *Controversies about Stuttering Therapy*. Baltimore: University Park Press.

SHEEHAN, J.D. (1984) Relapse and recovery from stuttering. In *Stuttering Therapy: Transfer and Maintenance*. Memphis, Tenn: Speech foundation of America, Publication No. 19.

ST. LOUIS, K.O. (1986) *The Atypical Stutterer*. Orlando, FL: Academic Press.

ST. LOUIS, K.O. and LASS, N.J. (1981) A survey of communicative disorders students' attitudes towards stuttering. *Journal of Fluency Disorders*, 6, 49–79.

ST. LOUIS, K.O. and WESTBROOK, J.B. (1987) The effectiveness of treatment for stuttering. In L. Rustin, H. Purser and D. Rowley (Eds), *Progress in the Treatment of Fluency Disorders*. London: Taylor and Francis.

STARKWEATHER, C.W. (1987) *Fluency and Stuttering*. Englewood-Cliffs, NJ: Prentice Hall.

STROMSTA, C. (1986) *Elements of Stuttering*. Oshtemo, Mich: Atsmorts Publishing.

TROWER, P., BRYANT, B. and ARGYLE, M. (1978) *Social Skills and Mental Health*. London: Methuen.

ULLIANA, L. and INGHAM, R. (1984) Behavioral and nonbehavioral variables in the measurement of stutterers' communication attitudes. *Journal of Speech and Hearing Disorders*, 49, 83–93.

VAN RIPER, C. (1982) *The Nature of Stuttering*. Englewood Cliffs, NJ: Prentice-Hall.

VAN RIPER, C. (1984) *The Treatment of Stuttering*. Englewood Cliffs, NJ: Prentice-Hall.

WEBSTER, R.L. (1979) Empirical considerations regarding stuttering therapy. In H. Gregory. (Ed.), *Controversies about Stuttering Therapy*. Baltimore: University Park Press.

WILKINSON, J. and CANTER, S. (1982) *Social Skills Training Manual*, Chichester: Wiley.

WINGATE, M.E. (1983) Speaking unassisted: comments on a paper by Andrews *et al.*, *Journal of Speech and Hearing Disorders*, 48, 255–63.

WOODS, C.L. and WILLIAMS, D.E. (1976) Traits attributed to stuttering and normally fluent males. *Journal of Speech and Hearing Disorders*, 19, 267–78.

17   Surgical Rehabilitation in Adults

Jerilyn Logemann

Rehabilitation of the patient with head and neck cancer begins with treatment selection. In laryngeal cancer, radiation therapy or conservation (partial) laryngectomy may cure the cancer while maintaining voice, swallowing and normal airway (DeSanto, 1974; Fletcher and Goepfert, 1981). Patients with smaller lesions of the larynx (that is T and T_2 lesions) are generally treated with radiotherapy for cure. These patients may exhibit some vocal changes after radiotherapy, but are able to maintain a normal airway and normal swallowing. Voice changes after radiotherapy have been described as mild. Only a few studies, however, have begun to quantify these voice changes (Karim, Snow, Skiek, and Njo, 1983; Stoicheff, 1975; Stoicheff, Campi, Pasi and Fredrickson, 1983).

Though some patients with T_3 lesions of the larynx may be treated with radiotherapy, cure rates are sometimes considered not as high compared with surgery (i.e., the total laryngectomy). Patients with the largest lesions (T_4) usually require total laryngectomy (Stell and Maran, 1978; Sven and Myers, 1981).

In the United States, an increasing number of patients with T_2 and occasionally T_3 lesions of the larynx are treated with what is known as a 'conservation' laryngectomy (Ogura and Mallen, 1965; Som, 1951). The term *conservation* indicates that function is preserved. The conservation laryngectomy procedures are also known as partial laryngectomies and fall into two categories: (1) the vertical or hemi-laryngectomy and (2) the horizontal or supraglottic laryngectomy. The surgical procedures in both types of partial laryngectomy vary from patient to patient, depending upon the exact location of the tumour and its size. Thus, the speech and language clinician working with any of these patients on their voice or swallowing must always ask the surgeon to describe exactly what tissues were resected and exactly how the reconstruction was accomplished.

Hemi-laryngectomy

Hemi-laryngectomy involves removal of one vertical half of the larynx, generally excluding the epiglottis, the hyoid bone and the arytenoid cartilages. The hemi-laryngectomy resection usually includes one true vocal fold, one ventricle, and one false vocal fold as well as the inner aspect of the thyroid lamina (Som, 1951). Following this resection, the surgeon generally rotates soft tissue into the surgical defect in order to provide a pad of tissue against which the normal vocal fold may make contact during swallow and voice production. In general, the hemi-laryngectomee has few difficulties swallowing, but does have significant changes in voice. Voice after hemi-laryngectomy is usually hoarse to some degree, varying from mild to severe. To date there have been no acoustic studies of voice in hemi-laryngectomised patients.

The hemi-laryngectomy procedure can also be extended beyond what would be considered a 'narrow-field' hemi-laryngectomy. The exact extent of the resection is always dictated by the tumour. Thus, if the tumour is located at the anterior commissure, the resection may be extended around the anterior commissure and well into the opposite vocal fold. Or, if the tumour extends posteriorly to the vocal process of the arytenoid, the resection may include the arytenoid cartilage itself as well as the rest of the vocal fold. In general, the larger the resection, the more severe the hoarseness which results and the longer it takes the patient to relearn to swallow. The swallowing problems of the hemi-laryngectomee involve reduced laryngeal closure. This problem can usually be managed with postural compensations: turning the patient's head to the operated side (which improves adduction), and by tilting the head forward (which puts the epiglottis in a more overhanging position to protect the airway).

Supraglottic laryngectomy

The supraglottic or vertical partial laryngectomy involves removal of the epiglottis and aryepiglottic folds, the false vocal folds, and the hyoid bone (Ogura and Mallen, 1965). Removal of the hyoid destroys the foundation of the tongue and the suspension of the larynx. Thus, in the reconstruction procedure, the remainder of the larynx is usually elevated and sutured under the base of the tongue (Calcaterra, 1971). This laryngeal re-elevation is designed to reconstruct the protection for the airway which is provided by the tongue base as it moves posteriorly and the larynx as it elevates under the tongue during the swallow. After a supraglottic laryngectomy, all patients must relearn to swallow by what is known as the 'supraglottic swallow technique' (Logemann, 1983). In this procedure, patients are taught to hold their breath at the height of their inhalation, to continue to hold their breath while they swallow, and to follow the swallow with a cough on the exhalation. This technique is designed to provide slightly improved vocal fold closure before and during the swallow, and to expectorate any residue which remains on the vocal folds or around the arytenoids after the swallow. Many supraglottic laryngectomees experience edema of the arytenoid after the surgery. Unless these patients cough after the swallow, they are likely to aspirate this residue when they inhale after the swallow.

In theory, the supraglottic laryngectomy should not have a voice problem, since the true vocal folds and arytenoids are left intact. Unfortunately, however, many supraglottic laryngectomees do exhibit some degree of hoarseness, probably related to edema, or to some degree of stiffness in the arytenoid after removal of the surrounding aryepiglottic folds and to possible damage of the superior laryngeal nerve. There are no acoustic studies of voice production after supraglottic laryngectomy.

If the supraglottic laryngectomy resection is extended into the tongue base, or into the arytenoid cartilage, the patient's chances of relearning to swallow are significantly reduced. If a larger amount of tongue base is removed, very often food runs directly off the tongue base and into the airway. If a portion of the arytenoid cartilage is removed, the last sphincter to protect the airway is damaged and the patient must attempt to compensate for this resection by tremendously increased adductor muscle effort. Though the exact extent of resection which results in functional versus nonfunctional swallowing has not been determined, it is clear that when the arytenoid cartilage is included in the resection, the chance of the patient relearning to swallow is reduced by at least 50 per cent. Voice quality is also severely impaired.

Total laryngectomy

Patients with very large laryngeal tumours (T_3 or T_4) or whose laryngeal cancer recurs after treatment with radiotherapy generally require total laryngectomy (Harrison, 1972; Stell and Maran, 1978; Sven and Myers, 1981). Total laryngectomy resection includes the hyoid bone, the entire larynx and some portion of the pharynx, and trachea. The exact extent of resection depends on the exact size and location of the tumour. Removal of the hyoid bone eliminates the foundation for the tongue, leaving the patient with slight changes in tongue function. After the entire larynx is removed, the tracheal stump is bent forward to the base of the neck, where a stoma or external hole is created with the tracheal stump sutured to the skin (see Figure 17.1).

In reconstruction of the pharyngo-oesophagus in the total laryngectomee, there is generally no attempt made to match fibres of the same muscle in the pharyngo-oesophagus. Once the larynx has been removed with whatever portion of

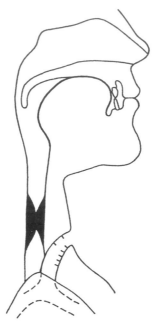

Figure 17.1 Location of stoma following total laryngectomy

the pharynx is necessary to eradicate the tumour, the remaining pharyngeal and oesophageal tissues are pulled together from each side and sutured. After studying four types of surgical reconstructions of the cricopharyngeal region, Simpson, Smith and Gordon (1972) concluded that re-approximating the cut ends of the pharyngo-oesophageal mucosa was highly correlated with proficiency of oesophageal speech. In many of their patients, the hyoid bone was preserved, unlike most total laryngectomees in the United States, in whom the hyoid bone is taken. It is reasonable to assume that such careful reconstruction might facilitate oesophageal voice learning. Because the extent of the resection in total laryngectomees varies from patient to patient and there is often no systematic reconstruction of pharyngeal or oesophageal musculature after total laryngectomy, there is wide variability in the location, size and shape of the pseudo-glottis, as demonstrated very clearly by Diedrich and Youngstrom's (1977) work. Their radiographic studies illustrate the variety of heights and configurations of the pseudo-glottis in a large number of total laryngectomees. The exact muscular composition of the pseudo-glottis is not understood. Though the pseudo-glottis is often called the presegment or pharyngo-oesophageal segment, there is no clear evidence that the pseudo-glottis is the cricopharyngeus muscle. After total laryngectomy, the pharynx and oesophagus form one continuous soft tissue tube. There is no longer any delineation of the end of the pharynx and the top of the cervical oesophagus. Somewhere along the pharyngo-oesophagus there is usually some flaccid tissue which is adiposed. This tissue comprises the pseudo-glottis, usually capable of vibrating in response to air flowing through it.

Vocal Rehabilitation in Total Laryngectomees

Separation of the airway from the pharyngo-oesophagus leaves no possibility that the patient will aspirate during eating. Unfortunately, this separation also precludes the patient from driving pulmonary air through the pseudoglottis in the pharyngo-oesophagus to create a vibrating airstream for speech.

Historically, vocal rehabilitation of the total laryngectomy began soon after the first laryngectomy was completed in 1876. The first attempts to restore voice to the total laryngectomee fell into four categories:

1　artificial larynges
2　oesophageal voice
3　surgical restoration methods involving the production of a tunnel or hole connecting the stoma with the oesophagus in order to allow pulmonary air into the pharyngo-oesophagus
4　surgical prosthetic methods to bring air from the stoma through a prosthesis and into a fistula in the patient's oesophagus below the pseudo-glottis.

Methods currently in use to rehabilitate laryngectomees still fall into these four categories.

Artificial Larynges

Artificial larynges provide the patient with an external vibratory (voice) source which are battery driven or pneumatic and are either held to the neck, as in cervical instruments, or introduced into the mouth, as in oral instruments (Lebrun, 1973; Salmon and Goldstein, 1978). Over the years, artificial larynges have improved in design and in vocal quality. Their overall effectiveness, however, is still hampered by their generally mechanical vocal quality, visibility, and the need to use at least one hand to hold the instrument.

Oesophageal Voice

Oesophageal voice requires that the patient learn to put air into the pharyngo-oesophagus voluntarily, trap it immediately below the pseudo-glottis and release the air back through the pseudo-glottis to produce voice. Two methods of air intake have been utilised: inhalation and injection (Damste, 1958; Edels. 1983). With the inhalation method of air intake, the patient rapidly expands his thoracic cavity, which drops the intra-thoracic pressure below atmospheric pressure. As the intra-thoracic pressure drops, so does the pressure in the oesophagus. Pressure above the segment (atmospheric pressure) is higher than intra-oesophageal pressure. This causes a suction effect that results in the patient's pulling air into the oesophagus, if the pressure in the segment or pseudo-glottis also drops below atmospheric pressure (i.e., if the segment relaxes).

With any of the 'injection' techniques, pre-injection or consonant injection, the patient must increase pressure above the pseudo-glottis sufficient to overcome the pressure in the pseudo-glottis and, thereby, drive air into the oesophagus. With consonant injection, the patient builds supra-segment pressure during articulation of speech sounds which are characterised by high intra-oral pressures (stops, affricates and fricatives). As the patient articulates these sounds, the intra-oral pressure pushes air into the oesophagus, which is then released to produce voice. During pre-injection techniques, the patient produces an oral gesture prior to speech which compresses air in the oropharynx and pushes air through the pseudo-glottis and into the oesophagus. These prespeech oral gestures may include compressing the tongue to the palate, closing the lips tightly or pulling the tongue base up and back.

As discussed earlier, there is a large amount of patient variability in the anatomy of the pharynx and the oesophagus after total laryngectomy. Most patients are able to introduce air into the cervical oesophagus through one of these air intake techniques, but not necessarily through all of them. The speech-language pathologist must identify which air intake technique best facilitates a particular patient's introduction of air into the oesophagus for oesophageal voice. As patients become proficient at oesophageal speech, they often use a combination of air intake techniques.

Once air has been put into the oesophagus, the patient must release the air through the pseudo-glottis in the cervical oesophagus to produce voice. This release of oesophageal air is usually, but not always, concurrent with a pulmonary exhalation (Snidecor and Isshiki, 1965; Isshiki and Snidecor, 1965). The pulmonary exhalation exerts pressure on the oesophagus and pushes air upward through the pseudo-glottis, usually creating voice. In general, when teaching the act of oesophageal voice, the patient first learns to put air into the cervical oesophagus and then to release that air. With the air release will come sound, if a pseudo-glottis is present. The requirement for a pseudo-glottis is that tissue in the pharyngo-oesophagus must be flaccid enough and adiposed in order to respond to the airflow with vibration and sound. Occasionally, some laryngectomees, particularly those who have had a large resection, such as cervical oesphagectomy, in addition to total laryngectomy, do not have a pseudo-glottis. That is, they do not have sufficient tissue, or tissue which is flaccid enough, to vibrate in response to the air stream. In these cases, digital pressure can be applied to the anterior neck in order to create a temporary pseudo-glottis (Damste, 1958; Duguay, 1979; Shanks, 1983). In some cases, the pseudo-glottis can be created by applying external pressure with a tight collar or elastic band.

Surgical and Surgical Prosthetic Voice Restoration

Because oesophageal voice requires learning and extensive therapy, and does not result in excellent speech in many patients, there have been both surgical and surgical-prosthetic attempts to restore voice to the total laryngectomy. Currently, one of the most successful voice restoration techniques, the tracheo-oesophageal puncture (TEP), falls into the surgical prosthetic category.

Surgical voice restoration

Almost as soon as the total laryngectomy surgery was devised, various surgeons attempted surgical reconstruction for vocal rehabilitation. In all cases, the intent was to surgically create a tunnel or tract to re-introduce pulmonary air into the patient's cervical oesophagus below the level of the pseudo-glottis in order to allow pulmonary airflow to activate the pseudo-glottis and produce voice. To speak, the patient inhaled and covered the stoma with a finger to drive air through the surgically created tract into the oesophagus. The concept, then, was that the patient could drive the pseudo-glottis with pulmonary air and thus produce sustained voicing without having to learn the air intake and release techniques necessary for oesophageal voice. Surgical attempts to create a tunnel between the stoma and the oesophagus have been fraught with numerous problems including: stenosis of the tract such that it would no longer conduct airflow, aspiration through the tract from the oesophagus to the trachea, surgical complications such as carotid blowout, and failure to produce consistent voice (Asai, 1965; Conley, DeAmesti and Pierce, 1958; Griffiths and Love, 1978; Guttman, 1935; Komorn, Weyer, Sessions and Malone, 1973).

Other surgical reconstruction procedures have attempted to reconstruct a valve at the top of the tracheal stump. This valve or pseudo larynx would have to prevent penetration of food into the airway, while shunting air into the pharyngo-oesophagus and servicing as the vibratory source (Serafini, 1980; Staffieri, 1980). These surgical reconstructions suffered from the same serious problems as the other surgically created shunts.

Surgical prosthetic voice restoration

The first surgical prosthetic attempts to cause re-entry of air from the stoma into the oesophagus included construction of cutaneous fistulae into the pharynx or cervical oesophagus which were fitted with prosthetic devices (Edwards, 1980; McConnel, Sisson, and Logemann, 1976; Taub and Bugner, 1973). These devices attached from the patient's stoma to the external fistula and served as a conduit for airflow back into the pharyngo-oesophagus.

These surgical prosthetic attempts to construct a cutaneous fistula to which a prosthesis would be connected from the stoma were fraught with problems including (1) poor prosthetic fit so that the prosthesis dislodged at either the stomal end or the fistula end, (2) leakage of food through the fistula onto the external skin, and (3) aspiration of food through the fistula down the prosthesis and into the stoma. Prosthetic devices tended to have complicated connections and were often awkward in fitting, requiring the patient to change or exchange dressings at least several times per day.

Tracheo-oesophageal puncture (TEP) restoration

Surgical prosthetic voice restoration attempts culminated in 1980 with the introduction of the tracheo-oesophageal puncture technique (Singer and Blom, 1980). In this technique, a small fistula tract is created from the posterior wall of the stoma to the oesophagus into which the patient places and wears a soft prosthesis containing a valve at the oesophageal end. This valve allows air flow from the stoma into the oesophagus, but prevents the backflow of food from the oesophagus to the stoma. To speak, the patient merely inhales and occludes the stoma with a finger to direct the exhaled air through the puncture prosthesis and into the oesophagus. Introduced by Mark Singer and Eric Blom (1980), this technique virtually revolutionised the surgical prosthetic voice rehabilitation of total laryngectomees. The puncture can be placed in a short operative procedure after laryngectomy or at the time of the total laryngectomy (i.e., primary puncture). If the patient dislikes the procedure, the puncture site will usually close spontaneously in 8-24 hours, when the prosthesis is removed. To create the puncture or fistula, an endoscope is introduced into the patient's oesophagus to the base of the cervical oesophagus. Another operator applies pressure to the posterior wall of the stoma at 12 o'clock. This pressure is visualised by the operator with the esophagoscope. When the proper position for the puncture is identified, a hole is created with a No. 18 gauge needle. The tract or fistula is created horizontally or slightly downgoing. A No. 14 French catheter is then placed through the puncture and down into the stomach. This catheter usually remains in place for at least 48 hours, after which the patient can be fitted for the proper length puncture prosthesis. A tracheostoma valve was developed to preclude the need for the patient to use a finger to occlude the stoma (Blom, Singer and Hamaker, 1982).

Since the introduction of the tracheo-oesophageal puncture procedure, the surgical procedure to construct the fistula tract has been modified only slightly by some clincians (Wolicki, Makielski and Olson, 1985). However, the prosthesis design has changed considerably. Initially, the prosthesis was a cylinder-shaped 'duck bill' prosthesis with a slit at the interior end (Singer and Blom, 1980; Singer, Blom and Hamaker, 1982). In the last several years, the prosthesis has been modified to a flap valve which reduces the resistance of the prosthesis to the air flow from the stoma into the oesophagus (Weinberg and Moon, 1982; 1984; 1986a,b).

Since the introduction of the Singer-Blom tracheo-oesophageal puncture technique, other head and neck surgeons have designed variations on the procedure (Ossoff, Lazarus and Sisson 1984; Perry, Cheesman and Eden, 1983; Shapiro and Ramanathan, 1982; Wood, Tucker, Rusnov and Levine, 1981). Panje (1981) introduced a similar technique in which the puncture wound was placed lower in the patient's stoma (just above the lower edge) and the prosthesis was shorter and biflanged to sit in the oesophageal wall. Examination of the resistance characteristics of the Panje prosthesis design indicated that the Panje prosthesis provided much higher resistance to the airflow than that of Singer-Blom prosthesis and that the Panje prosthesis was highly variable in its quality control (Moon and Weinberg, 1983, 1984; Smith, 1986; Weinberg, 1982; Weinberg and Moon, 1982, 1984, 1986a).

Acoustic characteristics of oesophageal voice

The introduction of the tracheo-oesophageal puncture technique spawned a number of other foci of research. First, a number of investigators began to assess the acoustic and perceptual properties of the voice produced with tracheo-oesophageal puncture speech as compared to oesophageal voice and to normal voice (Baggs and Pine 1983; Blood, 1984; Monaghan and Murry, 1986; Robbins 1984; Robbins, Fisher, Blom and Singer, 1984; Trudeau, 1986).

These studies indicated that tracheo-oesophageal puncture voice was superior to oesophageal speech in duration and intensity parameters, as well as in intelligibility. These studies have also determined that the range of individual differences in TEP speakers is less than those in oesophageal speakers. However, candidacy issues are important in all methods of alaryngeal communication. Many patients are unable to learn oesophageal voice because of such learning variables as motivation, ability to follow directions, memory, etc. Some patients are unable to comply with home practice programs given to them for oesophageal voice, or are simply not compliant in attending therapy sessions. Some of these same patients would also be poor candidates for the puncture procedure. To be a good candidate for the TEP procedure, patients need to be able to follow directions, to learn to change the prosthesis and to clean it. They must be motivated to wear a prosthesis and to maintain it, they must have adequate dexterity and vision to take care of the prosthesis and their stoma and they must be compliant to return to the surgeon or speech pathologist should there by any problem. Table 17.1 provides a summary of data from this comparative research and earlier work on the acoustic characteristics of oesophageal voice.

Table 17.1 Comparative Temporal Acoustic and Intensity Data on Esophageal and TEP Talkers

Measures	Esophageal Talkers	TEP Talkers
Reading rate	[1]90–124.2 wpm	[2]127-5–144.1 wpm
Fundamental frequency	[3]58.4–87.0 Hz	[4]82.8–109.2 Hz
Percent periodic	[5]41.6%–59.6%	[6]77.7%
Percent aperiodic	[5]1.9%–25.08%	[6]11.9%
Percent silence	[5]29.73%–38.5%	[6]10.5%
Mean phonation time	[8]1.9–4.82 sec	[7]10.99–14 sec
Mean intensity during sustained vowel	73.8 dB SPL (Robbins et al., 1984)	88.1 dB SPL (Robbins et al., 1984

1 Hoops and Noll, 1969; Horii, 1983; Robbins, Fisher, Blom and Singer, 1984; Shipp, 1967; Snidecor and Curry, 1959; 1960; snidecor and Isshiki, 1965.
2 Robbins, Fisher and Singer, 1984; Trudeau, 1986.
3 Smith, Weinberg, Feth and Horii, 1978; Weinberg and Bennett, 1972.
4 Blood, 1984; Robbins, Fisher, Blom and Singer, 1984; Trudeau, 1986.
5 Robbins, Fisher, Blom and Singer, 1984; Shipp, 1967; Weinberg and Bennett, 1972.
6 Robbins, Fisher, Blom and Singer, 1984.
7 Baggs and Pine, 1983; Robbins, Fisher, Blom and Singer, 1984; Wetmore, Krueger and Wesson, 1981.
8 Baggs and Pine, 1983; Berlin, 1963; Robbins, Fisher, Blom and Singer, 1984.

Pharyngo-oesophageal spasm

The tracheo-oesophageal puncture procedure has also triggered a group of studies on the anatomy and physiology of the pharyngo-oesophagus and the pseudo-glottis and their relationship to the ability to produce voice. One group of studies has looked at the compliance of the pseudo-glottis in response to air flow (Lewin, Baugh and Baker, 1987; McGarvey and Weinberg, 1984; Schuller, Jarrow, Kelly and Miglets, 1983). After the puncture had been utilised for several years, it became clear to Blom and Singer, as well as others, that the tracheo-oesophageal puncture did not always result in excellent voice. Some patients exhibited what Singer and Blom (1981) have called 'pharyngo esophageal spasm' in the pseudo-glottis. That is, when air was introduced below the pseudo-glottis, the pseudo-glottis went into spasm and failed to vibrate in response to the airflow. Instead of vibrating in response to the air stream, the pseudo-glottis closed tightly and did not allow any air to escape. This 'spasm' was not present during breathing or swallowing. Thus, it was a physiologic response to air, not an anatomic narrowing or stricture. Singer and Blom have called this spasm non-productive to voice restoration and have treated it with one or two procedures, a myotomy or neurectomy (Singer and Blom, 1981; Singer, Blom and Hamaker, 1986). In a myotomy, the pharyngeal constrictors and cricopharyngeal region of the laryngectomee are cut vertically to reduce the tone in this musculature in the pharyngo-oesophagus and prevent the musculature from going into spasm. In neurectomy, the innervation to the pharyngo-oesophagus is cut so that this musculature cannot contract to create the spasm. In both instances, the rationale for the surgical procedure is to produce a pseudo-glottis which is flaccid enough to respond to the airstream and produce voice rather than to contract in spasm and prevent vibration. In a study of normal talkers after introduction of air into the oesophagus, McGarvey and Weinberg (1984) described the spasmodic behaviour of the segment as a normal reaction of the oesophagus to the introduction of air flow. These normal data have created some controversy regarding the exact nature of the spasmodic activity seen in some laryngectomees in response to air introduced into the oesophagus below the pseudo-glottis. Clearly, however, whether or not this spasm is a normal reaction to the introduction of air, or is an abnormal response, it prevents the pseudo-glottis from vibrating in response to the airstream and is, therefore, unproductive to the successful acquisition of oesophageal or puncture voice. Thus, it is necessary to manage this spasm in the total laryngectomee in order for the patient to successfully produce voice. Whether neurectomy or myotomy produces better voice has yet to be determined.

Stricture

Some total laryngectomee patients exhibit a stricture in the pharyngo-oesophagus, in contrast to a spasm. A stricture is an area of narrowing which is anatomically present at all times, (i.e., during respiration, swallowing and phonation). Often, stricture occurs in patients who have had prior radiotherapy or whose surgical resection was large, requiring a tight surgical closure. Currently, if a large resection is required, surgeons will often introduce tissue from another site to prevent a tight closure and stricture (Bakamjian, 1965; Gowgher and Robin, 1954; Harrison, 1972; LeQuesne and Ranger, 1966; Slaney and Dalton, 1973).Such tissue may be from the chest wall, colon, or the stomach. When a stricture is present, it is observable on swallowing as well as on speech attempts. On swallowing, the stricture appears as a narrowed area in the pharyngo-oesophagus above which food will tend to collect (Logemann, 1983). Patients with a stricture will often complain that they have difficulty swallowing thicker foods. This occurs because liquids will drain through the narrowed area, while thicker food will tend to collect and build up above it. On voice attempts, the stricture again is seen as a narrowed area through which the patient may have difficulty putting air into the oesophagus for oesophageal voice. That is, the patient may have difficulty injecting or inhaling air into the oesophagus through the stricture. If the stricture extends into the region of the pseudo-glottis, it may reduce the flexibility of the vibrator and thus reduce its vibratory capability. In contrast to a stricture, a spasm is not present on swallowing, but only when air is introduced into the oesophagus below the pseudo-glottis. A patient with spasm will have normal swallowing with no obstruction. The spasm will be seen only during speech attempts.

Management of a stricture can be difficult. Often, a patient with a stricture must be dilated, which involves stretching the area by repeated swallowing of Mercury-filled soft tubes of increasing diameter. Generally, the effects of this dilation last one or two months and the procedure must be regularly repeated to facilitate swallowing and voice. A more permanent solution to a stricture is further surgical reconstruction, introducing tissue from another site such as the chest wall or the colon.

The airblowing test

The introduction of the tracheo-oesophageal puncture technique has also increased our understanding of oesophageal voice failures, i.e., those patients who attempt to learn oesophageal voice but are unable to do so for previously undetermined reasons (Chodosh, Giancario and Goldstein, 1984; Gates, Ryan, Cantu and Hearne 1982; Perry, 1983). Over the last five years, a number of clinicians have applied the evaluation techniques utilised in assessment of candidates for the TEP, to the total laryngectomee who is attempting to learn oesophageal voice. The first of these assessment techniques is what has been called 'the airblowing' test. First used by Vandenberg and Moolenaar-Bijl (1959) and Seeman (1967) to predict oesophageal voice production from measures of intra-oesophageal pressures, this test was re-introduced by Stanley Taub (1975; 1980), the creator of the Voice-Bak prosthesis, as a way to assess the patient's potential for successful use of his prosthesis. It has been adapted by Singer and Blom (1980) as a test for the successful use of the puncture. In the air blowing technique, a size 14 red rubber catheter is introduced through the patient's nose and from there down through the oro-pharynx into the thoracic-oesophagus. The end of the catheter is positioned below the pseudo-glottis, usually 23-25cm from the nose. The operator then blows air through the catheter into the patient's oesophagus, and subjectively assesses the resulting voice. If the voice is spasmodic rather than sustained, the patient may be unable to produce oesophageal voice because of the abnormality known as 'spasm' discussed earlier. If no voice results, the patient may have a spasm, a stricture, or an absent pseudo-glottis. A radiographic study (i.e., videofluoroscopy) is needed to determine which of these problems is present. In 1985, Blom, Singer and Hamaker introduced an improved air insufflation test in which the patient was able to self-inflate the oesophagus through a special tracheostoma housing fitted to the catheter.

Recently, a number of investigators have questioned the subjectivity of the air blowing assessment (Donegan, Gluckman and Singh, 1981; McGarvey and Weinberg, 1984; Panje, 1981). Variables such as catheter distance into the pharynx and amount of force of airflow needed to initiate and maintain vibration of the pseudoglottis have created controversy regarding the validity of the test. Recently, Lewin, Baugh and Baker (1987) have examined intra-oesophageal pressures in 27 laryngectomized patients prior to tracheoesophageal puncture in an attempt to predict TEP speech outcome. These investigators objectified the air blowing test by utilizing compressed air from a Thorpe flow meter at flow rates of 1 and 3l per minute and compared their results with air insufflation by the examiner. The catheter placement was standardised at 23 and 25 cm from the nares. Three groups of speakers were identified during air blowing: fluent speakers, nonfluent speakers, and nonspeakers. These groups demonstrated low, intermediate and high intra oesophageal pressures respectively. Patients with intermediate and high intra oesophageal pressures needed myotomy to achieve fluent speech with the TEP. Insufflation by the flow meter and by the examiner were both successful in identifying patients in whom fluent speech would not be achieved without myotomy.

Patients who have undergone extended resection of the larynx, pharynx and cervical oesophagus require the use of tissue from another site to facilitate the reconstruction (Bakamjian 1965; Gowgher and Robin, 1954; Harrison, 1972). If just the cervical oesophagus is resected with the larynx, tissue from the chest wall in the form of a pectoralis or deltal-pectoral flap may be introduced to reconstruct the pharynx and cervical oesophagus. Or, tissue from the colon may be introduced to reconstruct the pharyngo-oesophagus. If the entire oesophagus must be resected with the larynx, a stomach pull-up may be utilized to reconstruct the defect. In this procedure, the stomach is freed from its ligaments in the abdomen and stretched vertically until the top of the stomach is at the base of the tongue. The surgeon may attempt to reconstruct an upper gastric valve to help prevent reflux of stomach acid or food from the stomach into the mouth. Individuals with a stomach pull-up generally function best when taking four to six small meals a day rather than three large meals. They must remain upright after eating to reduce the change of reflux. Patients who have had these extensive reconstructions are able to learn oesophageal (i.e., gastric or colon) voice or undergo surgical prosthetic voice restoration techniques such as tracheo-oesophageal puncture. However, their voices are often not as good, perceptually, as patients who have a normal oesophagus. These vocal differences are apparent to the clinician, though they have not been studied objectively. The perceptual differences in voice quality in these patients probably result from the difference in elasticity in the tissues of the colon, the stomach or chest flap as compared to oesophageal mucosa.

While the tracheo-oesophageal puncture has enabled many total laryngectomees to produce fluent voice and highly intelligible speech, it is clear that some pieces of the puzzle are missing in our understanding of all of those factors which contribute to the production of excellent vocal quality and fluent speech. Continued research into prosthetic characteristics and tissue characteristics, such as flexibility and reaction to airflow within the pharyngo-oesophagus may provide us with additional answers needed to further improve rehabilitation of the total laryngectomee.

Clinical Care of the Total Laryngectomy with Surgical Prosthetic Voice Restoration

Pre-operatively, the patient who is about to undergo a total laryngectomy should receive counselling regarding his/her communication alternatives. In general, these alternatives include oesophageal voice, the surgical prosthetic speech rehabilitation techniques and artificial larynges. Usually, patients do not have detailed questions about each of these communication modes preoperatively, but are content to be aware that a speech-language pathologist will be available postoperatively for asistance in restoring their vocal communication. Generally, pre-operative patients are most concerned with their general survival. Immediately following surgery, many patients and their families have a number of questions regarding communication alternatives. It is in the first postoperative week that the speech-language pathologist should provide additional counselling, initial training with artificial larynges and discussion of oesophageal voice therapy. In most institutions, any surgical prosthetic voice restoration is provided as a secondary rehabilitation technique. The patient is usually given 6–8 weeks post-operatively to accommodate to the stoma and its care and to become familiar with the other voice restoration procedures, i.e. oesophageal voice and the artificial larynx. In general, within the first week of hospitalisation, the patient should be given a variety of artificial larynges to work with. In that time, with the help of the speech-language pathologist, patients can select the instrument best for them. When the nasogastric tube is removed, the patient can begin oesophageal voice therapy. If no healing problems exist, this therapy usually begins about 10–14 days postoperatively. Thus, by 6–8 weeks after surgery, the patient will have had at least one month of oesophageal voice therapy, and patient and clinician will be aware of the ease with which the patient is able to put air into the oesophagus, trap the air and release the air with voice.

Radiographic assessment

Within the first therapy session, perhaps the second, the speech language clinician should have a good idea of the patient's facility for putting air into the oesophagus and releasing it with voice. If, after trying all of the available techniques to put air into the oesophagus and release it with sound, the patient is unable to put air into the oesophagus or to produce sound, it is incumbent upon the clinician to assess the physiology of the total laryngectomy patient's pharyngo-oesophagus. This requires radiographic study of the oral cavity and pharyngo-oesophagus during swallowing and voice attempts. Radiographic asessment should begin with swallows of 1cc and 3ccs of liquid barium and paste barium. During the swallows, the clinician should assess the oral and pharyngo-oesophageal transit times of the bolus. Oral transit times should be no more than 1.5 secs, while pharyngo-oesophageal transit time should be 3–4 secs. There should be no obvious narrowing or obstruction of the flow of the food through the oral cavity or pharyngo-oesophagus. If there is an obvious narrowing or stricture, the patient may have difficulty in putting air into the oesophagus because of this. After assessing swallowing physiology, the clinician should assess the patient's pharyngo-oesophagus fluoroscopically while the patient attempts to put air into the oesophagus and release it with voice. On lateral radiographic view, the clinician should be able to see air entering the pharyngo-oesophagus below the adiposed tissue which comprises the patient's vibratory segment. When the patient releases the air with voice, the radiographic image will show the vibratory movement of the pseudo-glottis. If the patient produces oral gestures which are not productive to putting air into the oesophagus, this will be visible radiographically. If the patient puts air into the oesophagus, but the pseudo-glottis goes into spasm and clamps closed tightly in response to the air pressure beneath it, this will also be visible radiographically. If the patient has an anatomic deterrent to the air intake process, this, too, will be visible. Thus, the radiographic assessment of the pharyngo-oesophagus during swallowing and attempts at oesophageal voice production will enable the clinician to assess the patient's physiological potential for learning oesophageal voice and the patient's potential for surgical prosthetic voice restoration procedures.

Primary voice restoration

In some medical centres, surgical prosthetic voice restoration is offered to the patient as a part of the laryngectomy surgery. This is known as a primary voice restoration procedure. In this case, the puncture is produced at the time of the total laryngectomy. The surgeon generally places a catheter (to be used for non-oral feeding) through the puncture site. Thus, the feeding tube is placed through the puncture and down into oesophagus and stomach, replacing the nasogastric tube. The non-oral feeding is kept in place for approximately two weeks and acts as a tent in the puncture site to keep it open. When the stoma and puncture site have healed adequately and the patient is ready for oral feeding, the catheter is removed and a voice restoration prosthesis is fitted in the same way as is done with secondary puncture procedures. Clinically, a number of speech-language pathologists have noted the psychological difference in patients who receive a primary versus a secondary puncture. Patients who receive a secondary voice restoration procedure have experienced the frustration of voice loss and the difficulty in learning oesophageal voice and/or using artificial larynges as a communication mode. These patients have become accommodated to the voice quality of oesophageal voice and its limitations in intensity and phrasing. When they receive the surgical prosthetic voice restoration procedure, the improvement in vocal intensity and in phrasing duration is such that they are appreciative of the voice improvement.

Patients who receive the surgical voice restoration procedure as a primary modality with total laryngectomy have never experienced the difficulties of communication with any other alaryngeal modality. They have only their preoperative voice as a baseline for comparison. Thus, some of these patients do not like the voice quality of the surgical prosthetic voice, perceiving it as abnormally low pitched and rough as compared to their preoperative voice. Many of them also do not experience the anxiety of voice loss because they know that soon after their surgery they will be able to produce fluent speech. Thus, these patients are often less satisfied with their voice restoration procedure, and some elect to have their puncture closed rather than use that mode of communication. Preoperative counselling with these patients is extremely important in providing them with examples of surgical prosthetic voice and with the kind of care which the prosthesis requires.

Conclusion

While surgical voice restoration for total laryngectomees have provided improved voice for many patients, and has increased our knowledge regarding the physiology of oesophageal voice, it has also opened a number of questions regarding the interaction of airflows, pressures and pharyngo-oesophageal vibration.

References

ASAI, R. (1965) Laryngoplasty after total laryngectomy. *Archives of Otolaryngology*, 95, 114–19.

BAGGS, T. and PINE, S. (1983) Acoustic characteristics: Tracheoesophageal speech. *Journal of Communication Disorders*, 16, 299–307.

BAKAMJIAN, V. (1965) A two-staged method for pharyngo-oesophageal reconstruction with a primary pectoral skin flap. *Plastic Reconstructive Surgery*, 36, 173–84.

BERLIN, C. (1963) Clinical measurement of Oesophageal Speech: 1. Methodology and Curves of Skill Acquisition. *Journal of Speech and Hearing Disoders*, 28: 42–51.

BLOM, E., SINGER, M. and HAMAKER, R. (1982) Tracheostoma valve for postlaryngectomy voice rehabilitation. *Annals of Otology, Rhinology and Laryngectomy*, 91, 576–8.

BLOM, E., SINGER, M. and HAMAKER, R. (1985) An improved oesophageal insufflation test. *Archives of Otolaryngology*, 3, 211–2.

BLOOD, G. (1984) Fundamental frequency and intensity measurements in laryngeal and alaryngeal speakers. *Journal of Communication Disorders*, 17, 319–24.

CALCATERRA, T. (1971) Laryngeal suspension after supraglottic laryngectomy. *Archives of Otolaryngology*, 94, 306–9.

CHODOSH, P., GIANCARLO, H. and GOLDSTEIN, J. (1984) Pharyngeal myotomy for vocal rehabilitation post laryngectomy. *Laryngoscope*, 94, 52–7.

CLINE, M.J. and HASKELL, C.M. (1980) *Cancer Chemotherapy* (3rd ed.). Philadelphia: Saunders.

CONLEY, J., DEAMESTI, F. and PIERCE, M. (1958) A new surgical technique for vocal rehabilitation of the laryngectomized patient. *Annals of Otology, Rhinology, and Laryngology*, 67, 655–64.

DAMSTE, P.H. (1958) *Oesophageal Speech*. Groningen: Hoitsema.

DeSANTO, L.W. (1974) Selection of treatment for in situ and early invasive carcinoma of the glottis. *Canadian Journal of Otolaryngology*, 3, 552–6.

DIEDRICH, W. and YOUNGSTROM, K. (1977) *Alaryngeal Speech*. Springfield, IL: Charles Thomas.

DONEGAN, J., GLUCKMAN, J. and SINGH, J. (1981) Limitations of the Blom-Singer technique for voice restoration. *Annals of Otology, Rhinology, and Laryngology*, 90, 495–7.

DUGUAY, M. (1979) Speech problems of the alaryngeal speaker. In R.L. Keith and F.L. Darley (Eds), *Laryngectomee Rehabilitation*. San Diego: College Hill.

EDELS, Y. (1983) (Ed.) *Laryngectomy: Diagnosis to Rehabilitation*. London: Croom Helm.

EDWARDS, N. (1980) Vocal rehabilitation by external vocal fistula and valved prosthesis: Edwards Method. In D.P. Shedd and B. Weinberg (Eds), *Surgical and Prosthetic Approaches to Speech Rehabilitation*. Boston: G.K. Hall Medical Publishers.

FLETCHER, G.H. and GOEPFERT, H. (1981) Irradiation in the management of squamous cell carcinomas of the larynx. In G.M. English (Ed.). *Otolaryngology*, 3, 8–14.

GATES, G., RYAN, W., CANTU, E. and HEARNE, E. (1982) Current status of laryngectomy rehabilitation II. Causes of failure. *Journal of Otolaryngology*, 3, 8–14.

GOWGHER, J. and ROBIN, I. (1954) Use of left colon for reconstruction of pharynx and oesophagus after pharyngectomy. *British Journal of Surgery*, 42, 283–90.

GRIFFITHS, C. and LOVE, J. (1978) Neoglottis reconstruction after total laryngectomy. *Annals of Otology, Rhinology, and Laryngology*, 87, 180–6.

GUTTMAN, M. (1935) Tracheohypopharyngeal fistulization. *Transactions of the American Laryngology, Rhinology and Otology Society*, 41, 219–26.

HARRISON, D. (1972) Role of surgery in the management of post-cricoid and cervical oesophageal neoplasma. *Annals of Otolaryngology, Rhinology, and Laryngology*, 8, 465–8.

HOOPS, H. and NOLL, J. (1969) Relationship of Selective Acoustic Variables to Judgements of Oesophageal Speech. *Journal of Communication Disorders*, 2: 1–13.

HORII, Y. (1983) Utterance and Pause Lengths and Frequencies in Oral Readings by Superior Oesophageal Speakers and by Normal Speakers. *Computer and Biomedical Research*, 16: 446–53.

ISSHIKI, N. and SNIDECOR, J.C. (1965) Air intake and usage in esophageal speech. *Acta Otolaryngologica*, 59, 559–74.

KARIM, A., SNOW, J., SIEK, H. and NJO, K. (1983) The quality of voice in patients irradiated for laryngeal carcinoma. *Cancer*, 41, 47–9.

KOMORN, R., WEYER, J., SESSIONS, R. and MALONE, P. (1973) Vocal rehabilitation with a tracheo esophageal shunt. *Archives of Otolaryngology*, 97, 103–5.

LEBRUN, Y. (1973) *Neurolinguistics 1. The Artificial Larynx.* Amsterdam: Swets and Zeitlinger, B.V.

LEWIN, J., BAUGH, R. and BAKER, S. (1987) An objective method for prediction of tracheoesophageal speech production. *Journal of Speech and Hearing Disorders*, 52, 212–7.

LE QUESNE, L.P. and RANGER, D. (1966) Pharyngo-laryngectomy with immediate pharyngo-gastric anastomiosis. *British Journal of Surgery*, 53, 105–9.

LOGEMANN, J. (1983) *Evaluation and Treatment of Swallowing Disorders.* San Diego: College Hill.

McCONNEL, F.M.S., SISSON, G.A. and LOGEMANN, J. (1976) Three years experience with a hypopharyngeal pseudoglottis for vocal rehabilitation after total laryngectomy. *Transactions of the American Academy of Ophthalmology and Otolaryngology*, 84, 63–7.

McGARVEY, S.D. and WEINBERG, B. (1984) Esophageal insufflation testing in non-laryngectomized adults. *Journal of Speech and Hearing Disorders*, 49, 272–7.

MONAGHAN, C. and MURRY, T. (1986) *Sex identification of laryngeal, esophageal and tracheosophageal speakers.* Paper, ASHA convention, Detroit, MI.

MOON, J. and WEINBERG, B. (1983) Evaluations of Blom – Singer tracheoesophageal puncture prosthesis performance. Journal of Speech and Hearing Disorders, 26, 259–64.

MOON, J. and WEINBERG, B. (1984) Airway resistance characteristics of Voice Button tracheoesophageal prosthesis. *Journal of Speech and Hearing Disorders*, 49, 326–8.

OGURA, J. and MALLEN, R. (1965) Partial laryngectomy for supraglottic and pharyngeal carcinoma. *Transactions of the American Academy of Opthalmology and Otolaryngology*, 69, 832–45.

OSSOFF, R., LAZARUS, C. and SISSON, G. (1984) Tracheoesophageal puncture for voice restoration: Modification of the Blom-Singer technique. *Otolaryngology, Head and Neck Surgery*, 92, 418–32.

PANJE, W. (1981) Prosthetic vocal rehabilitation following laryngectomy. *Annals of Otology, Rhinology and Laryngology*, 90, 116–20.

PERRY, A. (1983) Difficulties in the acquisition of alaryngeal speech. In Y. Edels (Ed.), *Laryngectomy: Diagnosis to Rehabilitation*. London: Croom Helm.

PERRY, A., CHEESMAN, A.C. and EDEN, R. (1983) A modification of the Blom-Singer valve for restoration of voice after laryngectomy. *Journal of Laryngology Otology*, 96, 1005–11.

ROBBINS, J. (1984) Acoustic differentiation of laryngeal, oesophageal, and tracheo-oesophageal speech. *Journal of Speech and Hearing Research*, 27, 557–85.

ROBBINS, J., FISHER, H., BLOM, E. and SINGER, M. (1984) A comparative acoustic study of normal, esophageal and tracheoesophageal speech production. *Journal of Speech and Hearing Disorders*, 49, 202–10.

SALMON, S.J. and GOLDSTEIN, L.P. (Eds) (1978) *Artificial Larynx Handbook*. New York: Grune and Stratton.

SEEMAN, M. (1967) Rehabilitation of Laryngectomized Subjects. *Acta Oto-Laryngologica*, 64, 235–41.

SERAFINI, I. (1980) Reconstructive Laryngectomy. In D.P. Shedd and B. Weinberg (Eds), *Surgical and Prosthetic Approaches to Speech Rehabilitation*. Boston: G.K. Hall Medical Publishers.

SCHULLER, D.E., JARROW, J.E., KELLY, D.R. and MIGLETS, A.W. (1983) Prognostic factors affecting the success of duck-bill vocal restoration. *Otolaryngology — Head and Neck Surgery*, 91, 396–8.

SHANKS, J. (1983) Improving oesophageal communication. In Y., Edels (Ed.), *Laryngectomy: Diagnosis to Rehabilitation*. London: Croom Helm.

SHAPIRO, M. and RAMANATHAN, V. (1982) Trachea stoma vent voice prosthesis. *Laryngoscope*, 92, 1126–9.

SHIPP, T. (1967) Frequency, Duration and Perceptual Measures and Relation of Judgements of Alaryngeal Speech Acceptability. *Journal of Speech and Hearing Research*, 10: 417–27.

SIMPSON, I.C., SMITH, J.C.S. and GORDON, M.T. (1972) Laryngectomy: The influence of muscle reconstruction on the mechanism of oesophageal voice production. *Journal of Laryngology and Otology*, 82, 961–90.

SINGER, M. and BLOM, E. (1980) An endoscopic technique for restoration of voice after total laryngectomy. *Annals of Otology, Rhinology and Laryngology*, 89, 529–33.

SINGER, M. and BLOM, E. (1981) Selective myotomy for voice restoration after total laryngectomy. *Archives of Otolaryngology*, 107, 670–3.

SINGER, M., BLOM, E. and HAMAKER, R. (1981) Further experience with voice restoration after total laryngectomy. *Annals of Otolaryngology*, 90.

SINGER, M., BLOM, E. and HAMAKER, R. (1986) Pharyngeal plexus neurectomy for alaryngeal speech rehabilitation. *Laryngoscope*, 96, 50–3.

SLANEY, G. and DALTON, G.A. (1973) Problems of viscus replacement following pharyngo-laryngectomy. *Journal of Laryngology and Otolaryngology*, 87, 539–46.

SMITH, B. (1986) Aerodynamic characteristics of Blom-Singer Low Pressure Voice Prostheses. *Archives of Otolaryngology Head and Neck Surgery*, 112, 50–2.

SMITH, B., WEINBERG, B., FETH, L. and HORII, Y. (1978) Vocal Roughness and Jitter Characteristics of Vowels produced by Oesophageal Speakers. *Journal of Speech and Hearing Research*, 21: 240–49.

SNIDECOR, J. and CURRY, E. (1959) Temporal and Pitch Aspects of superior esophageal Speech. *Annals of Otology, Rhinology and Laryngology,* 68: 1–4.

SNIDECOR, J. and CURRY, E. (1960) How effectively can the laryngectomee expect to Speak? *Laryngoscope,* 70: 62–7.

SNIDECOR, J. and ISSHIKI, N. (1965) Air volume and airflow relationships of six male oesophageal speakers. *Journal of Speech and Hearing Disorders,* 30, 205–16.

SOM, M. (1951) Hemilaryngectomy — a modified technique for cordal carcinoma with extension posteriorly. *Archives of Otolaryngology,* 54, 524–33.

STAFFIERI, M. (1980) New surgical approaches for speech rehabilitation after total laryngectomy. In D.P. Shedd and B. Weinberg (Eds), *Surgical and Prosthetic Approaches to Speech Rehabilitation.* Boston: G.K. Hall Medical Publishers.

STELL, P.M. and MARAN, A.G.D. (1978) *Head and Neck Surgery.* London: Heinemann.

STOICHEFF, M., CAMPI, A, PASSI, J. and FREDRICKSON, J. (1983) The irradiated larynx and voice: A perceptual study. *Journal of Speech and Hearing Research,* 26, 482–5.

SVEN, J.Y. and MYERS, E.N. (1981) *Cancer of the Head and Neck.* Edinburgh: Churchill.

TAUB, S. (1980) Airbypass voice prosthesis: an 8-year experience, in D.P. Shedd and B. Weinberg (Eds), *Surgical and Prosthetic Approaches to Speech Rehabilitation.* Boston: G.K. Hall Medical Publishers.

TAUB, S. (1975) Airbypass voice prosthesis for vocal rehabilitation of laryngectomees. *Ear, Nose and Throat Journal,* 60, 42–54.

TAUB, S. and BUGNER, L.H. (1973) Air bypass voice prosthesis for vocal rehabilitation of laryngectomees. *American Journal of Surgery,* 125, 748–56.

TRUDEAU, M. (1986) *Characteristics of Female Tracheoesophageal-Speech.* Paper presented at ASHA Convention, Detroit, MI.

VANDENBERG, J. and MOOLENAAR-BIJL, A.J. (1959) Cricopharyngeal sphincter, pitch, intensity and fluency in oesophageal speech. *Practica Oto-rhino-laryngologica,* 21, 298–315.

WEINBERG, B. (1982) Airway resistance of the Voice Button. *Archives of Otolaryngology,* 108, 498–500.

WEINBERG, B. and BENNETT, S. (1972) Selected Acoustic Characteristics of Oesophageal Speech by Female Laryngectomees. *Journal of Speech and Hearing Research,* 15: 211–6.

WEINBERG, B. and MOON, J. (1982) Airway resistance characteristics of Blom–Singer tracheoesophageal puncture prostheses. *Journal of Speech and Hearing Disorders,* 47, 441–2.

WEINBERG, B. and MOON, J. (1984) Aerodynamic properties of four tracheo-esophageal puncture prostheses. *Archives of Otolaryngology,* 110, 673–5.

WEINBERG, B. and MOON, J. (1986a) Airway resistance characteristics of Blom-Singer and Panje low pressure tracheoesophageal puncture prostheses. *Journal of Speech and Hearing Disorders,* 51, 169–72.

WEINBERG, B. and MOON, J. (1986b) Impact of tracheoesophageal puncture prostheses airway resistance on in-vivo phonatory performance. *Journal of Speech and Hearing Disorders,* 51, 88–91.

WETMORE, S., KRUEGER, K. and WESSEN, K. (1981) The Singer-Blom Speech Rehabilitation Procedure. *Laryngoscope,* 91: 1109–17.

WOLIKI, K., MAKIELSKI, K. and OLSON, N. (1985) An improved technique for tracheoesophageal puncture using the urethral filiform and follower. Scientific poster presented at the American Academy of Otolaryngology — Head and Neck Surgery, Annual Meeting, Atlanta, GA.

WOOD, B., TUCKER, H., RUSNOV, M. and LEVINE, H. (1981) Tracheoesophageal puncture for alaryngeal voice restoration. *Annals of Otolaryngology,* 90, 492–6.

Conclusion:
Developing the Science of Intervention

Margaret M. Leahy

Previous drafts of this conclusion attempted to synthesise all that had gone before, integrating the scope of the work done in different divisions of communication disorders. But that work could not be satisfactorily encompassed in the space available. Since the authors have already posed questions in the individual chapters, a re-statement or a re-interpretation of these questions is not necessary. Rather, this conclusion will attempt to focus on some important aspects of the profession and its development.

Discomforting Aspects of Science

Anyone scanning this book would have no doubt that speech and language clinicians have a broad base of knowledge from which to work as well as a strong set of paradigms within which to use this knowledge. The fact that questions arise about the nature of the knowledge and its use reflects a basic uncertainty that is an essential aspect of science. This uncertainty that derives from dealing with so-called established facts leads to the exploration and testing of new alternatives and, without it, scientific progress would be halted. But there is no great comfort in this: on the contrary, it is very discomforting. It may be so discomforting that traditional views and methods may be adhered to even when they have become inadequate. Or, it may spur some to formulate new dogmas prematurely (Kahn and Earle, 1982). In either of these instances, it is not only the person being served that suffers because the best possible service is not provided, but also the profession because of the threat to its development and acceptability by other professions and by the public. The vital and most demanding aspect of the discomfort of uncertainty is to be able to use it creatively.

Spreading the Word and Increasing Visibility

Work which is centred on improving communication ability is generally well recognised as being of vital importance. But how many of our colleagues know about the scope of our work? How much does the general public know? There is an impetus in this area with the establishment of community-based programmes to develop public awareness (e.g., 'Speak Week' or 'Speech and Language Month'), but the profession remains undervalued and rarely regarded as an autonomous discipline. Various explanations have been proposed to account for this low visibility (e.g., the high proportion of female members, the notion that the average clinician is so preoccupied with patient care that there is 'not enough time' for either research or for disseminating knowledge, or the fact that we have been traditionally linked with elocutionists). Whatever the reason, the inability of those working in communication disorders to communicate knowledge about the profession and the scope of our work suggests a basic flaw in organisation that must be corrected if the profession is to gain its rightful status.

The profession cannot develop without the active involvement of its members. Each clinician will agree that the care of the person with a communication disorder is the primary consideration, but can the provision of care be adequate when the profession itself is not recognised or valued for its worth? Individual development is arguably where professional development begins. Development of personal skills and expertise in specialisation within the field is a prerequisite of a profession wishing to become autonomous. The achievement of higher degrees, particularly professional doctorates, will not only improve research but will lead to improved recognition by others.

Education

A second level of involvement is in education. Many clinicians are actively involved in clinical supervision of students and this is essential work. But educational alternatives need to be discussed with future service provision given priority. The question of whether specialisation should begin at undergraduate level, with perhaps a course offered for those wishing to specialise in working with children only, or alternatively with adults only, needs to be addressed. There are many viable alternatives, even at undergraduate level, and the scope for specialisation at postgraduate level is virtually unlimited.

Local development

Professional organisation at local levels is necessary for supporting the clinician who feels isolated, not only from other disciplines but from members of their own profession. Sharing of knowledge and expertise within the profession, between professions and with the community will improve the visibility and acceptance of those with a communication disorder as well as those professionally concerned with their care. Community education is a vital preventive measure and there is much that the clinician can do in working in the community to increase local awareness, knowledge and involvement.

National Organisation

Involvement in national organisation of the profession too often reflects the apathy that individual clinicians come to experience when their service is undervalued and they are not recognised as professionals whose education and expertise is of a high standard. National organisations stand or fall on the strength of their members. The clinician who wants to improve the status of the profession has an obligation to become involved. Better organisation means better service. The development of the profession ultimately depends on *you,* the individual clinician.

Reference

KAHN, J. and EARLE, E. (1982) *The Cry for Help and the Professional Response.* London: Pergamon.

Index